STATE OF THE ART OF THERAPEUTIC ENDOCRINOLOGY

Edited by **Sameh Magdeldin**

State of the Art of Therapeutic Endocrinology
http://dx.doi.org/10.5772/2906
Edited by Sameh Magdeldin

Contributors

Henrik Ortsäter, Åke Sjöholm, Alex Rafacho, Ignacio Jáuregui Lobera, Imre Zoltán Kun, Zsuzsanna Szántó, Ildikó Kun, Béla Szabó, Marie-Odile Soyer-Gobillard, Charles Sultan, Masoumeh Mehdipour, Ali Taghavi Zenouz, Antonio C. Boschero, Ilhan Satman, Sazi Imamoglu, Candeger Yilmaz, ADMIRE Study Group, Andrew John Pask, Nooshin Bagherani

Published by InTech

Janeza Trdine 9, 51000 Rijeka, Croatia

Notice

Publishing Process Manager Vedran Greblo
Technical Editor InTech Prepress, Novi Sad
Cover InTech Design team

Additional hard copies can be obtained from orders@intechopen.com

State of the Art of Therapeutic Endocrinology, Edited by Sameh Magdeldin
p. cm.
ISBN 978-953-51-0772-9

For EU product safety concerns:
IN TECH d.o.o., Prolaz Marije Krucifikse Kozulić 3, 51000 Rijeka, Croatia,
info@intechopen.com or visit our website at intechopen.com.

Meet the editor

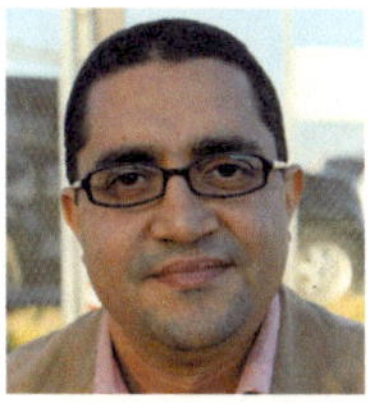

Sameh Magdeldin is currently a research associate at The Scripps Research Institute (TSRI), La Jolla. CA in the United States of America. He is a senior postdoctoral researcher in the Medical School, Niigata University, Japan and academic associate professor (Lecturer) in Physiology Dept. Suez Canal University, Egypt. He received his M.V.Sc and Ph.D in Physiology (2007) and 2nd Ph.D in proteomics (2012). Dr. Magdeldin is expert in shotgun proteomics analysis, reversed-phase chromatography and label-free comparative proteomic approaches. Dr. Magdeldin created an outstanding "All and None" methodology for analyzing large throughput proteomic data published in a highly respected proteomics journal. Beside his published articles, he currently serves as a guest editor, associate editor and a peer-reviewer in several international journals. Dr. Magdeldin received several grants and honorary prizes such as 8th HUPO Congress Young Investigator Award, JSN Award, Grant-in–Aid for young scientist, and Young Researcher Overseas Grant from Japan society for the promotion of science

Contents

Preface

The book in your hands respresents a concise research of an up-to-date frontier in therapeutic endocrinology. While the book title is no doubt broad, we selected limited related topics focusing on corticosteroid treatment and others. The book contains nine separate chapters.

State of the Art of Therapeutic Endocrinology is aimed at mainly those interested in physiology, endocrinology, medicine and pharmacology with different specialities such as biochemists, biologists, pharmacists, advanced graduate students and post graduate researchers.

Finally, I am grateful to the working team in InTech and all the experts who participated and contributed to this book with their valuable experience. Indeed, without their participation, this book would not come to light.

Sameh Magdeldin, M.V.Sc, Ph.D (Physiology), Ph.D (Proteomics)
Research Associate, The Scripps Research Institute (TSRI), La Jolla,
USA

Senior post-doc researcher and Proteomics team leader
Medical School, Niigata University,
Japan

Ass. Prof. (Lecturer), Physiology Dept.
Suez Canal University,
Egypt

Chapter 1

Regulation of Glucocorticoid Receptor Signaling and the Diabetogenic Effects of Glucocorticoid Excess

Henrik Ortsäter, Åke Sjöholm and Alex Rafacho

Additional information is available at the end of the chapter

http://dx.doi.org/10.5772/51759

1. Introduction

Glucocorticoids (GCs), such as cortisol, are key hormones to regulate carbohydrate metabolism (Wajchenberg et al., 1984). Furthermore, CG-based drugs are effective in providing anti-inflammatory and immunosuppressive effects (Stahn & Buttgereit, 2008). Their clinical desired effects are generally associated with adverse effects that include muscle atrophy, hypertension, osteoporosis, increased central fat deposition, and metabolic disturbance such as induction of peripheral insulin resistance (IR) and glucose intolerance (Schacke et al., 2002). In this context, we aim, in this chapter, to present and discuss the different factors that control tissue sensitivity towards GCs. These factors include expression levels of the GC receptor (GR), GR interacting proteins, GR phosphorylation and pre receptor regulation of GC availability. In this chapter we will also present some clinical manifestations of endogenous or exogenous CG excess on glucose homeostasis. Latter, in the coming chapter a special focus will be placed on GC effects on the endocrine pancreas.

1.1. General aspects of the glucocorticoid

GCs, like cortisol and dehydroepiandrosterone (DHEA), are produced and released from the *zona fasciculata* of the adrenal gland cortex. Especially cortisol secretion has an inherent rhythm over a 24 hours sleeping-wake period. The most pronounced feature of the diurnal cortisol cycle is a burst of secretory activity following awakening with a diurnal decline thereafter. Like other steroid hormones, GCs are derived from cholesterol via pregnenolone by a series of enzymatic reactions. Moreover, with the exception of vitamin D, they all contain the same cyclopentanophenanthrene ring and atomic numbering system as cholesterol. Common names of the steroid hormones are widely recognized, but systematic nomenclature is gaining acceptance and familiarity with both nomenclatures is increasingly important. Steroids with 21 carbon atoms are known systematically as pregnanes, whereas those containing 19 and 18 carbon atoms are known as androstanes (male sex hormones, *e.g.* testosterone) and estranes (female sex hormones, *e.g.* estrogen), respectively. Figure 1 depicts the pathways for biosynthesis of pregnanes, androstanes and estranes.

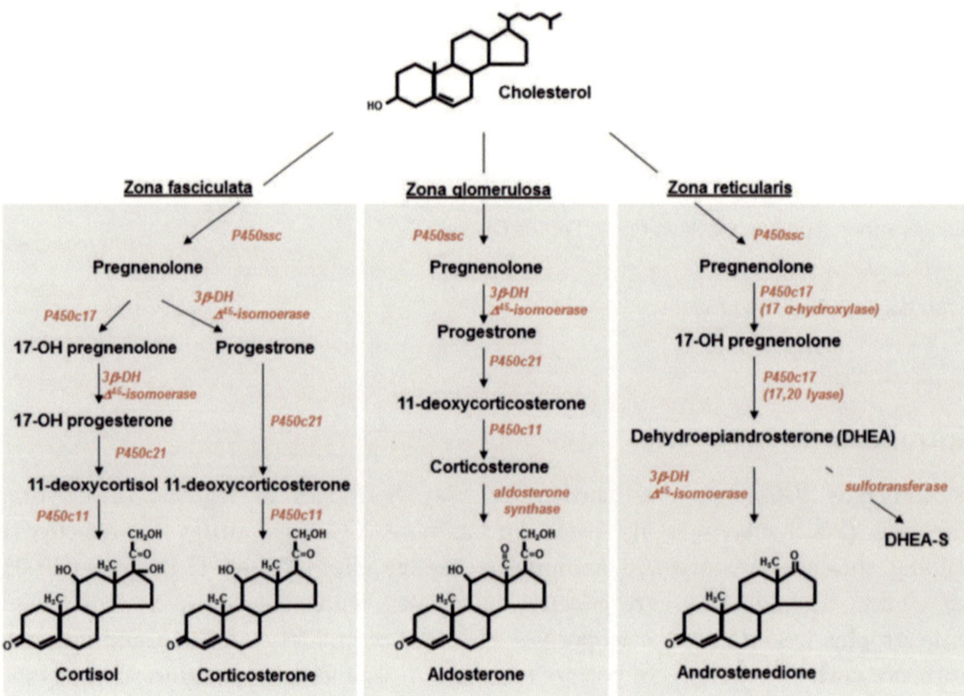

Figure 1. Synthesis of steroid hormones in the adrenal cortex. Synthesis of the adrenal steroid hormones from cholesterol. Steroid synthesis originates from cholesterol. In *zona fasciculata, zona glomerulosa* and *zona reticularis,* a series of enzymatic reactions give rise to glucocorticoids, mineralocorticoids and androgens, respectively. P450ssc enzyme (also called 20,22-desmolase or cholesterol desmolase) is identified as CYP11A1. 3β-DH and Δ4,5-isomerase are the two activities of 3β-hydroxysteroid dehydrogenase type 1 (gene symbol HSD3B2), P450c11 is 11β-hydroxylase (CYP11B1), P450c17 is CYP17A1. CYP17A1 is a single microsomal enzyme that has two steroid biosynthetic activities: 17α-hydroxylase which converts pregnenolone to 17-hydroxypregnenolone (17-OH pregnenolone) and 17,20-lyase which converts 17-OH pregnenolone to DHEA. P450c21 is 21-hydroxylase (CYP21A2, also identified as CYP21 or CYP21B). Aldosterone synthase is also known as 18α-hydroxylase (CYP11B2). The gene symbol for sulfotransferase is SULT2A1.

Secretion of cortisol and other GCs by the adrenal cortex are under the control of a prototypic neuroendocrine feedback system, the hypothalamic-pituitary-adrenal (HPA) axis. GCs are secreted in response to a single stimulator, adrenocorticotropic hormone (ACTH) from the anterior pituitary (Feek et al., 1983). ACTH is itself secreted mainly under control of the hypothalamic peptide corticotropin-releasing hormone (CRH). Secreted GC has a negative influence on both CRH and ACTH release; hence, the steroid regulates its own release in a negative feedback loop. The central nervous system (CNS) is thus the commander and chief of GC responses, providing an excellent example of close integration between the nervous and endocrine systems (Vegiopoulos & Herzig, 2007).

The GCs are a class of hormones that is primarily responsible for modulating carbohydrate metabolism (Wajchenberg et al., 1984). In principle, GCs mobilize glucose to the systemic circulation. In the liver cortisol induces gluconeogenesis, potentiates the action of other hyperglycemic hormones (*e.g.* glucagon, catecholamines and growth hormone) on glycogen breakdown, which culminates in release of glucose from hepatocytes. Cortisol inhibits uptake and utilization of glucose in skeletal muscle and adipose tissue by interfering with insulin signaling. The hormone also promotes muscle wasting via reduction of protein synthesis and degradation of protein and release of amino acids. The effect of cortisol on blood glucose levels is further enhanced through the increased breakdown of triglycerides (TG) in adipose tissues, which provide energy and substrates for gluconeogenesis. The increased rate of protein metabolism leads to increased urinary nitrogen excretion and the induction of urea cycle enzymes.

In addition to its metabolic effects, GCs have strong immunomodulatory properties for which they now are used as standard therapy for reducing inflammation and immune activation. At supraphysiological concentrations (greater than normally present in the body), GCs display strong clinical applications. In this regard, the relevant properties are the immunosuppressive, anti-inflammatory and anti-allergic effects that GCs exert on primary and secondary immune cells, tissues and organs (Stahn & Buttgereit, 2008), and the alleviation of the emesis associated with chemotherapy (Maranzano et al., 2005). GCs are used in virtually all medical specialties for both systemic and topical therapy. To have an idea of GCs relevance on clinical therapies, approximately 10 million new prescriptions for oral corticosteroids are issued in the United States annually (Schacke et al., 2002). The most prescribed synthetic GCs (*e.g.*, prednisolone, methylprednisolone, dexamethasone [DEX] and betamethasone – agents with high GC potency and low mineralocorticoid activities) are relatively inexpensive drugs, but due to the large volume prescribed they achieve a market size of about 10 billion US$ per year (Schacke et al., 2002). In dermatology, GCs are the most widely used therapy to, for example, treat atopic eczema. Inhalation of GCs is used to treat allergic reactions in airways and to dampen bronchial hyperreactivity in asthma. Systemically, GCs are used to combat inflammations in connective tissue, rheumatoid arthritis, bowel diseases as well as in allotransplantation. The anti-inflammatory activity of the GCs is exerted, in part, through inhibition of phospholipase A2 (PLA2) activity with a consequent reduction in the release of arachidonic acid from membrane phospholipids. Arachidonic acid serves as the precursor for the synthesis of various eicosanoids. GCs also affect circulation and migration of leukocytes. For more detailed information on the immunomodulatory properties of GCs the reader is kindly referred to reference (Löwenberg et al., 2008). Despite their excellent effects for the treatment of inflammatory and allergic diseases, GCs use is limited by their side effects on several systems, organs and/or tissues (Table 1), which are dependent on the dose and duration of the GC treatment. Among these adverse effects are the endocrine derangements that include increase in central fat deposition (Rockall et al., 2003; Asensio et al., 2004), hyperphagia (Debons et al., 1986), hepatic steatosis (Rockall et al., 2003), dyslipidemia characterized by increased TG and nonesterified fatty acid (NEFA) levels (Taskinen et al., 1983; Rafacho et al., 2008), muscle atrophy (Prelovsek et al., 2006), IR and/or glucose intolerance (Stojanovska et al., 1990; Binnert et al., 2004; Rafacho et al., 2008), as well as overt diabetes in susceptible individuals (Schacke et al., 2002).

ORGANS AND/OR TISSUES AND THE RESPECTIVE ALTERATIONS
Skin: atrophy, delayed wound healing
Skeleton and muscle: osteoporosis, muscle atrophy/myopathy
Eye: glaucoma, cataract
Central nervous system: disturbance in mood, behavior, memory, and cognition
Endocrine system/metabolism: dyslipidemia, insulin resistance and/or glucose intolerance, β-cell dysfunction (susceptible individuals)
Cardiovascular system: hypertension
Immune system: increased risk of infection, re-activation of viruses
Gastrointestinal system: peptic ulcer, pancreatitis

Table 1. Some typical side effects in GC-treated patients ordered by the affected organs. Modified from Schäcke et al., 2002 (Schacke et al., 2002).

2. Factors controlling tissue sensitivity towards glucocorticoids

2.1. The Glucocorticoid Receptor

The GC receptor (GR), a ligand-regulated transcription factor that belongs to the superfamily of nuclear receptors, binds GCs and regulates transcription of target genes after binding specific DNA sequences in their promoters or enhancers regions (Mangelsdorf et al., 1995).

The human GR ([NCBI Reference Sequence: NM_000176, Uniprot identifier P04150]) cDNA was isolated by expression cloning in 1985 (Hollenberg et al., 1985). The hGR gene consists of 9 exons and is located on chromosome 5. The mouse GR gene (NCBI Reference Sequence: NM_008173, Uniprot identifier P06537) maps to chromosome 18 and the rat GR gene (NCBI Reference Sequence: NM_012576, Uniprot identifier P06536]) to chromosome 18.

Alternative splicing of the human GR gene in exon 9 generates two highly homologous receptor isoforms, termed α and β. These are identical through amino acid 727 but then diverge, with the α isoform having an additional 50 amino acids and the β isoform having an additional, nonhomologous, 15 amino acids. In addition, different translation initiation sites increase the number of possible isoforms of the GR to 16 (8 α isoforms + 8 β isoforms) (Duma et al., 2006). All these variants have different transcriptional activity in response to DEX, varies in the subcellular distribution, and display distinct transactivation or transrepression patterns on gene expression as judged by cDNA microarray analyses (Lu &

Cidlowski, 2005). The relative expression of different GRs isoforms in pancreatic β-cells is not known but it is conceivable that differences in the expression pattern might predispose certain individuals to develop glucose intolerance upon GC exposure. The molecular weights of the canonical α and β receptor isoforms are 97 and 94 kilo-Dalton, respectively. The α isoform of human GR resides primarily in the cytoplasm of cells and represents the classic GR that functions as a ligand-dependent transcription factor. The β isoform of the human GR, on the other hand, does not bind GC agonists, may or may not bind the synthetic GC antagonist RU38486 (mifepristone), has intrinsic, α isoform-independent, gene-specific transcriptional activity, and exerts a dominant negative effect upon the transcriptional activity of the α isoform (Oakley et al., 1999; Zhou & Cidlowski, 2005; Kino et al., 2009).

The human GR is a modular protein composed of distinct regions, as illustrated in Figure 2. In the N-terminal part of the receptor, is the A/B domain that contains transcription activation function-1 (AF-1) that in many cases acts synergistically with ligand-dependent AF-2 located in the ligand binding domain (LBD) of the receptor (Ma et al., 1999). In addition, this domain harbours several phosphorylation sites and is the target of various signaling kinases, such as mitogen-activated protein kinases (MAPK) and cyclin-dependent kinases (Cdk) (Ismaili & Garabedian, 2004). Thereafter follows the DNA binding domain (DBD) and a hinge region (HR). In the C-terminal part is the LBD that starts with the important site for interaction with heat-shock proteins (Hsp) and ends with a second transcription activation function (AF-2).

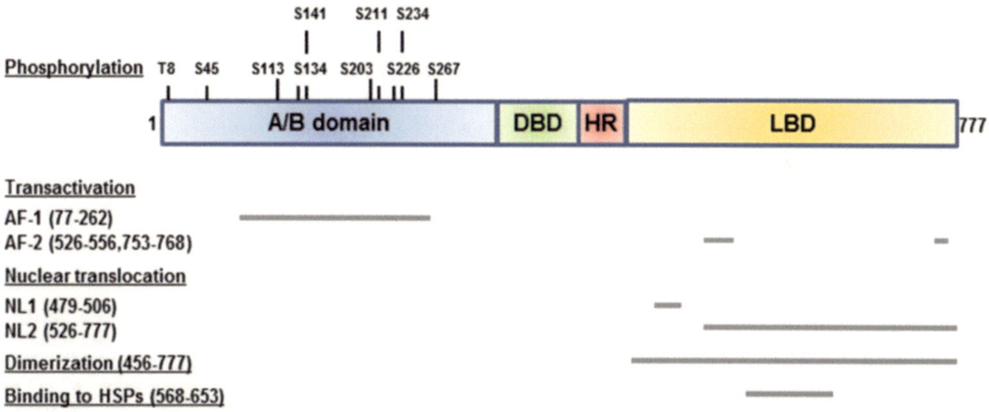

Figure 2. Structure and domains in the human GR α isoform. The human GR (Uniprot identifier P04150) isoform α is considered to be the canonical version. This isoform is made up of 777 amino acids. The β isoform is similar to α variant up amino acid 727 but then contain only 15 more amino acids that are non-homologous to those in the α isoform. The human GR is a modular protein composed of distinct regions. In the N-terminal part of the receptor is the A/B domain that contains transcription activation function-1 (AF-1) that in many cases acts synergistically with ligand-dependent AF-2 located in the ligand binding domain (LBD) of the receptor. In addition, this domain harbours several phosphorylation sites. Thereafter follows the DNA binding domain (DBD) and a hinge region (HR). In the C-terminal part is the LBD that starts with the important site for interaction with heat-shock proteins (Hsp) and ends with a second transcription activation function AF-2. This last domain also contains amino acid sequences responsible for receptor dimerization and nuclear translocation.

Ligand-activated GR exerts its classic transcriptional activity by binding via zinc finger motifs in the DBD to the promotor region, a GC-responsive element (GRE), of GC-responsive genes. To initiate transcription, the GR uses its transcriptional activation domains (AF-1 and AF-2) to interact with various transcriptional coactivators that bridges to RNA polymerase II (McKenna et al., 1999; Auboeuf et al., 2002; McKenna & O'Malley, 2002).

2.2. GR interacting proteins

The GR is expressed in virtually all tissues, yet it has the capacity to regulate genes in a cell-specific manner, indicating that the response to GCs is regulated by factors beyond receptor expression. Steroid hormones, such as cortisol, act as the primary signal in activating the receptor's transcriptional regulatory functions. But, GRs do not proceed through their signaling pathway alone. They are guided from the moment of their synthesis, through signal transduction and until they decay by a variety of molecular chaperones, which facilitate their encounter with various fates (Grad & Picard, 2007; Sanchez, 2012). In addition, GR-mediated transcriptional activation is modulated both positively and negatively by phosphorylation (Ismaili & Garabedian, 2004) exerted by kinases and phosphatases. These interacting proteins have profound implications for GC action as they regulate folding, maturation, phosphorylation, trafficking and degradation of the GR. An overview of these different proteins is given in Table 2.

Protein name	Uniprot ID (Human)	Function	Phenotypic effects in genetic mouse knock out models	References
Hsp90	P07900 (α) P08238 (β)	Molecular chaperone involved in GR maturation and trafficking. Binds to cochaperones.	Hsp90α knock mice are viable and healthy but male have defective spermatogenesis resulting in male sterility. Hsp90β knock out generates embryonic lethality at E9 in the mouse due to defective placental development.	(Brehmer et al., 2001; Pearl & Prodromou, 2006)
Hsp70	P08107	Molecular chaperone involved in GR folding. Binds to cochaperones.	Male infertility. At the cellular level, mice homozygous for a knock out allele exhibit impaired thermotolerance and increased sensitivity to heat stress-induced apoptosis.	(Brehmer et al., 2001; Pearl & Prodromou, 2006)
Hsp40	P25685	Cochaperone of Hsp70, activate Hsp70 ATPase activity.	Mice homozygous for a knock out allele are viable, fertile, and overtly normal; however, homozygous null peritoneal macrophages display impaired thermotolerance in the early (but not in the late) phase after mild heat treatment.	(Laufen et al., 1999)
Hip	P50502	Cochaperone of Hsp70, catalyzes folding.	Not described	(Höhfeld et al., 1995)
Bag-1	Q99933	Cochaperone of Hsp70, promotes	Homozygous null mice display embryonic lethality and liver hypoplasia.	(Ballinger et al., 1999;

Protein name	Uniprot ID (Human)	Function	Phenotypic effects in genetic mouse knock out models	References
		GR degradation.		Kanelakis et al., 2000)
Hop	P31948	Cochaperone of both Hsp70 and Hsp90, contains three TPR domains, transfers GR from Hsp70 to Hsp90.	Not described	(Chen & Smith, 1998; Odunuga et al., 2004)
CHIP	Q9UNE7	Cochaperone of Hsp70, promotes GR degradation.	Homozygous null mice develop normally but are susceptible to stress-induced apoptosis of multiple organs. Increased peri- and postnatal lethality.	(Ballinger et al., 1999; Kanelakis et al., 2000)
p23	Q15185	Cochaperone of Hsp90, stabilizes Hsp90 to catalyze ligand binding,	Disruption of gene function results in neonatal lethality, respiratory system abnormalities, as well as skin morphological and physiological defects.	(Grad et al., 2006; Lovgren et al., 2007; Nakatani et al., 2007)
FKBP51	Q13451	Cochaperone of Hsp90, contains TPR domain.	Mice homozygous for a null allele are normal and fertile. Mice homozygous for another knock out allele exhibit decreased depression-related behavior and increased anxiety-related behavior.	(O'Leary et al., 2011)
FKBP52	Q02790	Cochaperone of Hsp90, contains TPR domain, interacts with dynein to support nuclear translocation via mirotubuli.	*Fkb52*$^{-/-}$ mice display a high rate of embryonic mortality. *Fkb52*$^{+/-}$ mice placed on a high-fat diet demonstrate a susceptibility to hyperglycemia and hyperinsulinemia that correlate with reduced insulin clearance.	(Warrier et al., 2010)
PP5	P53041	Cochaperone of Hsp90, contains TPR domain, protein phosphatase.	Reduced body weight, and improved glucose clearance. Mice homozygous for a null allele exhibit a decrease in cell cycle check-point arrest following treatment with ionizing radiation.	(Hinds et al., 2011; Grankvist et al., 2012)

Uniprot ID (http://www.uniprot.org/) are given for the human version.
Information on phenotypes are partly taken from the Mouse Genome Informatics (MGI) database http://www.informatics.jax.org/.

Table 2. Proteins interacting with the GR.

2.2.1. Heat shock proteins

Over its entire lifespan, the GR is tightly associated with Hsp, mostly notably Hsp70 and Hsp90. Hsp70 and Hsp90 are ATP-dependent and their interaction with either ATP or ADP controls the binding and release of client proteins. Their activities are regulated via interaction with cochaperones that can act as modulators of the ATPase activity or as nucleotide exchange factors (Brehmer et al., 2001; Pearl & Prodromou, 2006). Several of these regulators are proteins containing so called tetratricopeptide repeat (TPR) domains. Via their TPR domains they bind to conserved C-terminal parts of Hsp70 (EEVD) and Hsp90 (MEEVD), respectively (Liu et al., 1999; Scheufler et al., 2000). Notably, only one species of these TPR containing protein can bind to one Hsp at any given time, leading to a competition among the TPR proteins for Hsp binding. This means that in any given cell at given time the actual levels of TPR proteins will determine the cellular response to GCs. This is an open arena for new research, both in pancreatic β-cells as well as in other types of cells.

The nascent translation product of GR mRNA is brought to Hsp70 by Hsp40 that at the same time accelerates ATP hydrolysis (Laufen et al., 1999). ADP-bound Hsp70 forms a tight complex with unfolded GR. In this configuration the receptor undergoes conformational changes, which results in a tertiary structure with low hormone affinity. A cochaperone, Hip, then binds to the ATPase domain of Hsp70 and catalyzes the folding process by keeping ADP bound to Hsp70 (Höhfeld et al., 1995). During the folding process, Hsp70 undergoes cycles of client binding and client release in conjunction with ADP and ATP interaction, respectively. Once the GR is correctly folded, Hip is exchanged for yet another cochaperone, Hop, which binds Hsp70 via one of its TPR domains (Odunuga et al., 2004). In fact, Hop contains three TPR domains that allows for simultaneous binding of Hsp70 and Hsp90 and can therefore transfer the newly folded GR from Hsp70 to Hsp90 (Chen & Smith, 1998). Before moving on to the function of the GR-Hsp90 complex, we need to acknowledge that Hsp70 also plays a role for proteosomal degradation of the GR. The two proteins Bag-1 and CHIP compete with Hip and Hop in their binding to Hsp70 (Ballinger et al., 1999; Kanelakis et al., 2000). In a configuration with either Bag-1 or CHIP, Hsp70 interaction with client protein does not promote folding but rather facilitates ubiquitination and subsequent proteosomal degradation of unfolded GR. Thus, increased cellular levels of Bag-1 and CHIP would negatively impact cellular responses to GC exposure by enhancing GR degradation.

While Hsp70 is the molecular chaperone that is essential for folding in nascent GR polypeptide chains, it is Hsp90 that is required for obtaining a mature GR with high affinity for GCs. Hsp90 interact with GR as a homodimer. The receptor's affinity for ligands is 100-fold lowered in the absence of Hsp90 as was investigated in cell-free steroid binding assays (Nemoto et al., 1990). Transfer of GR from the Hsp70 to the Hsp90 complex is facilitated by Hop (Chen & Smith, 1998). Hsp90 binds to Hop in an ADP state but, once Hsp70 is released, ADP is exchanged for ATP. The Hsp90 – GR complex, in its ATP-bound form, recruits the protein p23 that stabilizes this configuration (Figure 3). According to the model proposed by Pratt et al. (Pratt et al., 2006), unligated GR constantly undergoes cycles of rapid opening and closing of the ligand binding site. When stabilized by p23, the opening time is prolonged and therefore p23 expression can augment GC action by facilitating ligand binding to GR. Different versions of p23-deficient mice have been generated (Grad et al., 2006; Lovgren et al., 2007; Nakatani et al., 2007) and these mice display pathologies similar to those seen in GR knock out mice (Cole et al., 1995; Bayo et al., 2008), including atelectatic lungs and skin defects, indicating that p23 is essential for GC signaling.

The exchange of ADP for ATP in the Hsp90–GR complex also decreases Hsp90's affinity for Hop. As a result, Hop is released and the binding site for other TPR domain containing protein is made available. The net result of this folding and maturation processes, orcheestrated by first Hsp70 and then Hsp90, is a receptor that has high affinity for steroid hormones. In addition, the Hsp90 protein is ready to interact with a new set of cochaperones that will regulate future GC action.

2.2.2. *Immunophilin-related cochaperones*

Immunophilins are members of a highly conserved family of proteins, all of which are cis-trans peptidyl-prolyl isomerases (PPI) (Marks, 1996). The prototypic members of the immunophilin family, cyclophilin A and FKPB12, were discovered on the basis of their ability to bind and mediate the immunosuppressive effects of the drugs cyclosporin, FK506, and rapamycin. However, the prolyl isomerase activity of these proteins is not involved in any of the immunosuppressive effects. Two other of members of this family, FKBP51 and FKBP52, play a fundamental role during cytosol to nucleus translocation of activated GR (Figure 3). Before stimulation with a GC hormone, the majority of Hsp90–GR complexes coprecipitates with FKBP51 but upon ligand binding there is a rapid shift of FKBP51 in favour of FKBP52 (Davies et al., 2002). In contrast to FKBP51, the PPI domain of FKBP52 interacts with the microtubule motor protein dynein via protein-protein binding. This is a function of the PPI domain that is independent of its enzymatic activity and is not affected by FK506 (Galigniana et al., 2004). Interestingly, swapping of the PPI domains between FKBP51 and FKBP52 reverses their respective function, indicating that the true function of FKBP52 is, via dynein, to make a bridge between the Hsp90–GR complex and the microtubuli system. FKBP52 immunoprecipitates with dynein and the FKBP52 co-localizes to the microtubule system in the cytosol (Czar et al., 1994; Galigniana et al., 2002). In accordance with these observations, ligand-activated GR rapidly accumulates in the nucleus (half time = 4-5 minutes) and this rate is slowed by injection of FKBP52 neutralizing antibodies (Czar et al., 1995). In addition, overexpression of a FKBP52 fragment that contained the dynein-interacting PPI domain, but not the TPR domain, disrupted the interaction of full length FKBP52 protein with dynein and delayed nuclear translocation of GR (Wochnik et al., 2005). The same type of reduced speed for GR translocation (half time = 40-60 minutes) is seen after treatment with the Hsp90 inhibitor geldanamycin (Czar et al., 1997) or after disruption of the microtubule network (Czar et al., 1995). However, nuclear GR translocation is not completely inhibited during these conditions. Thus, there is a possibility for GR translocation and, hence, signaling that is independent of Hsp90, FKBP52 and a functional microtubuli system (Figure 3); however, it is not clear if this pathway is of any physiological relevance.

From the information presented above, we can conclude that in the absence of steroid ligand the GR resides in the cytosol in a complex with Hsp90 and FKBP51 but, upon ligand binding, FKPB51 is replaced by FKBP52 that will interact with dynein and promote nuclear translocation via the microtubuli system (Figure 3). It is not clear whether Hsp90 is released from the complex during transportation or if Hsp90 sticks on to the receptor during nuclear translocation. There are also some indications that the GR can translocate to the nucleus independent of Hsp90, FKBP52 and a functional microtubuli system.

This model would imply that the binding of FKBP51 to Hsp90 has a suppressive impact on GC signaling, whereas FKBP52 serves as an enhancer. Indeed, FKBP52 selectively potentiated hormone-dependent gene activation in *Saccharomyces cereviviae* by as much as 20-fold at limiting concentrations and this potentiation was blocked when FKBP51 was co-expressed (Riggs et al., 2003). Another striking example on how GR-interacting proteins can regulate GC signaling comes from studies of new world primates, like the Squirrel monkeys (*Genus Saimiri*). Many new world primates have high circulating levels of cortisol to compensate for GC resistance. A role for changes in immunophilins, causing GC resistance in neotropical primates, is supported by enhanced protein levels of FKBP51 and reduced levels FKBP52 in these neotropical primates with GC resistance (Reynolds et al., 1999; Scammell et al., 2001).

Mice lacking FKBP52 display a high, but not total, rate of embryonic lethality, especially when backcrossed on the C57BL/6 background (Cheung-Flynn et al., 2005; Yang et al., 2006; Warrier et al., 2010). The exact cause for mortality in FKBP52 null mice has not been established but notably FKBP52 null mice do not appear to die from the atelectaisa that is typical for GR knock out mice. However, surviving mice of both sexes grow into healthy adults except for reduced fertility due to defective penis development in males and sterility due to failure of uterus to support oocyte implantation in females.

FKBP52 does seem to have a role in GC control of metabolism (Warrier et al., 2010). *Fkb52*$^{+/-}$ mice placed on a high-fat demonstrated a propensity to hyperglycemia and hyperinsulinemia. Livers of high-fat diet fed mutant mice were steatotic and showed elevated expression of lipogenic genes and pro-inflammatory markers. Interestingly, mutant mice on high-fat diet showed elevated serum corticosterone but their steatotic livers had reduced expression of gluconeogenic genes, whereas muscle and adipose tissue expressed normal to elevated levels of GC markers. These findings suggest a state of GC resistance mainly affecting hepatocytes.

To this date, no metabolic studies have been performed in mice lacking FKBP51. However, with respect to metabolism FKBP51 null mice would be expected to have elevated GR activity, presumably leading to increased susceptibility towards GC-induced glucose intolerance and diabetes. But, such *a priori* assumption should be made with caution. GCs affect virtually every type of mammalian cell and therefore the overall effect of a global knock out is difficult to anticipate. Indeed, tissue-specific deletion of both FKBP51 and FKBP52 would be vital tools to dissect the role played by these GR-interacting proteins.

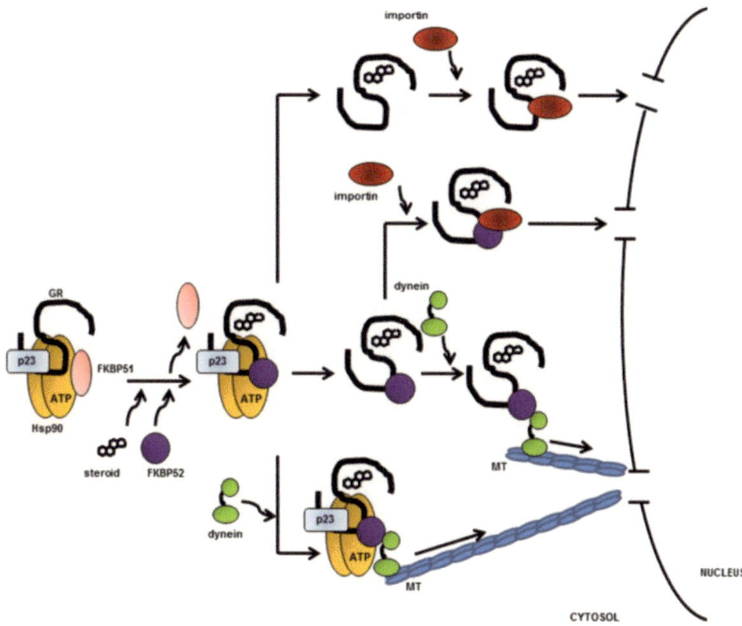

Figure 3. Cytosol to nucleus transportation of activated GR. Glucocorticoids exert their effects after binding to an intracellular receptor that, upon ligand binding, is translocated to the nucleus. Before ligand binding the GR is held in a complex with Hsp90, p23 and FKBP51. After ligand binding, FKBP51 is replaced by FKBP52 and Hsp90 and p23 detaches or can be kept bound to the GR. FKBP52 stimulates interaction with dynein and translocation to the nucleus via the microtubuli (MT) system. However, some experimental evidence suggests that GR can be translocated to the nucleus independent on the MT system. Figure adopted from Grad and Picard 2007 (Grad & Picard, 2007).

2.3. GR phosphorylation

As depicted in Figure 2, the GR contains several phosphorylation sites within the C-terminal A/B-domain. The receptor is phosphorylated in the absence of hormone and additional phosphorylation events occur in conjunction with agonist, but not antagonist, binding (Almlof et al., 1995; Webster et al., 1997; Wang et al., 2002). The hormone-dependent increase in receptor phosphorylation has led to the hypothesis that phosphorylation may modulate GR transcriptional regulatory functions.

Consistent with this notion is the finding that GR is phosphorylated at three serine residues, S203, S211 and S226, which are particularly associated with activation of the GR (Wang et al., 2002). Serine to alanine mutations of S203 and S211, individually or in combination, decrease transcriptional activation in mammalian cells, indicating that phosphorylation of these residues are required for full GR activity (Almlof et al., 1995; Webster et al., 1997; Miller et al., 2005). In contrast, an alanine substitution for S226 increases GR transcriptional activity relative to the wild-type receptor, suggesting that phosphorylation of S226 is inhibitory to GR function (Rogatsky et al., 1998; Itoh et al., 2002). Thus, phosphorylation appears to provide both positive and negative regulatory inputs with respect to GR transcriptional activation. In an analysis of the relative contribution of the different phosphorylation sites within the GR, it was found that GR-mediated transcriptional activation was greatest when the relative phosphorylation of S211 exceeded that of S226 (Krstic et al., 1997).

Two different Cdks have been identified as responsible for phosphorylation of S203 and S211; cyclin E/Cdk2 and cyclin A/Cdk2 phosphorylate S203 and, S203 and S211, respectively (Krstic et al., 1997). Mammalian cells lacking $p27^{KIP1}$ demonstrate a concomitant rise in cyclin/Cdk2 activity and increased GR phosphorylation at S203 and S211, as well as enhanced receptor transcriptional activity, further strengthening the role for Cdks in GR phosphorylation and activity (Wang & Garabedian, 2003). In addition, it was recently shown that the phosphorylation site S211 is a substrate for p38 MAPK (Miller et al., 2005), an observation that provides a mechanistic link as to why inhibitors of p38 MAPK protect pancreatic β-cells against cytotoxic effects of DEX (Reich et al., 2012).

The c-Jun N-terminal kinase (JNK) is the kinase primarily responsible for phosphorylation of S226 (Rogatsky et al., 1998). Thus, inhibitors of JNK can be expected to have a negative impact on GR activity. JNK phosphorylation of GR has also been reported to increase receptor nuclear export under conditions of hormone withdrawal (Itoh et al., 2002). Thus, JNK phosphorylation inhibits receptor activity by at least two distinct mechanisms; in the presence of hormone GR phosphorylation by JNK affects receptor interaction with factors involved in transcriptional activation, whereas in the absence of hormone it enhances receptor nuclear export.

Perturbations in protein phosphatase activity have also been shown to affect GR function. Treatment of cells with okadaic acid, a general serine/threonine protein phosphatase inhibitor, results in receptor hyperphosphorylation, retaining of the receptor in the cytosol but also a transcriptional activation in mammalian cells (DeFranco et al., 1991; Somers & DeFranco, 1992). Endogenous phosphatase activity of the GR is catalyzed by serine/threonine protein phosphatase 5 (PP5). Like FKBP51 and FKBP52, the PP5 protein contains TPR domains (Chen et al., 1994), is a major component of the Hsp90–GR complex and has also been shown to be associated with ligand-free receptor in the nucleus (Silverstein et al., 1997).

In vitro experiments with A549 cells showed that suppression of PP5 expression through antisense oligonucleotides increased GR transcriptional activity both in the absence and presence of hormone (Zuo et al., 1999). Embryonic fibroblasts generated from a line of PP5 knock out mice were used to study the balance between lipolysis and lipogenesis. In these studies, embryonic fibroblasts from mice lacking PP5 demonstrated resistance to lipid accumulation in response to adipogenic stimuli, which was due to elevated GR phosphorylation and reduced peroxisome proliferator activated receptor (PPAR)γ activity on genes controlling lipid metabolism (Hinds et al., 2011). In line with these observation, PP5 null mice have reduced body weight (Amable et al., 2011). Interestingly, PP5 null mice have improved glucose tolerance when subjected to a glucose tolerance test, despite having normal insulin sensitivity, indicating enhanced insulin secretion capacity (Grankvist et al., 2012).

2.4. 11β-hydroxysteroid dehydrogenase

In humans, circulating GCs exist in two forms. The plasma levels of the inactive form, cortisone, are around 50-100 nM and the hormone is largely unbound to plasma proteins (Walker et al., 1992). In contrast, approximately 95% of the active form, cortisol, is bound to corticosteroid-binding globulin. In the rat and mouse, the plasma concentration of 11-dehydrocorticosterone (DHC), which is the rodent equivalent to cortisone, is also around 50 nM (Kotelevtsev et al., 1997). As has been discussed above, tissue response to GCs is regulated both by the expression level of the GR, cochaperones interacting with the receptor and by the intracellular concentration of the active form of the hormone. But for GCs there is a possibility for an additional level of control that involves intracellular pre-receptor regulation of inactive and active forms of GCs. Conversion between the inactive and active forms of GCs is performed by the enzyme 11β-hydroxysteroid dehydrogenase (11β-HSD; EC 1.1.1.146). In rodents, 11β-HSD type 1 (11β-HSD1, Uniprot identifier for the human form P28845) works as a NADPH-dependent reductase converting inactive DHC to active corticosterone (Low et al., 1994; Voice et al., 1996; Davani et al., 2000). The type 2 (11β-HSD2, Uniprot identifier for the human form P80365) isoform works as a NAD^+-dependent dehydrogenase catalyzing the opposite reaction (Brown et al., 1993). 11β-HSD2 expression is particularly abundant in kidney and placenta where the enzyme modulates intracellular GC levels, thus protecting the non-selective mineralocorticoid receptor from occupancy by GCs (Albiston et al., 1994). Thus, cellular activities of 11β-HSD1 and 11β-HSD2 function as pre-receptor regulators of GC action. The former enzyme is widely expressed, most notably in liver, lung, adipose tissue, vascular tissue, ovary and the CNS (Stewart & Krozowski, 1999). Sequence analysis of the cloned 11β-HSD1 gene revealed a putative GC-responsive element in the promoter region (Tannin et al., 1991), suggesting that corticosterone or cortisol can regulate the transcription of 11β-HSD1. Evidence for such a mechanism was obtained in human skeletal muscle biopsy, where cortisol induced elevated levels of 11β-HSD1 mRNA (Whorwood et al., 2001). Also in rat and human hepatocytes, it was demonstrated that carbenoxolone (CBX), an inhibitor of both type 1 and type 2 11β-HSD, reduced 11β-HSD1 reductase activity (Ricketts et al., 1998).

It has been proposed that local variations in tissue cortisol levels can occur in the absence of any discernible changes in circulating cortisol (Walker & Andrew, 2006). Although cortisol plasma levels are slightly elevated in patients with the metabolic syndrome or in obese subjects of cortisol (Phillips et al., 1998; Duclos et al., 2005; Misra et al., 2008; Sen et al., 2008; Weigensberg et al., 2008) they are within the normal range (Walker, 2006). This would imply that tissue-specific expression levels 11β-HSD1 and 11β-HSD2 are determinants of the local cellular concentration of active steroid that can influence the metabolic effects of GC. In agreement with this concept, in a study of 101 obese patients (BMI 34.4 ± 4.3 kg/m^2) of both sexes, impaired glucose tolerance and IR was associated with increased adipose 11β-HSD1 expression (Tomlinson et al., 2008). Furthermore, transgenic mice over-expressing 11β-HSD1 selectively in adipose tissue faithfully recapitulate the phenotype of the metabolic syndrome (Masuzaki et al., 2001; Masuzaki et al., 2003). These mice had increased adipose levels of corticosterone and developed visceral obesity that was exaggerated by a high-fat diet. The transgenic mice also exhibited profound insulin-resistant diabetes and hyperlipidemia. As these studies suggest that local GC excess perturbs glucose homeostasis via 11β-HSD1, attempts have been made to pharmacologically inhibit 11β-HSD1 (Tomlinson & Stewart, 2007). In this respect, carbenoxolone, an inhibitor of both 11β-HSD1 and 11β-HSD2, increases hepatic insulin sensitivity in man (Walker et al., 1995). Selective inhibition of 11β-HSD1 decreases glycemia and improves hepatic insulin sensitivity in hyperglycemic mouse strains (Alberts et al., 2002; Alberts et al., 2003). Clinical studies in humans with selective 11β-HSD1 inhibitors are ongoing, for a review see reference (Pereira et al., 2012).

Finally, 11β-HSD1 mRNA and enzyme activity has been detected in both human and mouse islets (Davani et al., 2000), indicating that 11β-HSD1 might regulate GC action in the endocrine pancreas. Indeed, islets treated with DHC had a suppressed glucose-stimulated insulin secretion (GSIS) (Davani et al., 2000) and this aspect will be further discussed in the coming chapter.

3. Diabetogenic effects of glucocorticoid excess

Hyperglycemia and diabetes mellitus are important causes of mortality and morbidity worldwide. The number of people with impaired glucose tolerance or type 2 diabetes (T2DM) is rising in all regions of the world. A systemic analysis of health examination surveys and epidemiological studies showed that between 1980 and 2008 there were nearly 194 million new cases of diabetes (Danaei et al., 2011). Of these, 70% could be attributed to population growth and ageing but the cause for the remaining 30% most be found among environmental changes that support the increased disease prevalence. Indeed, lifestyle changes including a higher caloric intake and decreased energy expenditure play a large part to explain increased prevalence of T2DM. However, as will be discussed in this chapter, the impact of GCs shall not be neglected.

GC-induced diabetes is a special form of glucose intolerance that can occur when endogenous GC activity is enhanced or during treatment with GC-based drugs (Raul Ariza-Andraca et al., 1998; Vegiopoulos & Herzig, 2007; van Raalte et al., 2009). Perhaps the most clear cut case is endogenous over production of GCs by adrenal cortex as it occurs in Cushing's syndrome. In 80-85 % of the cases the syndrome is caused by a pituitary tumour (referred as Cushing's disease) and is ACTH-dependent. Symptoms include rapid weight gain, particularly of the trunk and face with sparing of the limbs (central obesity). Other signs include persistent hypertension (due to activation of the mineralocorticoid receptor leading to increased sodium retention and expanded plasma volume) and IR (due to insulin signaling defects), which in turn may lead to hyperglycemia. In patients with hypercortisolism due to Cushing's syndrome, the incidence of T2DM is 30-40% (Biering et al., 2000). The similar phenotypes in patients with Cushing's syndrome and in patients with the metabolic syndrome has led to the hypothesis that cortisol can play a pathological role in the metabolic syndrome (Anagnostis et al., 2009).

Subclinical Cushing's syndrome is also observed and it is defined as alterations of the HPA axis that result in elevated circulating cortisol levels without those gross adverse metabolic effects of GC excess as mentioned above. In a study including patients of both sexes (aged 18-87 years), diagnosed with adrenal incidentaloma via imaging techniques, participants were classified according to levels of cortisolemia after administration of 1 mg DEX (Di Dalmazi et al., 2012). DEX is a synthetic GC analogue that will suppress endogenous cortisol production via the existing negative feedback loop. Patients with cortisol levels above 138 nM on the morning after administration of 1 mg DEX were classified as subclinical Cushing's syndrome that can be compared with those diagnosed with non-secreting adenoma, whose cortisol levels were below 50 nM. Among these patients, T2DM was over represented as were coronary heart disease and osteoporosis.

Yet, a third example of GC excess, and a much more common one, is during pharmacological treatment. Low-dose GC is considered when the daily dose is less than 7.5 mg prednisolone or equivalent (van der Goes et al., 2010). When such a dose is administrated orally, plasma prednisolone levels peaks 2-4 hours after intake at about 400-500 nM (~150-200 ng/ml) and returns to baseline within 12 hours after steroid administration (Wilson et al., 1977; Tauber et al., 1984). These values are in the same range as normal endogenous cortisol values, reference values for samples taken between 4:00 am and 8:00 am are 250-750 nM and for samples taken between 8:00 pm and 12:00 pm are 50-300 nM. This indicates that the absolute cortisol values are not as important for developing adverse effects during low-dose GC therapy as is the diurnal variation. Current knowledge gives at hand that developing diabetes after starting low-dose GC treatment seems rare but progression of already impaired glucose tolerance to overt diabetes is possible (van der Goes et al., 2010). Therefore, clinical recommendation states that baseline fasting glucose should be monitored before initiating therapy and during following up according to standard patient care.

Certainly, the adverse effects are more pronounced during high-dose GC therapies (>30 mg prednisolone or equivalent daily). In a retrospective study of hemoglobin A1c (HbA1c) levels in patients with rheumatic diseases subjected to prednisolone treatment, it was found that around 82% had HbA1c levels higher than 48 mmol/mol (given in IFCC standard, corresponding to 6.7% in DCCT standard). Serum HbA1c levels higher than 52 mmol/mol (7.1%), were seen in 46% of the patients and 23% of the patients had HbA1c levels as high as 57 mmol/mol (7.6%) which should be considered as a high risk factor for diabetes. Taken together, it was found that the cumulative prednisolone dose was the only factor significantly associated with the development of steroid induced diabetes among rheumatic patients (Origuchi et al., 2011).

Inhaled GCs are the mainstay of therapy in asthma, but their use raises certain safety concerns. In a study of 21,645 elderly subjects using inhaled beclomethasone, an increased risk of developing diabetes was found (Dendukuri et al., 2002). However, when adjusting for the simultaneous use of oral GCs no evidence was found for an increased risk of diabetes among users of inhaled GCs. In contrast, a more recent study of 388,584 patients treated for respiratory disease identified that inhaled GC use is associated with modest increases in the risks of diabetes onset and diabetes progression (Suissa et al., 2010). The risks are more pronounced at the higher doses (equivalent to 1.0 g or more per day of fluticasone) currently prescribed for the treatment of chronic obstructive pulmonary disease. Therefore, diabetes should be considered as a risk factor during treatment with inhaled GCs and especially in those cases when higher doses are used or when GCs are taken orally at the same time.

Diabetogenic effects of GCs include the induction or aggravation of preexisting IR in peripheral tissues (Grill et al., 1990; Larsson & Ahren, 1999; Nicod et al., 2003; Besse et al., 2005). The molecular base for IR was studied in rodent models or in primary cells subjected to GC treatment (Olefsky et al., 1975; Caro & Amatruda, 1982; Saad et al., 1993; Ishizuka et al., 1997; Sakoda et al., 2000; Burén et al., 2002; Ruzzin et al., 2005; Burén et al., 2008). DEX-treated rats (1.5 mg/kg *b.w.* for 6 consecutive days) exhibit around 50-70% and 40-50% reduction of insulin binding to its receptors in hepatocytes and adipocytes, respectively (Olefsky et al., 1975). Significant reduction in insulin receptor density was also observed in hepatocytes from rats chronically treated with DEX (1.0 mg/kg *b.w.*) (Caro & Amatruda, 1982). Previous studies demonstrated that especially post-receptor events are involved on the reduction of peripheral insulin action after GC treatment *in vivo*. Diminished tyrosine phosphorylation in either insulin receptor and insulin receptor substrate (IRS)-1 was observed in liver from rats treated with DEX for 5 consecutive days (1.0 mg/kg *b.w.*) (Saad et al., 1993). Decreased insulin-stimulated association of IRS-1/phosphatidylinositol 3-kinase (PI3K) in skeletal muscle tissue was also observed. These *in vivo* data are in accordance with *in vitro* findings. Adipocytes and myocytes cultured in the presence of DEX show reduction of insulin-stimulated glucose uptake, which is associated with impairment of post-insulin receptor signaling transduction and/or reduction of glucose transporter protein content (Ishizuka et al., 1997; Sakoda et al., 2000; Burén et al., 2002). Rats treated with DEX for 11 consecutive days (1.0 mg/kg *b.w.*) have around 40% and 70% reduction in insulin-induced glucose uptake in adipose and muscle tissues, respectively (Burén et al., 2008). The authors also observed increased lipolysis in response to 8-bromo-AMP and reduced antilipolytic insulin effects. These alterations are associated with diminished total protein kinase B (PKB) content and insulin-stimulated PKB serine/threonine phosphorylation in muscle and white adipose tissue (Burén et al., 2008). It is interesting to note that DEX-induced IR may occur through GR independent mechanisms. It was demonstrated that DEX induces reduction in insulin action in adipocytes even in the presence of the GR antagonist RU38486 or even in the presence of a protein synthesis inhibitor (cycloheximide) (Ishizuka et al., 1997; Kawai et al., 2002). It was also demonstrated that inhibition of protein kinase C (PKC) isoform β improves glucose uptake into adipocytes cultured in the presence of DEX (Kawai et al., 2002). Subsequent studies have demonstrated this GR- and/or transcription factor-independent mechanisms of GC action on insulin signaling, which leads to impairment of insulin action (Löwenberg et al., 2006).

Finally, when considering situations of GC excess, it is important to keep in mind that cortisol is a stress hormone with a diurnal secretion pattern that peaks at the time of wakening. Various stressful situations, including low socioeconomic status, chronic work stress (Eller et al., 2006; Maier et al., 2006), anxiety and depression (Chrousos, 2000; Kinder et al., 2004) may stimulate neuroendocrine responses. These conditions are all associated with disturbed sleeping patterns that often result in interrupted sleeping sessions and hence, wakening. In this latter condition, not only increased circulating cortisol levels are found, but also enhanced sympathetic nervous drive. Sleep deprivation alters hormonal glucose regulation and is especially affecting pancreatic insulin secretion (Schmid et al., 2007). Activation of the HPA axis works together with increased sympathetic nervous tone to mediate the effects of stress on various organ systems and may disturb glucose homeostasis (Buren & Eriksson, 2005).

4. Conclusions

Prolonged therapies based on moderate or high GC doses are clearly diabetogenic for healthy individuals. In susceptible subjects (obese, low-insulin responders, first-degree relatives of patients with T2DM, pregnant, etc) even low doses GC treatment may disrupt glucose homeostasis. These adverse effects of the CGs vary according to the specific tissue responses to the hormone. Tissue sensitivity towards GCs is regulated at several points from 11β-HSD1 activity to GR phosphorylation. The impact of various cochaperones that regulate GR function on the effects of GCs is an open field for coming research. Tissue specific knock-out models for the different GR interacting proteins would provide valuable tools to elucidate the roles played by these proteins in various tissues. Development of novel drugs with desirable GC activity (gene transrepression) without undesirable side effects (gene transactivation) are in progress and hold promise as good pharmacological options for GC-based therapies (Stahn et al., 2007).

Author details

Henrik Ortsäter and Åke Sjöholm
Department of Clinical Science and Education, Södersjukhuset, Karolinska Insititutet, Sweden

Alex Rafacho
Department of Physiological Sciences, Centre of Biological Sciences, Universidade Federal de Santa Catarina, Brazil

Acknowledgement

H. Ortsäter is funded by the Swedish Society for Medical Research. A. Rafacho is funded by CNPq and FAPESC. The authors have no conflict of interest to disclose.

5. References

Alberts, P., Engblom, L., Edling, N., Forsgren, M., Klingstrom, G., Larsson, C., Ronquist-Nii, Y., Ohman, B., & Abrahmsen, L. (2002). Selective inhibition of 11β-hydroxysteroid dehydrogenase type 1 decreases blood glucose concentrations in hyperglycaemic mice. *Diabetologia* Vol. 45, No. 11, pp. 1528-1532

Alberts, P., Nilsson, C., Selen, G., Engblom, L.O., Edling, N.H., Norling, S., Klingstrom, G., Larsson, C., Forsgren, M., Ashkzari, M., Nilsson, C.E., Fiedler, M., Bergqvist, E., Ohman, B., Bjorkstrand, E., & Abrahmsen, L.B. (2003). Selective Inhibition of 11β-Hydroxysteroid Dehydrogenase Type 1 Improves Hepatic Insulin Sensitivity in Hyperglycemic Mice Strains. *Endocrinology* Vol. 144, No. 11, pp. 4755-4762

Albiston, A.L., Obeyesekere, V.R., Smith, R.E., & Krozowski, Z.S. (1994). Cloning and tissue distribution of the human 11β-hydroxysteroid dehydrogenase type 2 enzyme. *Mol Cell Endocrinol* Vol. 105, No. 2, pp. R11-17

Almlof, T., Wright, A.P., & Gustafsson, J.A. (1995). Role of acidic and phosphorylated residues in gene activation by the glucocorticoid receptor. *J Biol Chem* Vol. 270, No. 29, pp. 17535-17540

Amable, L., Grankvist, N., Largen, J.W., Ortsäter, H., Sjöholm, A., & Honkanen, R.E. (2011). Disruption of Serine/Threonine Protein Phosphatase 5 (PP5:PPP5c) in Mice Reveals a Novel Role for PP5 in the Regulation of Ultraviolet Light-induced Phosphorylation of Serine/Threonine Protein Kinase Chk1 (CHEK1). *J Biol Chem* Vol. 286, No. 47, pp. 40413-40422

Anagnostis, P., Athyros, V.G., Tziomalos, K., Karagiannis, A., & Mikhailidis, D.P. (2009). Clinical review: The pathogenetic role of cortisol in the metabolic syndrome: a hypothesis. *J Clin Endocrinol Metab* Vol. 94, No. 8, pp. 2692-2701

Asensio, C., Muzzin, P., & Rohner-Jeanrenaud, F. (2004). Role of glucocorticoids in the physiopathology of excessive fat deposition and insulin resistance. *Int J Obes Relat Metab Disord* Vol. 28 Suppl 4, No., pp. S45-52

Auboeuf, D., Honig, A., Berget, S.M., & O'Malley, B.W. (2002). Coordinate regulation of transcription and splicing by steroid receptor coregulators. *Science* Vol. 298, No. 5592, pp. 416-419

Ballinger, C.A., Connell, P., Wu, Y., Hu, Z., Thompson, L.J., Yin, L.Y., & Patterson, C. (1999). Identification of CHIP, a novel tetratricopeptide repeat-containing protein that interacts with heat shock proteins and negatively regulates chaperone functions. *Mol Cell Biol* Vol. 19, No. 6, pp. 4535-4545

Bayo, P., Sanchis, A., Bravo, A., Cascallana, J.L., Buder, K., Tuckermann, J., Schutz, G., & Perez, P. (2008). Glucocorticoid receptor is required for skin barrier competence. *Endocrinology* Vol. 149, No. 3, pp. 1377-1388

Besse, C., Nicod, N., & Tappy, L. (2005). Changes in insulin secretion and glucose metabolism induced by dexamethasone in lean and obese females. *Obes Res* Vol. 13, No. 2, pp. 306-311

Biering, H., Knappe, G., Gerl, H., & Lochs, H. (2000). Prevalence of diabetes in acromegaly and Cushing syndrome. *Acta Med Austriaca* Vol. 27, No. 1, pp. 27-31

Binnert, C., Ruchat, S., Nicod, N., & Tappy, L. (2004). Dexamethasone-induced insulin resistance shows no gender difference in healthy humans. *Diabetes Metab* Vol. 30, No. 4, pp. 321-326

Brehmer, D., Rudiger, S., Gassler, C.S., Klostermeier, D., Packschies, L., Reinstein, J., Mayer, M.P., & Bukau, B. (2001). Tuning of chaperone activity of Hsp70 proteins by modulation of nucleotide exchange. *Nat Struct Biol* Vol. 8, No. 5, pp. 427-432

Brown, R.W., Chapman, K.E., Edwards, C.R., & Seckl, J.R. (1993). Human placental 11β-hydroxysteroid dehydrogenase: evidence for and partial purification of a distinct NAD-dependent isoform. *Endocrinology* Vol. 132, No. 6, pp. 2614-2621

Buren, J., & Eriksson, J.W. (2005). Is insulin resistance caused by defects in insulin's target cells or by a stressed mind? *Diabetes Metab Res Rev* Vol. 21, No. 6, pp. 487-494

Burén, J., Lai, Y.C., Lundgren, M., Eriksson, J.W., & Jensen, J. (2008). Insulin action and signalling in fat and muscle from dexamethasone-treated rats. *Arch Biochem Biophys* Vol. 474, No. 1, pp. 91-101

Burén, J., Liu, H.X., Jensen, J., & Eriksson, J.W. (2002). Dexamethasone impairs insulin signalling and glucose transport by depletion of insulin receptor substrate-1, phosphatidylinositol 3-kinase and protein kinase B in primary cultured rat adipocytes. *Eur J Endocrinol* Vol. 146, No. 3, pp. 419-429

Caro, J.F., & Amatruda, J.M. (1982). Glucocorticoid-induced insulin resistance: the importance of postbinding events in the regulation of insulin binding, action, and degradation in freshly isolated and primary cultures of rat hepatocytes. *J Clin Invest* Vol. 69, No. 4, pp. 866-875

Chen, M.X., McPartlin, A.E., Brown, L., Chen, Y.H., Barker, H.M., & Cohen, P.T. (1994). A novel human protein serine/threonine phosphatase, which possesses four tetratricopeptide repeat motifs and localizes to the nucleus. *Embo J* Vol. 13, No. 18, pp. 4278-4290

Chen, S., & Smith, D.F. (1998). Hop as an adaptor in the heat shock protein 70 (Hsp70) and hsp90 chaperone machinery. *J Biol Chem* Vol. 273, No. 52, pp. 35194-35200

Cheung-Flynn, J., Prapapanich, V., Cox, M.B., Riggs, D.L., Suarez-Quian, C., & Smith, D.F. (2005). Physiological role for the cochaperone FKBP52 in androgen receptor signaling. *Mol Endocrinol* Vol. 19, No. 6, pp. 1654-1666

Chrousos, G.P. (2000). The role of stress and the hypothalamic-pituitary-adrenal axis in the pathogenesis of the metabolic syndrome: neuro-endocrine and target tissue-related causes. *Int J Obes Relat Metab Disord* Vol. 24 Suppl 2, No., pp. S50-55

Cole, T.J., Blendy, J.A., Monaghan, A.P., Krieglstein, K., Schmid, W., Aguzzi, A., Fantuzzi, G., Hummler, E., Unsicker, K., & Schutz, G. (1995). Targeted disruption of the glucocorticoid receptor gene blocks adrenergic chromaffin cell development and severely retards lung maturation. *Genes Dev* Vol. 9, No. 13, pp. 1608-1621

Czar, M.J., Galigniana, M.D., Silverstein, A.M., & Pratt, W.B. (1997). Geldanamycin, a heat shock protein 90-binding benzoquinone ansamycin, inhibits steroid-dependent translocation of the glucocorticoid receptor from the cytoplasm to the nucleus. *Biochemistry* Vol. 36, No. 25, pp. 7776-7785

Czar, M.J., Lyons, R.H., Welsh, M.J., Renoir, J.M., & Pratt, W.B. (1995). Evidence that the FK506-binding immunophilin heat shock protein 56 is required for trafficking of the glucocorticoid receptor from the cytoplasm to the nucleus. *Mol Endocrinol* Vol. 9, No. 11, pp. 1549-1560

Czar, M.J., Owens-Grillo, J.K., Yem, A.W., Leach, K.L., Deibel, M.R., Jr., Welsh, M.J., & Pratt, W.B. (1994). The hsp56 immunophilin component of untransformed steroid receptor complexes is localized both to microtubules in the cytoplasm and to the same nonrandom regions within the nucleus as the steroid receptor. *Mol Endocrinol* Vol. 8, No. 12, pp. 1731-1741

Danaei, G., Finucane, M.M., Lu, Y., Singh, G.M., Cowan, M.J., Paciorek, C.J., Lin, J.K., Farzadfar, F., Khang, Y.H., Stevens, G.A., Rao, M., Ali, M.K., Riley, L.M., Robinson, C.A., & Ezzati, M. (2011). National, regional, and global trends in fasting plasma glucose and diabetes prevalence since 1980: systematic analysis of health examination surveys and epidemiological studies with 370 country-years and 2.7 million participants. *Lancet* Vol. 378, No. 9785, pp. 31-40

Davani, B., Khan, A., Hult, M., Martensson, E., Okret, S., Efendic, S., Jornvall, H., & Oppermann, U.C. (2000). Type 1 11β-hydroxysteroid dehydrogenase mediates glucocorticoid activation and insulin release in pancreatic islets. *J Biol Chem* Vol. 275, No. 45, pp. 34841-34844.

Davies, T.H., Ning, Y.M., & Sanchez, E.R. (2002). A new first step in activation of steroid receptors: hormone-induced switching of FKBP51 and FKBP52 immunophilins. *J Biol Chem* Vol. 277, No. 7, pp. 4597-4600

Debons, A.F., Zurek, L.D., Tse, C.S., & Abrahamsen, S. (1986). Central nervous system control of hyperphagia in hypothalamic obesity: dependence on adrenal glucocorticoids. *Endocrinology* Vol. 118, No. 4, pp. 1678-1681

DeFranco, D.B., Qi, M., Borror, K.C., Garabedian, M.J., & Brautigan, D.L. (1991). Protein phosphatase types 1 and/or 2A regulate nucleocytoplasmic shuttling of glucocorticoid receptors. *Mol Endocrinol* Vol. 5, No. 9, pp. 1215-1228

Dendukuri, N., Blais, L., & LeLorier, J. (2002). Inhaled corticosteroids and the risk of diabetes among the elderly. *Br J Clin Pharmacol* Vol. 54, No. 1, pp. 59-64

Di Dalmazi, G., Vicennati, V., Rinaldi, E., Morselli-Labate, A.M., Giampalma, E., Mosconi, C., Pagotto, U., & Pasquali, R. (2012). Progressively increased patterns of subclinical cortisol hypersecretion in adrenal incidentalomas differently predict major metabolic and cardiovascular outcomes: a large cross-sectional study. *Eur J Endocrinol* Vol. 166, No 4, pp. 669-677

Duclos, M., Marquez Pereira, P., Barat, P., Gatta, B., & Roger, P. (2005). Increased cortisol bioavailability, abdominal obesity, and the metabolic syndrome in obese women. *Obes Res* Vol. 13, No. 7, pp. 1157-1166

Duma, D., Jewell, C.M., & Cidlowski, J.A. (2006). Multiple glucocorticoid receptor isoforms and mechanisms of post-translational modification. *J Steroid Biochem Mol Biol* Vol. 102, No. 1-5, pp. 11-21

Eller, N.H., Netterstrom, B., & Hansen, A.M. (2006). Psychosocial factors at home and at work and levels of salivary cortisol. *Biol Psychol* Vol. 73, No. 3, pp. 280-287

Feek, C.M., Marante, D.J., & Edwards, C.R. (1983). The hypothalamic-pituitary-adrenal axis. *Clin Endocrinol Metab* Vol. 12, No. 3, pp. 597-618

Galigniana, M.D., Harrell, J.M., Murphy, P.J., Chinkers, M., Radanyi, C., Renoir, J.M., Zhang, M., & Pratt, W.B. (2002). Binding of hsp90-associated immunophilins to cytoplasmic dynein: direct binding and in vivo evidence that the peptidylprolyl isomerase domain is a dynein interaction domain. *Biochemistry* Vol. 41, No. 46, pp. 13602-13610

Galigniana, M.D., Harrell, J.M., O'Hagen, H.M., Ljungman, M., & Pratt, W.B. (2004). Hsp90-binding immunophilins link p53 to dynein during p53 transport to the nucleus. *J Biol Chem* Vol. 279, No. 21, pp. 22483-22489

Grad, I., McKee, T.A., Ludwig, S.M., Hoyle, G.W., Ruiz, P., Wurst, W., Floss, T., Miller, C.A., 3rd, & Picard, D. (2006). The Hsp90 cochaperone p23 is essential for perinatal survival. *Mol Cell Biol* Vol. 26, No. 23, pp. 8976-8983

Grad, I., & Picard, D. (2007). The glucocorticoid responses are shaped by molecular chaperones. *Mol Cell Endocrinol* Vol. 275, No. 1-2, pp. 2-12

Grankvist, N., Amable, L., Honkanen, R.E., Sjöholm Å & Ortsäter H (2012). Serine/threonine protein phosphatase 5 regulates glucose homeostasis in vivo and apoptosis signalling in mouse pancreatic islets and clonal MIN6 cells. *Diabetologia* Vol. 55, No 7, pp. 2005-2015

Grill, V., Pigon, J., Hartling, S.G., Binder, C., & Efendic, S. (1990). Effects of dexamethasone on glucose-induced insulin and proinsulin release in low and high insulin responders. *Metabolism* Vol. 39, No. 3, pp. 251-258

Hinds, T.D., Jr., Stechschulte, L.A., Cash, H.A., Whisler, D., Banerjee, A., Yong, W., Khuder, S.S., Kaw, M.K., Shou, W., Najjar, S.M., & Sanchez, E.R. (2011). Protein phosphatase 5 mediates lipid metabolism through reciprocal control of glucocorticoid receptor and peroxisome proliferator-activated receptor-gamma (PPARgamma). *J Biol Chem* Vol. 286, No. 50, pp. 42911-42922

Hollenberg, S.M., Weinberger, C., Ong, E.S., Cerelli, G., Oro, A., Lebo, R., Thompson, E.B., Rosenfeld, M.G., & Evans, R.M. (1985). Primary structure and expression of a functional human glucocorticoid receptor cDNA. *Nature* Vol. 318, No. 6047, pp. 635-641

Höhfeld, J., Minami, Y., & Hartl, F.U. (1995). Hip, a novel cochaperone involved in the eukaryotic Hsc70/Hsp40 reaction cycle. *Cell* Vol. 83, No. 4, pp. 589-598

Ishizuka, T., Nagashima, T., Kajita, K., Miura, A., Yamamoto, M., Itaya, S., Kanoh, Y., Ishizawa, M., Murase, H., & Yasuda, K. (1997). Effect of glucocorticoid receptor antagonist RU 38486 on acute glucocorticoid-induced insulin resistance in rat adipocytes. *Metabolism* Vol. 46, No. 9, pp. 997-1002

Ismaili, N., & Garabedian, M.J. (2004). Modulation of glucocorticoid receptor function via phosphorylation. *Ann N Y Acad Sci* Vol. 1024, No., pp. 86-101

Itoh, M., Adachi, M., Yasui, H., Takekawa, M., Tanaka, H., & Imai, K. (2002). Nuclear export of glucocorticoid receptor is enhanced by c-Jun N-terminal kinase-mediated phosphorylation. *Mol Endocrinol* Vol. 16, No. 10, pp. 2382-2392

Kanelakis, K.C., Murphy, P.J., Galigniana, M.D., Morishima, Y., Takayama, S., Reed, J.C., Toft, D.O., & Pratt, W.B. (2000). hsp70 interacting protein Hip does not affect glucocorticoid receptor folding by the hsp90-based chaperone machinery except to oppose the effect of BAG-1. *Biochemistry* Vol. 39, No. 46, pp. 14314-14321

Kawai, Y., Ishizuka, T., Kajita, K., Miura, A., Ishizawa, M., Natsume, Y., Uno, Y., Morita, H., & Yasuda, K. (2002). Inhibition of PKCbeta improves glucocorticoid-induced insulin resistance in rat adipocytes. *IUBMB Life* Vol. 54, No. 6, pp. 365-370

Kinder, L.S., Carnethon, M.R., Palaniappan, L.P., King, A.C., & Fortmann, S.P. (2004). Depression and the metabolic syndrome in young adults: findings from the Third

National Health and Nutrition Examination Survey. *Psychosom Med* Vol. 66, No. 3, pp. 316-322

Kino, T., Manoli, I., Kelkar, S., Wang, Y., Su, Y.A., & Chrousos, G.P. (2009). Glucocorticoid receptor (GR) β has intrinsic, GRα-independent transcriptional activity. *Biochem Biophys Res Commun* Vol. 381, No. 4, pp. 671-675

Kotelevtsev, Y., Holmes, M.C., Burchell, A., Houston, P.M., Schmoll, D., Jamieson, P., Best, R., Brown, R., Edwards, C.R., Seckl, J.R., & Mullins, J.J. (1997). 11β-hydroxysteroid dehydrogenase type 1 knockout mice show attenuated glucocorticoid-inducible responses and resist hyperglycemia on obesity or stress. *Proc Natl Acad Sci U S A* Vol. 94, No. 26, pp. 14924-14929

Krstic, M.D., Rogatsky, I., Yamamoto, K.R., & Garabedian, M.J. (1997). Mitogen-activated and cyclin-dependent protein kinases selectively and differentially modulate transcriptional enhancement by the glucocorticoid receptor. *Mol Cell Biol* Vol. 17, No. 7, pp. 3947-3954

Larsson, H., & Ahren, B. (1999). Insulin resistant subjects lack islet adaptation to short-term dexamethasone-induced reduction in insulin sensitivity. *Diabetologia* Vol. 42, No. 8, pp. 936-943

Laufen, T., Mayer, M.P., Beisel, C., Klostermeier, D., Mogk, A., Reinstein, J., & Bukau, B. (1999). Mechanism of regulation of hsp70 chaperones by DnaJ cochaperones. *Proc Natl Acad Sci U S A* Vol. 96, No. 10, pp. 5452-5457

Liu, F.H., Wu, S.J., Hu, S.M., Hsiao, C.D., & Wang, C. (1999). Specific interaction of the 70-kDa heat shock cognate protein with the tetratricopeptide repeats. *J Biol Chem* Vol. 274, No. 48, pp. 34425-34432

Low, S.C., Chapman, K.E., Edwards, C.R., & Seckl, J.R. (1994). 'Liver-type' 11β-hydroxysteroid dehydrogenase cDNA encodes reductase but not dehydrogenase activity in intact mammalian COS-7 cells. *J Mol Endocrinol* Vol. 13, No. 2, pp. 167-174

Lovgren, A.K., Kovarova, M., & Koller, B.H. (2007). cPGES/p23 is required for glucocorticoid receptor function and embryonic growth but not prostaglandin E2 synthesis. *Mol Cell Biol* Vol. 27, No. 12, pp. 4416-4430

Lu, N.Z., & Cidlowski, J.A. (2005). Translational regulatory mechanisms generate N-terminal glucocorticoid receptor isoforms with unique transcriptional target genes. *Mol Cell* Vol. 18, No. 3, pp. 331-342

Löwenberg, M., Stahn, C., Hommes, D.W., & Buttgereit, F. (2008). Novel insights into mechanisms of glucocorticoid action and the development of new glucocorticoid receptor ligands. *Steroids* Vol. 73, No. 9-10, pp. 1025-1029

Löwenberg, M., Tuynman, J., Scheffer, M., Verhaar, A., Vermeulen, L., van Deventer, S., Hommes, D., & Peppelenbosch, M. (2006). Kinome analysis reveals nongenomic glucocorticoid receptor-dependent inhibition of insulin signaling. *Endocrinology* Vol. 147, No. 7, pp. 3555-3562

Ma, H., Hong, H., Huang, S.M., Irvine, R.A., Webb, P., Kushner, P.J., Coetzee, G.A., & Stallcup, M.R. (1999). Multiple signal input and output domains of the 160-kilodalton nuclear receptor coactivator proteins. *Mol Cell Biol* Vol. 19, No. 9, pp. 6164-6173

Maier, R., Egger, A., Barth, A., Winker, R., Osterode, W., Kundi, M., Wolf, C., & Ruediger, H. (2006). Effects of short- and long-term unemployment on physical work capacity and on serum cortisol. *Int Arch Occup Environ Health* Vol. 79, No. 3, pp. 193-198

Mangelsdorf, D.J., Thummel, C., Beato, M., Herrlich, P., Schutz, G., Umesono, K., Blumberg, B., Kastner, P., Mark, M., Chambon, P., & Evans, R.M. (1995). The nuclear receptor superfamily: the second decade. *Cell* Vol. 83, No. 6, pp. 835-839

Maranzano, E., Feyer, P., Molassiotis, A., Rossi, R., Clark-Snow, R.A., Olver, I., Warr, D., Schiavone, C., & Roila, F. (2005). Evidence-based recommendations for the use of antiemetics in radiotherapy. *Radiother Oncol* Vol. 76, No. 3, pp. 227-233

Marks, A.R. (1996). Cellular functions of immunophilins. *Physiol Rev* Vol. 76, No. 3, pp. 631-649

Masuzaki, H., Paterson, J., Shinyama, H., Morton, N.M., Mullins, J.J., Seckl, J.R., & Flier, J.S. (2001). A transgenic model of visceral obesity and the metabolic syndrome. *Science* Vol. 294, No. 5549, pp. 2166-2170.

Masuzaki, H., Yamamoto, H., Kenyon, C.J., Elmquist, J.K., Morton, N.M., Paterson, J.M., Shinyama, H., Sharp, M.G., Fleming, S., Mullins, J.J., Seckl, J.R., & Flier, J.S. (2003). Transgenic amplification of glucocorticoid action in adipose tissue causes high blood pressure in mice. *J Clin Invest* Vol. 112, No. 1, pp. 83-90

McKenna, N.J., Lanz, R.B., & O'Malley, B.W. (1999). Nuclear receptor coregulators: cellular and molecular biology. *Endocr Rev* Vol. 20, No. 3, pp. 321-344

McKenna, N.J., & O'Malley, B.W. (2002). Combinatorial control of gene expression by nuclear receptors and coregulators. *Cell* Vol. 108, No. 4, pp. 465-474

Miller, A.L., Webb, M.S., Copik, A.J., Wang, Y., Johnson, B.H., Kumar, R., & Thompson, E.B. (2005). p38 Mitogen-activated protein kinase (MAPK) is a key mediator in glucocorticoid-induced apoptosis of lymphoid cells: correlation between p38 MAPK activation and site-specific phosphorylation of the human glucocorticoid receptor at serine 211. *Mol Endocrinol* Vol. 19, No. 6, pp. 1569-1583

Misra, M., Bredella, M.A., Tsai, P., Mendes, N., Miller, K.K., & Klibanski, A. (2008). Lower growth hormone and higher cortisol are associated with greater visceral adiposity, intramyocellular lipids, and insulin resistance in overweight girls. *Am J Physiol Endocrinol Metab* Vol. 295, No. 2, pp. E385-392

Nakatani, Y., Hokonohara, Y., Kakuta, S., Sudo, K., Iwakura, Y., & Kudo, I. (2007). Knockout mice lacking cPGES/p23, a constitutively expressed PGE2 synthetic enzyme, are perinatally lethal. *Biochem Biophys Res Commun* Vol. 362, No. 2, pp. 387-392

Nemoto, T., Ohara-Nemoto, Y., Denis, M., & Gustafsson, J.A. (1990). The transformed glucocorticoid receptor has a lower steroid-binding affinity than the nontransformed receptor. *Biochemistry* Vol. 29, No. 7, pp. 1880-1886

Nicod, N., Giusti, V., Besse, C., & Tappy, L. (2003). Metabolic adaptations to dexamethasone-induced insulin resistance in healthy volunteers. *Obes Res* Vol. 11, No. 5, pp. 625-631

O'Leary, J.C., 3rd, Dharia, S., Blair, L.J., Brady, S., Johnson, A.G., Peters, M., Cheung-Flynn, J., Cox, M.B., de Erausquin, G., Weeber, E.J., Jinwal, U.K., & Dickey, C.A. (2011). A new anti-depressive strategy for the elderly: ablation of FKBP5/FKBP51. *PLoS ONE* Vol. 6, No. 9, pp. e24840

Oakley, R.H., Jewell, C.M., Yudt, M.R., Bofetiado, D.M., & Cidlowski, J.A. (1999). The dominant negative activity of the human glucocorticoid receptor α isoform. Specificity and mechanisms of action. *J Biol Chem* Vol. 274, No. 39, pp. 27857-27866

Odunuga, O.O., Longshaw, V.M., & Blatch, G.L. (2004). Hop: more than an Hsp70/Hsp90 adaptor protein. *Bioessays* Vol. 26, No. 10, pp. 1058-1068

Olefsky, J.M., Johnson, J., Liu, F., Jen, P., & Reaven, G.M. (1975). The effects of acute and chronic dexamethasone administration on insulin binding to isolated rat hepatocytes and adipocytes. *Metabolism* Vol. 24, No. 4, pp. 517-527

Origuchi, T., Yamaguchi, S., Inoue, A., Kazaura, Y., Matsuo, N., Abiru, N., Kawakami, A., & Eguchi, K. (2011). Increased incidence of pre-diabetes mellitus at a department of rheumatology: a retrospective study. *Mod Rheumatol* Vol. 21, No. 5, pp. 495-499

Pearl, L.H., & Prodromou, C. (2006). Structure and mechanism of the Hsp90 molecular chaperone machinery. *Annu Rev Biochem* Vol. 75, No., pp. 271-294

Pereira, C.D., Azevedo, I., Monteiro, R., & Martins, M.J. (2012). 11β-Hydroxysteroid dehydrogenase type 1: relevance of its modulation in the pathophysiology of obesity, the metabolic syndrome and type 2 diabetes mellitus. *Diabetes Obes Metab* Vol., No., pp.

Phillips, D.I., Barker, D.J., Fall, C.H., Seckl, J.R., Whorwood, C.B., Wood, P.J., & Walker, B.R. (1998). Elevated plasma cortisol concentrations: a link between low birth weight and the insulin resistance syndrome? *J Clin Endocrinol Metab* Vol. 83, No. 3, pp. 757-760

Pratt, W.B., Morishima, Y., Murphy, M., & Harrell, M. (2006). Chaperoning of glucocorticoid receptors. *Handb Exp Pharmacol* Vol., No. 172, pp. 111-138

Prelovsek, O., Mars, T., Jevsek, M., Podbregar, M., & Grubic, Z. (2006). High dexamethasone concentration prevents stimulatory effects of TNF-alpha and LPS on IL-6 secretion from the precursors of human muscle regeneration. *Am J Physiol Regul Integr Comp Physiol* Vol. 291, No. 6, pp. R1651-1656

Rafacho, A., Giozzet, V.A., Boschero, A.C., & Bosqueiro, J.R. (2008). Functional alterations in endocrine pancreas of rats with different degrees of dexamethasone-induced insulin resistance. *Pancreas* Vol. 36, No. 3, pp. 284-293

Raul Ariza-Andraca, C., Barile-Fabris, L.A., Frati-Munari, A.C., & Baltazar-Montufar, P. (1998). Risk factors for steroid diabetes in rheumatic patients. *Arch Med Res* Vol. 29, No. 3, pp. 259-262

Reich, E., Tamary, A., Sionov, R.V., & Melloul, D. (2012). Involvement of thioredoxin-interacting protein (TXNIP) in glucocorticoid-mediated beta cell death. *Diabetologia* Vol. 55, No. 4, pp. 1048-1057

Reynolds, P.D., Ruan, Y., Smith, D.F., & Scammell, J.G. (1999). Glucocorticoid resistance in the squirrel monkey is associated with overexpression of the immunophilin FKBP51. *J Clin Endocrinol Metab* Vol. 84, No. 2, pp. 663-669

Ricketts, M.L., Shoesmith, K.J., Hewison, M., Strain, A., Eggo, M.C., & Stewart, P.M. (1998). Regulation of 11β-hydroxysteroid dehydrogenase type 1 in primary cultures of rat and human hepatocytes. *J Endocrinol* Vol. 156, No. 1, pp. 159-168

Riggs, D.L., Roberts, P.J., Chirillo, S.C., Cheung-Flynn, J., Prapapanich, V., Ratajczak, T., Gaber, R., Picard, D., & Smith, D.F. (2003). The Hsp90-binding peptidylprolyl isomerase FKBP52 potentiates glucocorticoid signaling in vivo. *Embo J* Vol. 22, No. 5, pp. 1158-1167

Rockall, A.G., Sohaib, S.A., Evans, D., Kaltsas, G., Isidori, A.M., Monson, J.P., Besser, G.M., Grossman, A.B., & Reznek, R.H. (2003). Computed tomography assessment of fat distribution in male and female patients with Cushing's syndrome. *Eur J Endocrinol* Vol. 149, No. 6, pp. 561-567

Rockall, A.G., Sohaib, S.A., Evans, D., Kaltsas, G., Isidori, A.M., Monson, J.P., Besser, G.M., Grossman, A.B., & Reznek, R.H. (2003). Hepatic steatosis in Cushing's syndrome: a radiological assessment using computed tomography. *Eur J Endocrinol* Vol. 149, No. 6, pp. 543-548

Rogatsky, I., Logan, S.K., & Garabedian, M.J. (1998). Antagonism of glucocorticoid receptor transcriptional activation by the c-Jun N-terminal kinase. *Proc Natl Acad Sci U S A* Vol. 95, No. 5, pp. 2050-2055

Ruzzin, J., Wagman, A.S., & Jensen, J. (2005). Glucocorticoid-induced insulin resistance in skeletal muscles: defects in insulin signalling and the effects of a selective glycogen synthase kinase-3 inhibitor. *Diabetologia* Vol. 48, No. 10, pp. 2119-2130

Saad, M.J., Folli, F., Kahn, J.A., & Kahn, C.R. (1993). Modulation of insulin receptor, insulin receptor substrate-1, and phosphatidylinositol 3-kinase in liver and muscle of dexamethasone-treated rats. *J Clin Invest* Vol. 92, No. 4, pp. 2065-2072

Sakoda, H., Ogihara, T., Anai, M., Funaki, M., Inukai, K., Katagiri, H., Fukushima, Y., Onishi, Y., Ono, H., Fujishiro, M., Kikuchi, M., Oka, Y., & Asano, T. (2000). Dexamethasone-induced insulin resistance in 3T3-L1 adipocytes is due to inhibition of glucose transport rather than insulin signal transduction. *Diabetes* Vol. 49, No. 10, pp. 1700-1708

Sanchez, E.R. (2012). Chaperoning steroidal physiology: Lessons from mouse genetic models of Hsp90 and its cochaperones. *Biochim Biophys Acta* Vol. 1823, No. 3, pp. 722-729

Scammell, J.G., Denny, W.B., Valentine, D.L., & Smith, D.F. (2001). Overexpression of the FK506-binding immunophilin FKBP51 is the common cause of glucocorticoid resistance in three New World primates. *Gen Comp Endocrinol* Vol. 124, No. 2, pp. 152-165

Schacke, H., Docke, W.D., & Asadullah, K. (2002). Mechanisms involved in the side effects of glucocorticoids. *Pharmacol Ther* Vol. 96, No. 1, pp. 23-43

Scheufler, C., Brinker, A., Bourenkov, G., Pegoraro, S., Moroder, L., Bartunik, H., Hartl, F.U., & Moarefi, I. (2000). Structure of TPR domain-peptide complexes: critical elements in the assembly of the Hsp70-Hsp90 multichaperone machine. *Cell* Vol. 101, No. 2, pp. 199-210

Schmid, S.M., Hallschmid, M., Jauch-Chara, K., Bandorf, N., Born, J., & Schultes, B. (2007). Sleep loss alters basal metabolic hormone secretion and modulates the dynamic counterregulatory response to hypoglycemia. *J Clin Endocrinol Metab* Vol. 92, No. 8, pp. 3044-3051

Sen, Y., Aygun, D., Yilmaz, E., & Ayar, A. (2008). Children and adolescents with obesity and the metabolic syndrome have high circulating cortisol levels. *Neuro Endocrinol Lett* Vol. 29, No. 1, pp. 141-145

Silverstein, A.M., Galigniana, M.D., Chen, M.S., Owens-Grillo, J.K., Chinkers, M., & Pratt, W.B. (1997). Protein phosphatase 5 is a major component of glucocorticoid receptor.hsp90 complexes with properties of an FK506-binding immunophilin. *J Biol Chem* Vol. 272, No. 26, pp. 16224-16230

Somers, J.P., & DeFranco, D.B. (1992). Effects of okadaic acid, a protein phosphatase inhibitor, on glucocorticoid receptor-mediated enhancement. *Mol Endocrinol* Vol. 6, No. 1, pp. 26-34

Stahn, C., & Buttgereit, F. (2008). Genomic and nongenomic effects of glucocorticoids. *Nat Clin Pract Rheumatol* Vol. 4, No. 10, pp. 525-533

Stahn, C., Löwenberg, M., Hommes, D.W., & Buttgereit, F. (2007). Molecular mechanisms of glucocorticoid action and selective glucocorticoid receptor agonists. *Mol Cell Endocrinol* Vol. 275, No. 1-2, pp. 71-78

Stewart, P.M., & Krozowski, Z.S. (1999). 11β-Hydroxysteroid dehydrogenase. *Vitam Horm* Vol. 57, No., pp. 249-324

Stojanovska, L., Rosella, G., & Proietto, J. (1990). Evolution of dexamethasone-induced insulin resistance in rats. *Am J Physiol* Vol. 258, No. 5 Pt 1, pp. E748-756

Suissa, S., Kezouh, A., & Ernst, P. (2010). Inhaled corticosteroids and the risks of diabetes onset and progression. *Am J Med* Vol. 123, No. 11, pp. 1001-1006

Tannin, G.M., Agarwal, A.K., Monder, C., New, M.I., & White, P.C. (1991). The human gene for 11β-hydroxysteroid dehydrogenase. Structure, tissue distribution, and chromosomal localization. *J Biol Chem* Vol. 266, No. 25, pp. 16653-16658

Taskinen, M.R., Nikkila, E.A., Pelkonen, R., & Sane, T. (1983). Plasma lipoproteins, lipolytic enzymes, and very low density lipoprotein triglyceride turnover in Cushing's syndrome. *J Clin Endocrinol Metab* Vol. 57, No. 3, pp. 619-626

Tauber, U., Haack, D., Nieuweboer, B., Kloss, G., Vecsei, P., & Wendt, H. (1984). The pharmacokinetics of fluocortolone and prednisolone after intravenous and oral administration. *Int J Clin Pharmacol Ther Toxicol* Vol. 22, No. 1, pp. 48-55

Tomlinson, J.W., Finney, J., Hughes, B.A., Hughes, S.V., & Stewart, P.M. (2008). Reduced glucocorticoid production rate, decreased 5alpha-reductase activity, and adipose tissue insulin sensitization after weight loss. *Diabetes* Vol. 57, No. 6, pp. 1536-1543

Tomlinson, J.W., & Stewart, P.M. (2007). Modulation of glucocorticoid action and the treatment of type-2 diabetes. *Best Pract Res Clin Endocrinol Metab* Vol. 21, No. 4, pp. 607-619

Wajchenberg, B.L., Prestes Cesar, F., Okada, H., Torres de Toledo e Souza, I., Lerario, A.C., Borghi, V.C., Malerbi, D.A., Giurna Filho, A., Liberman, B., & Gianella, D. (1984). Glucocorticoids, glucose metabolism and hypothalamic-pituitary-adrenal axis. *Adv Exp Med Biol* Vol. 171, No., pp. 25-44

Walker, B.R. (2006). Cortisol--cause and cure for metabolic syndrome? *Diabet Med* Vol. 23, No. 12, pp. 1281-1288

Walker, B.R., & Andrew, R. (2006). Tissue production of cortisol by 11beta-hydroxysteroid dehydrogenase type 1 and metabolic disease. *Ann N Y Acad Sci* Vol. 1083, No., pp. 165-184

Walker, B.R., Campbell, J.C., Fraser, R., Stewart, P.M., & Edwards, C.R. (1992). Mineralocorticoid excess and inhibition of 11β-hydroxysteroid dehydrogenase in patients with ectopic ACTH syndrome. *Clin Endocrinol (Oxf)* Vol. 37, No. 6, pp. 483-492

Walker, B.R., Connacher, A.A., Lindsay, R.M., Webb, D.J., & Edwards, C.R. (1995). Carbenoxolone increases hepatic insulin sensitivity in man: a novel role for 11-oxosteroid reductase in enhancing glucocorticoid receptor activation. *J Clin Endocrinol Metab* Vol. 80, No. 11, pp. 3155-3159

van der Goes, M.C., Jacobs, J.W., Boers, M., Andrews, T., Blom-Bakkers, M.A., Buttgereit, F., Caeyers, N., Cutolo, M., Da Silva, J.A., Guillevin, L., Kirwan, J.R., Rovensky, J., Severijns, G., Webber, S., Westhovens, R., & Bijlsma, J.W. (2010). Monitoring adverse events of low-dose glucocorticoid therapy: EULAR recommendations for clinical trials and daily practice. *Ann Rheum Dis* Vol. 69, No. 11, pp. 1913-1919

van Raalte, D.H., Ouwens, D.M., & Diamant, M. (2009). Novel insights into glucocorticoid-mediated diabetogenic effects: towards expansion of therapeutic options? *Eur J Clin Invest* Vol. 39, No. 2, pp. 81-93

Wang, Z., Frederick, J., & Garabedian, M.J. (2002). Deciphering the phosphorylation "code" of the glucocorticoid receptor in vivo. *J Biol Chem* Vol. 277, No. 29, pp. 26573-26580

Wang, Z., & Garabedian, M.J. (2003). Modulation of glucocorticoid receptor transcriptional activation, phosphorylation, and growth inhibition by p27Kip1. *J Biol Chem* Vol. 278, No. 51, pp. 50897-50901

Warrier, M., Hinds, T.D., Jr., Ledford, K.J., Cash, H.A., Patel, P.R., Bowman, T.A., Stechschulte, L.A., Yong, W., Shou, W., Najjar, S.M., & Sanchez, E.R. (2010). Susceptibility to diet-induced hepatic steatosis and glucocorticoid resistance in FK506-binding protein 52-deficient mice. *Endocrinology* Vol. 151, No. 7, pp. 3225-3236

Webster, J.C., Jewell, C.M., Bodwell, J.E., Munck, A., Sar, M., & Cidlowski, J.A. (1997). Mouse glucocorticoid receptor phosphorylation status influences multiple functions of the receptor protein. *J Biol Chem* Vol. 272, No. 14, pp. 9287-9293

Vegiopoulos, A., & Herzig, S. (2007). Glucocorticoids, metabolism and metabolic diseases. *Mol Cell Endocrinol* Vol. 275, No. 1-2, pp. 43-61

Weigensberg, M.J., Toledo-Corral, C.M., & Goran, M.I. (2008). Association between the metabolic syndrome and serum cortisol in overweight Latino youth. *J Clin Endocrinol Metab* Vol. 93, No. 4, pp. 1372-1378

Whorwood, C.B., Donovan, S.J., Wood, P.J., & Phillips, D.I. (2001). Regulation of glucocorticoid receptor α and β isoforms and type I 11β-hydroxysteroid dehydrogenase expression in human skeletal muscle cells: a key role in the pathogenesis of insulin resistance? *J Clin Endocrinol Metab* Vol. 86, No. 5, pp. 2296-2308

Wilson, C.G., May, C.S., & Paterson, J.W. (1977). Plasma prednisolone levels in man following administration in plain and enteric-coated forms. *Br J Clin Pharmacol* Vol. 4, No. 3, pp. 351-355

Wochnik, G.M., Ruegg, J., Abel, G.A., Schmidt, U., Holsboer, F., & Rein, T. (2005). FK506-binding proteins 51 and 52 differentially regulate dynein interaction and nuclear translocation of the glucocorticoid receptor in mammalian cells. *J Biol Chem* Vol. 280, No. 6, pp. 4609-4616

Voice, M.W., Seckl, J.R., Edwards, C.R., & Chapman, K.E. (1996). 11β-hydroxysteroid dehydrogenase type 1 expression in 2S FAZA hepatoma cells is hormonally regulated: a model system for the study of hepatic glucocorticoid metabolism. *Biochem J* Vol. 317, No. Pt 2, pp. 621-625.

Yang, Z., Wolf, I.M., Chen, H., Periyasamy, S., Chen, Z., Yong, W., Shi, S., Zhao, W., Xu, J., Srivastava, A., Sanchez, E.R., & Shou, W. (2006). FK506-binding protein 52 is essential to uterine reproductive physiology controlled by the progesterone receptor A isoform. *Mol Endocrinol* Vol. 20, No. 11, pp. 2682-2694

Zhou, J., & Cidlowski, J.A. (2005). The human glucocorticoid receptor: one gene, multiple proteins and diverse responses. *Steroids* Vol. 70, No. 5-7, pp. 407-417

Zuo, Z., Urban, G., Scammell, J.G., Dean, N.M., McLean, T.K., Aragon, I., & Honkanen, R.E. (1999). Ser/Thr protein phosphatase type 5 (PP5) is a negative regulator of glucocorticoid receptor-mediated growth arrest. *Biochemistry* Vol. 38, No. 28, pp. 8849-8857

Chapter 2

Neurophysiological Basis of Food Craving

Ignacio Jáuregui Lobera

Additional information is available at the end of the chapter

http://dx.doi.org/10.5772/48717

1. Introduction

Craving is defined as an irresistible urge to consume a substance and its study was initiated in the field of drugs, considering that it constituted an important base for maintaining addictions (Tiffany, 1990, 1995). From a psychophysiological point of view it would be a motivational state that encourages consumption of both, drugs or food (Cepeda-Benito & Gleaves, 2001).

Psychological explanations based on learning theories, being appropriate, are insufficient to explain the irresistible desire for food. That food craving seems to share the neurophysiological basis with the craving for drugs.

The addictive substances share some ability to induce lasting structural changes in the central nervous system, specifically in regions implicated in reinforcement-motivation. Situational elements associated with the intake of these substances become attractive or outgoing incentives. In short, sensitization maintains the addictive behaviour, beyond or independently of other motivational elements (e.g., the rewarding effect of substances) or aversive properties specific to the situation of abstinence. This model of Robinson and Berridge (2003) would be different from the proposed theories of incentive or homeostatic theories.

Craving for drugs and food craving have differences, which seem to lie in the ability of the drug to sensitize, more intensely, the dopaminergic systems, although the process, in both cases is similar, sharing the same brain structures. In craving for drugs, incentive properties of substances (which tend to increase gradually) and the subjective pleasurable effects (which usually decrease) are usually differentiated. In order to understand the phenomenon of food craving it must be distinguished between what one likes and what one wants. Usually one wants what one likes and one likes what one wants, but both (wanting and liking) do not always go together. It seems that the neural substrates are different in each case. The taste, pleasure or enjoyment of food is determined by the opioid system and the system of neurotransmitters gamma-amino-butyric acid/ benzodiazepines, GABA/BZD), anatomically located in the ventral pallidum and primary gustatory areas of the brainstem. On the other hand, the desire for food (appetitive aspect, incentive) is determined by the mesencephalic dopaminergic system anatomically located in the nucleus accumbens and amygdala.

Neurotransmitter	**Effect**
Dopamine decrease	Dysphoria *
Serotonin decrease	Dysphoria
γ-Aminobutyric acid decrease	Anxiety **
Neuropeptide Y decrease	Anti-stress
Dynorphin increase	Dysphoria
Corticotropin-releasing factor increase	Stress
Norepinephrine increase	Stress

Table 1. Aversive emotional effects caused by neurotransmitter changes in abstinence of substances (From Koob & Le Moal, 2008)

* Any unpleasant or uncomfortable mood (dissatisfaction, irritableness)

** A combination of edgy symptoms, difficulty in concentration, muscular tension, sleep disturbances, etc.

Taste and desire for food may occur outside of subjective consciousness. As a result, it may be difficult for humans to distinguish between what they like (pleasure) and what they want (craving). Pelchat et al., (2004) identified a specific brain activation in subjects with food craving, located in the hippocampus, insula and caudate. The activation of such structures has been shown in experimental induction studies on the desire for food or drugs. It has been suggested that hippocampus and insula evoke the memory of craving precipitators reinforcing stimuli, whereas the dopamine released in the caudate nucleus is related to the incentive to these stimuli. The desire, as craving, liking or both, has been linked to the parahippocampal and fusiform gyrus, putamen, anterior cingulate cortex, amygdala and orbitofrontal cortex. These last two structures seem to be a key for the motivational control of eating behaviour. What is the role of those extrinsic determinants of the desire for food (learned) that are capable of arousing the desire for it without the homeostatic deficit related with hunger? It seems that the amygdala would be a meeting point of the value of the food given by hunger with the hedonic properties (learning) of that food. We also know that hunger is able to modulate orbitofrontal activity related to the information of the food (sensory, affective value, previous experience) to guide the subsequent behaviour.

The prefrontal cortex mediates complex executive functions (e.g., self-control). It is known that orbitofrontal damage causes behavioural disinhibition and perseveration, with failure in the assessment of the consequences of one's own actions. In addition, dorsolateral lesions cause cognitive deficits such as reduced ability to relate stimuli, less capacity for abstraction and rigidity of thought. Finally, a global damage at the level of medial frontal cortex and anterior cingulate is associated with apathy and lack of future planning.

If craving is associated with brain changes induced by substances, such changes, in turn, will cause a psychological change. Thus, a dysfunction of the cortical systems, that govern decision-making and behavioural inhibition, leads to emotional and cognitive deregulation. A reduced prefrontal activity may increase the activity of subcortical dopamine systems by raising the appetite awareness. In summary, dopaminergic hyperactivity may cause a low activity of prefrontal cortex related to impulse control deficits.

Different substances and food are not the only factors that may sensitize dopaminergic mesocortical system resulting in an "isolation" of the prefrontal cortex to devote itself to less rational behaviours. Daily environmental stressors causing anxiety may sensitize chronically subcortical areas (nucleus accumbens, amygdala and striatum), which are the basis of impulse or acquired appetite manifested as craving (for drugs or food). The mesocortical dopaminergic system hyperactivity (caused by drugs, food or anxiety) increases sensitivity to craving (with relapse, in the case of food, in form of binge eating). The experience of craving is irrational, and there is a deficit of frontal inhibitory control over subcortical systems that mediate incentive appetitive responses and automated and unconscious behaviours.

But the irrational overwhelming desire (craving) is often accompanied by an attempt of rational avoidance. Thus, the first pre-attentive attraction for food (craving) is often accompanied by attempts to avoid its use (restriction), thus emerging an approach-avoidance motivational conflict. The approach would be automatic, pre-attentive, involuntary, emotional, impulsive and irrational (craving) with a subcortical base, and avoidance would be aware, attentive, voluntary, cognitive, planned and rational (control) with a cortical base.

To some extent, it would be correct to say that an aberrant functioning of a body homeostatic system occurs. This system would have the hypothalamus as its brain structure, which receives hormonal signals of hunger and satiety (e.g., leptin released by adipocytes during satiety or ghrelin secreted in the stomach during hunger). The system seems to be perfect to respond to signals of hunger and satiety, when to eat and when to stop eating.

However, paradoxically, human beings can eat while satiated and, therefore, they have other reasons (pleasure) to eat beyond hunger. That brings to mind a second system involved in food motivation, the motivational or reward system. This reward system seems to be constituted by a neural network of cortical and mesolimbic structures with a core role of the nucleus accumbens of the striatum. This reward system has been evolutionarily modified so that pleasurable stimuli (essential for survival such as food, sex and other natural rewards) are attended, desired and wanted, while aversive stimuli (predators, poisons) are also attended but as a result avoided and unwanted. Therefore, the system responds to motivationally relevant cues.

Regarding the food, the reward system regulates the experience or desire to eat (craving) and hedonic responses to food (liking). The desire or craving is associated with dopamine release while liking is also modulated by the release of endogenous opioids such as endorphins.

Eating behaviour results from the interaction of both systems, assuming that motivational-hedonic mechanisms might nullify purely homeostatic mechanisms. Thus, the mere presence of food-related stimuli would become more powerful than the usual satiety signals facing the intake of food.

The role of the motivational system is of interest in understanding both the normal and pathological eating behaviour. Based on animal experiments it is known that rats make less effort to obtain food and eat less when their dopaminergic activity is eliminated. Similarly, human neuroimaging research has shown that dopamine is directly involved in food craving. Using positron emission tomography (PET) an increased release of dopamine has been observed in the striatum in hungry participants compared with satiated participants, both exposed to food stimuli. Furthermore, the amount of dopamine correlated positively with the subjective experience of food craving. On the other hand, it is well known that antipsychotic drugs (blockers of the dopamine D2-receptor binding) increase appetite and often lead to weight gain (sometimes important), while amphetamines (which increase dopamine activity in the brain) reduce appetite.

Wang et al., (2004) found by means of PET, a significant reduction in the density of dopamine-D2 receptors in the striatum of obese patients compared with individuals of normal weight. The number of dopamine-D2 receptors negatively correlated with BMI in obese participants, so that the higher the degree of obesity the lower the number of these receptors. Previously, other authors have found a higher prevalence of the Taq1-A1 allele in obese patients. This allele is also associated with fewer dopamine-D2 receptors. More recent studies have confirmed the relationship between overweight/obesity and a depression of the dopaminergic reward system.

Returning to the beginning, it should be noted that the finding of a lower density of these receptors in obesity has also been found in drug addiction. The question arises whether this reduction in D2-dopamine receptors density is a cause or a consequence of both obesity and substance dependencies. Some authors state that it would be a down-regulation caused by overstimulation of the reward system due to the chronic use of a substance or a sustained overeating. For others, the reduction in receptors density would be an indicator of an innate vulnerability to reach an addiction. Blum et al. (2000) speak of a "reward deficiency syndrome" in which people with fewer dopamine receptors lack the ability to enjoy the simple and routine rewards of everyday life (for lack of adequate dopamine release in response to these stimuli). Therefore, these people are driven to seek more potent stimuli of reward, like food or drugs.

At this point it is worth mentioning some differences with respect to hunger, appetite and craving. Hunger is the basic, very physical need for food. It happens around three to four hours after eating the last meal once the stomach has emptied. The muscular walls of the stomach begin to contract and grind, sending neurohormonal messages to the brain, indicating that it is time to eat again. Meanwhile, dipping levels of blood sugar send similar signals to the brain.

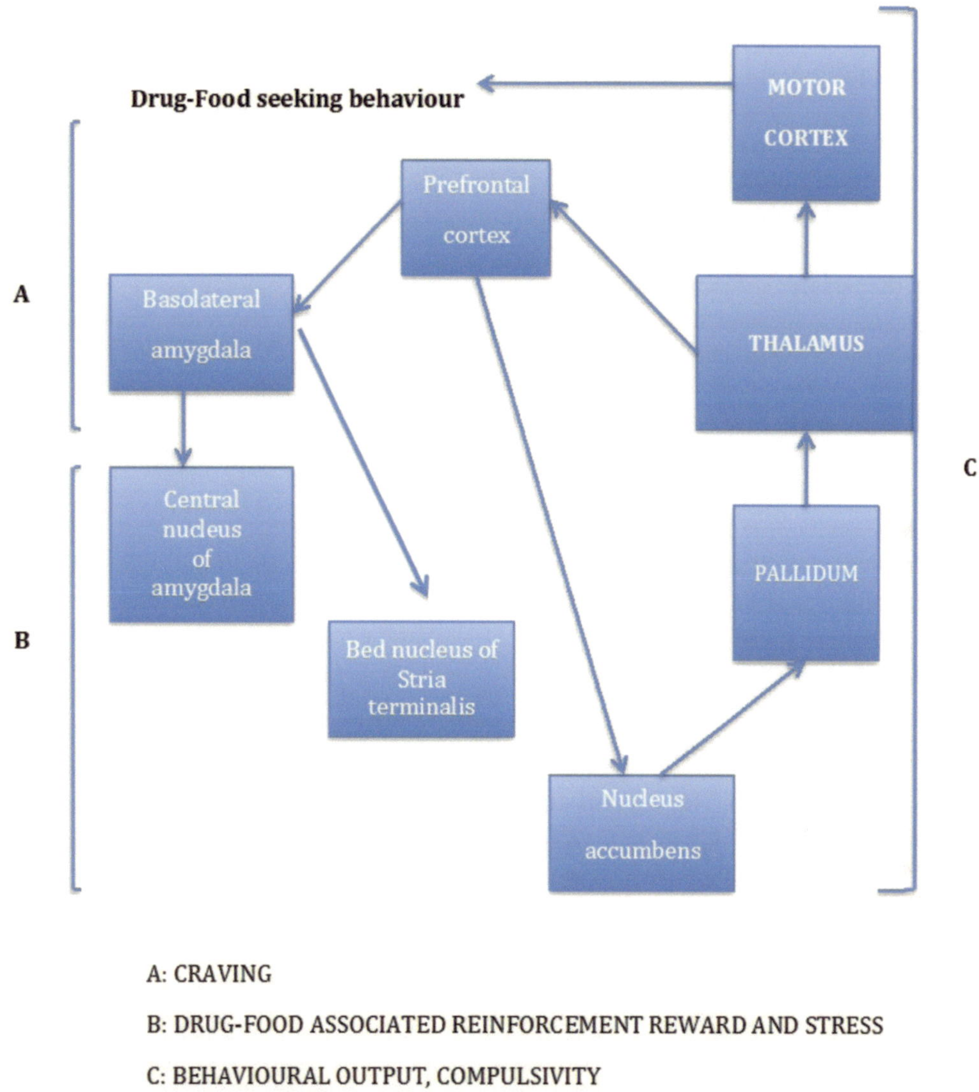

Figure 1. Neural circuits involved in addiction. Modified from Le Moal and Koob (2007)

Appetite is all about the desire for food triggered by anything from the thought, smell and sight of it. One can have an appetite for something even when physically full. The list of things that stimulate, tempt and perpetuate appetite are highly personal and almost endless, and it's easy to see how one can mix them up with genuine cues of physical hunger.

In addition to hunger and appetite, many people experience cravings, a powerful longing for one particular type of food. In practice, cravings are usually emotionally based or simply down to habit.

1.1. Summarizing

- From a psychophysiological point of view, food craving can be defined as a motivational state that encourages the consumption of food.
- Although it appears that in drug craving, drugs sensitize more intensely the dopaminergic systems, the craving for drugs and food share brain structures.
- Taste, pleasure or enjoyment of food is determined by the opioid system and by the system GABA/BZD neurotransmitters. On the other hand, the desire for food is determined by the mesencephalic dopaminergic system.
- The amygdala would be the meeting point between the value of food caused by hunger and the hedonic properties of food.
- Craving is associated with brain changes produced by food, and such changes in turn cause psychological changes.
- Everyday stressors that cause anxiety can chronically sensitize the subcortical areas, which are the base of the impulse or acquired appetite (craving).
- Humans can eat being satiated, so there may be other motives (pleasure) to eat beyond hunger. This suggests a second system involved in food motivation, namely motivational or reward system.
- The "reward deficiency syndrome" (Blum et al., 2000) assumes that people with fewer dopamine receptors do not properly enjoy the regular and simple rewards of everyday life (due to a lack of an adequate release of dopamine after these stimuli), which would lead them to search for more powerful stimuli of reward as, for example, food.

2. Obesity and addiction

Once the link between craving for substances or food is analysed, it is easy to assume that it could be a link between intake and addiction. In fact, there are some similarities between obesity and substance dependencies. In both cases there is a problematic central behaviour: the intake of something repeatedly, excessively, uncontrollably, causing an immediate strengthening effect but which has long-term dire consequences on both physical and psychosocial health. In treatment programs for both obesity and substance dependence, relapses are frequent, the usual relapse trigger being an intense craving that leads to loss of control. It seems that in both cases there is an excessive response to stimuli associated with the substance (drug or food).

In addictions, the responses to signals of substances (craving) are essential for the persistence of dependence. The release of dopamine in the reward system is associated with cognitive reactivity (e.g., attention bias), physiological (e.g., tachycardia), subjective (craving) and behavioural (e.g., approach behaviour) to the perception of signals related to substances. To explain the relationship between the perception of stimuli and substance use different models have been proposed as, for example, the model of Robinson and Berridge (1993), which considers that due to the sensitization of the dopaminergic system of reward (for the repeated use of a substance) certain qualities (incentives) are attributed not only to the substance but to the entire set of stimuli associated with it (by a process of classical conditioning). Thus, the mere perception of such stimuli would induce a classically conditioned dopamine release in the mesolimbic reward system. The consequence is that such stimuli catch the attention, cause craving and lead to the search for the substance. The model of Robinson and Berridge (1993) was modified by Franken (2003) who added the idea that attention bias and craving have mutually excitatory interactions.

These neurocognitive models related with substances may be applied to eating behaviour, especially in overweight/obesity. The first models of addiction applied to eating behaviour focused on physiological reactivity of food signals (brain response), while more recent models focus on attention bias to stimuli associated with food. The basis of these models is that in obese people there is an increased reactivity to stimuli associated with food compared with people at normal weight.

Our relationship with food presents a clear difference with the relationship with drugs: we need food and we cannot do without it, as we can do with drugs. Therefore, our reward system responds to the food as something attractive, attention grabber and desired. In this sense all persons may be "addicted" to food. However, due to sensitization and hyperresponsiveness (innate or acquired) of the reward system obese people have a greater attention bias than people at normal weight.

This attention bias toward food-related stimuli would be greater in obese people in situations of hunger and satiety. This seems to be contrary to the internality-externality theory of Schachter (1968, 1971), which assumes that obese people would be insensitive to internal cues of hunger and satiety.

Attention bias to stimuli associated with food is related to energy intake and this energy intake is also related with food craving. The reciprocal stimulation between the attention to food and food craving leads people to seek food. This behavioural response is enhanced as it may be seen in obese people compared with persons at normal weight.

People with an intake based on external stimuli usually show greater reactivity to food-related signals. This reactivity is expressed as attention bias, food craving and energy intake.

As obesity, it has been suggested that binge eating disorder has common aspects with addictions. The experience of bingeing is accompanied by the feeling of loss of control and other negative feelings, and often occurs after a previous period of more or less restriction. In patients with binge eating disorder some attention biases have been found (e.g., with the Stroop test) and comparing obese women with binge eating disorder with obese women without that disorder, the first group report more craving related with food stimuli. Therefore it seems that there would be a relationship between the presence of binge eating and the responsiveness to food-related stimuli.

Negative affects have also been analysed in relation to overeating. For example, it was found that patients with overweight/obesity without associated eating disorders and with high negative affect show a tendency to binge in response to negative mood induction and food exposure, while patients with overweight/obesity without associated eating disorders and with low negative affect and normal weight participants usually eat a similar amount of food under the same experimental conditions. The conclusion is that obese or overweight patients with high negative affectivity present extra difficulties to resist the temptation to eat.

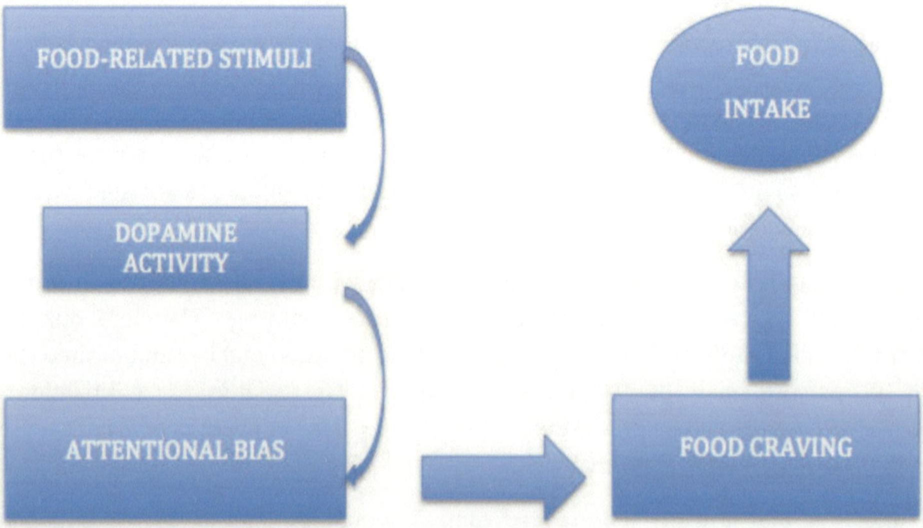

Figure 2. Neurocognitive model derived from Franken (2003).

Something similar occurs with stress, which could increase the vulnerability to eat after being exposed to food signals. Indeed both acute and chronic stresses are related with the maintenance of obesity and with relapse (presence of binge eating) as well as with a greater appetite for hypercaloric foods. It seems that stress signals enter into interaction with the reward system.

2.1. Summarizing

- The neurocognitive models related with substances may be applied to eating behaviour, especially in overweight/obesity.
- The base of these models is that in obese people there is an increased reactivity to stimuli associated with food compared with people at normal weight
- Due to sensitization and hyperresponsiveness (innate or acquired) of the reward system obese people have a greater attention bias than people at normal weight.
- As obesity, it has been suggested that binge eating disorder has common aspects with addictions.
- In patients with binge eating disorder some attention biases have been found and comparing obese women with binge eating disorder with obese women without that disorder, the first group report more craving related with food stimuli.
- Overweight/obese patients without associated eating disorders and with high negative affect show a tendency to binge in response to negative mood induction and food

exposure, while overweight/obese patients without associated eating disorders and with low negative affect and normal weight participants usually eat.

- Both acute and chronic stresses are related with the maintenance of obesity and with relapse (presence of binge eating) as well as with a greater appetite for hypercaloric foods. It seems that stress signals enter into interaction with the reward system.

3. Psychophysiology of craving

As it has been seen before, the current basic model of study focuses on the reactivity to stimuli or signals (cue reactivity). Studies are based on exposing the presence of food and recording the physiological and subjective responses of participants. The response to a substance-related stimuli and the response to the substance itself are different (opposite) for the so called homeostatic theories. However, theories based on the incentive effects of the substances indicate that physiological responses will be consistent with the reinforcing capacities of the substances. Cognitive models also predict different results depending on the different theories of these models. For some authors (Baker et al., 1987) it would be two motivational systems involved in craving, the appetitive and the aversive. According to Baker et al., both can be activated directly by the substances thus contributing to the compulsive consumption of them. Being two reciprocally inhibitory systems, the response to the substance is given by the system that prevails: appetitive response (as indicated by the theories of incentive) or aversive response (as suggested by the homeostatic theories). Tiffany (1990) states that the responses associated with the substance and the contextual stimuli related to their consumption are linked to the consequent behaviour. Faced with substance-related stimuli, it is possible to observe, for example, an increase in the heart rate.

But what does this physiological response mean? It could indicate a preparation for physical action (Obrist et al., 1970), a cognitive effort to process the desire of the substance (Tiffany, 1990) or a negative affect resulting from the frustration of not being able to consume the substance (Drobes et al., 2001). Therefore, faced with a substance, the physiological responses may indicate different aspects to consider. There is a good example of the complexity of the meaning of the responses. Thus, an increase in skin conductance as a response to the smell and the presence of alcohol in alcoholics has been found (Staiger et al., 1999) as well as a response to the presence of chocolate cookies in people with food craving (Wilson & Mercer, 1990). However, the presentation of stimuli-related and not related to alcohol causes a similar skin conductance in alcoholics (Stormak et al., 1993), and considering the psychophysiological responses to food, restrictive and not restrictive people, have similar responses (Overduin et al., 1997).

Other psychophysiological measures such as heart rate and blood pressure have been considered as powerful psychophysiological predictors of eating behaviour. For example, induction of stress (with increased heart rate and blood pressure) may inhibit food intake in non-restrictive females (but not in restrictive). In some diseases, such as bulimia nervosa, an increased attention to pictures of food accompanied by slow heart rate has been observed (Laberg et al., 1991).

The psychophysiological measures of food craving highlights the anticipation of eating (cognitive development), the knowledge of the responses to food signals and the knowledge of affective responses to such stimuli (Cavallo & Pinto, 2001; Lang et al., 1993, Overduin et al., 1997).

The response to food craving in the form of binge eating (not necessary but usual) has led to analyse its triggers, both on the basis of food deprivation as well as postulating negative moods at the origin. The homeostatic model argues that food restriction produces biological effects (e.g., changes in brain neurotransmitters) that cause the uncontrollable desire to eat (craving). Binge eating would be the way to restore the lost balance, in many cases all that happens as well. In patients with eating disorders, the onset of binge eating episodes is frequently preceded by dieting (Green, 2001; Polivy & Herman, 2002; Stice, 2001).

As homeostatic theories, cognitive theories consider that food restriction is a food craving trigger. Thoughts about food, body image and weight are usual explanations that people give about their restrictions or overeating. The restriction involves feelings of psychophysiological deprivation (craving) that lead to loss of behavioural control and possible binge episodes. Moreover if it is likely possible the use of compensatory behaviours, the probability of chaos increases (Gendall & Joyce, 2001; Jansen, 2001). Models based on physiological deprivation (homeostatic) and psychological deprivation (cognitive), as triggers of craving and binge eating, have empirical support. Nevertheless it is well known that only the feeling of hunger does not completely explain the uncontrolled episodes. In addition, the fact that negative emotional states (anxiety, boredom, sadness) may also cause uncontrolled episodes suggests that food deprivation is not a sufficient explanation for the presence of craving and bingeing (Moreno, 2003: Stice & Fairburn, 2003). Considering the distinction between objective and subjective binge eating, it was found that food deprivation with a negative emotional state may raise the former, while negative mood is capable, by itself, to elicit subjective binge eating (Agras & Telch, 1998). The relationship between negative mood and eating behaviour leads to talk about emotional eating, which takes the value of food to alleviate these negative moods. Craving implies a link between emotional states and food intake, although craving does not always lead to the intake (Hetherington & Macdiarmid, 1993). In regards to the relationship between craving and binge eating, the influence of two fundamental variables such as hunger and stress have been suggested. It has even been shown that the craving-binge relationship increases when the sensation of hunger is lower but the feeling of tension is highest. In short, even with less hunger if there is a high tension, the probability that craving will end up in a binge episode increases (Waters, Hill, & Waller, 2001).

3.1. Summarizing

- It would be two motivational systems involved in craving, the appetitive and the aversive, and both can be activated directly by substances/food thus contributing to the compulsive consumption of them.

- Being two reciprocally inhibitory systems, the response to the substance is given by the system that prevails: appetitive response (as indicated by the theories of incentive) or aversive response (as suggested by the homeostatic theories).
- Faced with a substance, the physiological responses may indicate different aspects to consider.
- Induction of stress (with increased heart rate and blood pressure) may inhibit food intake in non-restrictive females (but not in restrictive).
- In some diseases, such as bulimia nervosa, an increased attention to pictures of food accompanied by slow heart rate has been observed.
- The response to food craving in the form of binge eating (not necessary but usual) has led to analyse its triggers, both on the basis of food deprivation as well as postulating negative moods at the origin.
- Models based on physiological deprivation (homeostatic) and psychological deprivation (cognitive), as triggers of craving and binge eating, have empirical support.
- Only the feeling of hunger does not explain completely the uncontrolled episodes. In addition, the fact that negative emotional states (anxiety, boredom, sadness) may also cause uncontrolled episodes suggests that food deprivation is not a sufficient explanation for the presence of craving and bingeing.

4. Conclusions

Theories focused on the psychophysiological mechanisms of food craving (e.g., Robinson & Berridge, 1993, 2003) argue that reinforcement and appetitive motivation that causes food can cause lasting changes in the brain structures involved, as the nucleus accumbens and amygdala. It would be a sensitization of dopaminergic systems that may explain the maintenance of craving regardless of the pleasurable effects of food (as suggested by the theories of incentive) or the aversive effects of food deprivation (as homeostatic theories propose). As noted by Garavan et al. (2000) and Wexler et al. (2001), craving needs the prefrontal and limbic structures involved in cognitive and emotional processes. Therefore, negative emotional states such as anxiety or depression, and those related to food stimuli that cause negative affective reactions can stimulate the mesocortical dopaminergic system and reduce the inhibitory control that the prefrontal and frontal cortex have on the subcortical structures, increasing the vulnerability to food craving. As a result, the sequence represented in Figure 3 would be triggered.

The approach to food can be done as an unconscious, automatic and preattentive level (appetitive motivational system) and avoidance could occur later as an attentional, conscious and controlled level (defence motivational system). Hyperactivation of the amygdala would explain the defensive style and the greater negative affect of people with high food craving and bulimia nervosa.

Overall, the theories that attempt to explain food craving emphasize the role of food deprivation (with the consequent psychological and physical discomfort) or the role of the relationship between dietary restraint and negative moods (eg, Polivy & Herman, 2002 ; Stice & Fairburn, 2003).

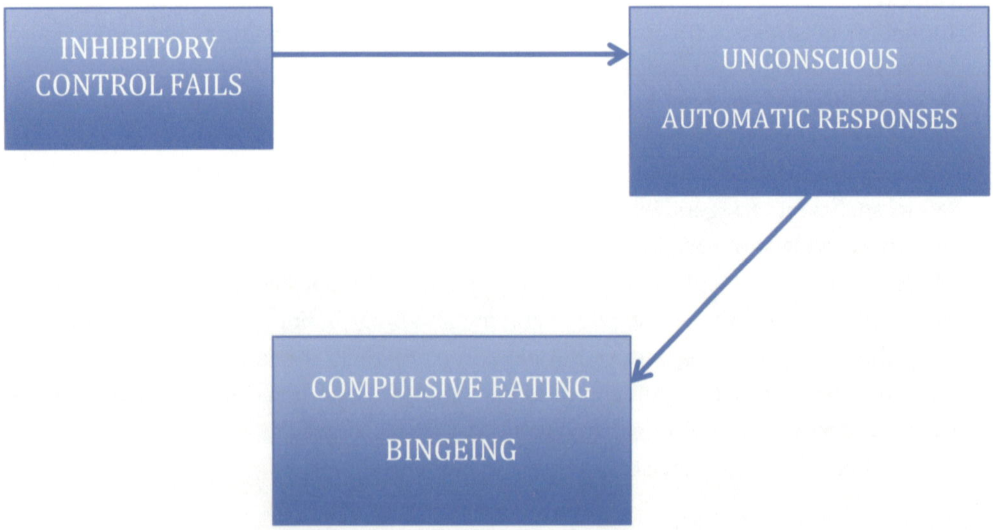

Figure 3. Cortical inhibitory control failure and its consequences.

Certain negative affects reduce the ability to control food intake, resulting in loss of control (binge). Deprivation of food should be accompanied by a negative mood in relation to craving and uncontrolled behaviour. In fact, among patients with bulimia nervosa, the combination of food craving without food deprivation (hunger) and negative affect seems to be the best predictor of binge eating (Moreno, 2003). In summary, the approach-avoidance motivational conflict related to food would be modulated by mood and food deprivation.

In the case of bulimia nervosa, an autonomic hyporeactivity, a defensive style and high negative affect have been reported (e.g., Legenbauer, Vögele, & Ruddel, 2004). This hyporresponsiveness is more characteristic of diffuse anxiety than of fear, and it must be taken into account that anxiety and fear have different neural basis. Thus, the central nucleus of the amygdala is responsible for fear and the bed nucleus of the stria terminalis is responsible for anxiety (Lang et al., 2000), both structures having similar efferent connections and being prepared to respond to significant emotional stimuli when well developed information comes from the basolateral nucleus of the amygdala (Davis, 1992). These subcortical structures can take the emotional control when the prefrontal cortex does not properly inhibit emotional stimuli, with consequent automatic and defensive responses.

The main ideas of this chapter would be summarised as indicated in Figure 4.

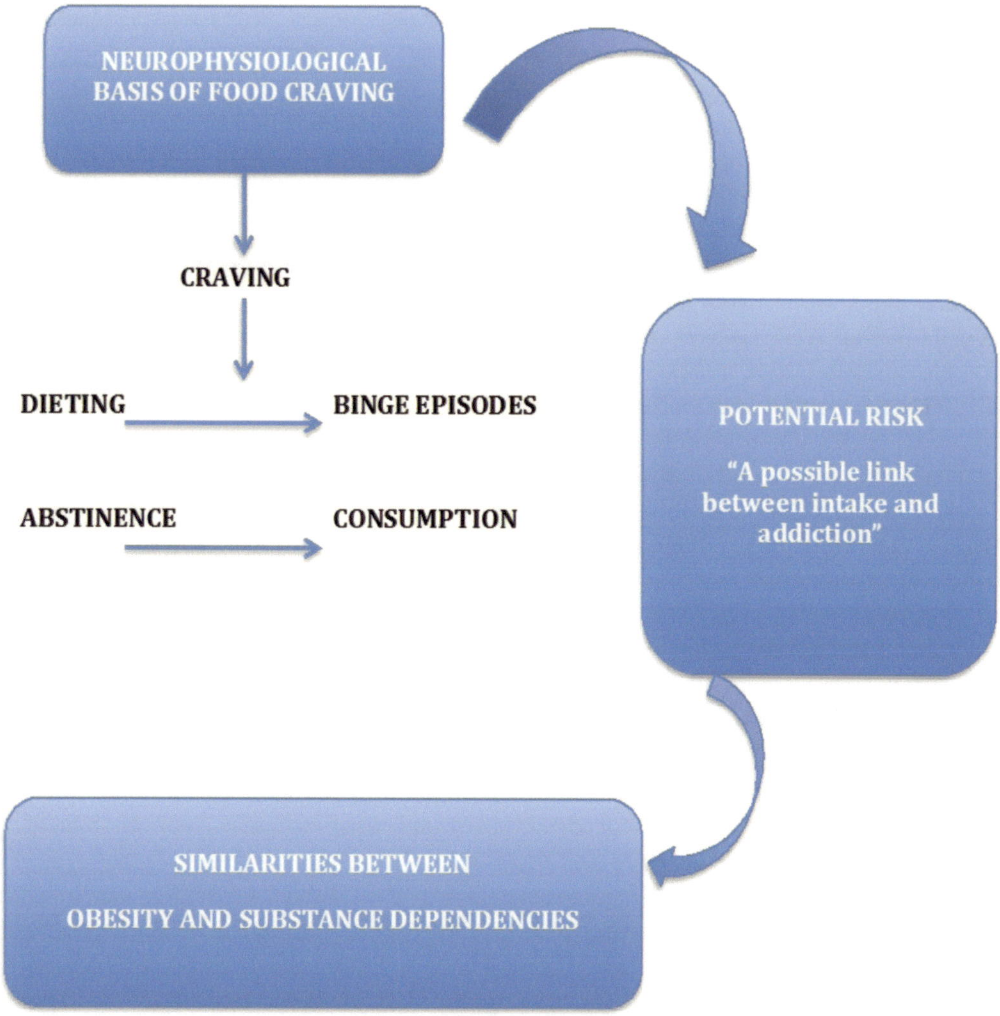

Figure 4. Main relationships with respect to neurophysiological basis of food craving, intake and addiction, and obesity and substance dependencies.

Author details

Ignacio Jáuregui Lobera
Department of Nutrition and Bromatology, Pablo de Olavide University, Seville, Spain

5. References

Agras, W.S. & Telch, C.F. (1998). The effects of caloric deprivation and negative affect on binge-eating in obese binge-eating disordered women. *Behavior Therapy, 29*, 491-503. ISSN 0005-7894.

Baker, T., Morse, E., & Sherman, J. (1987). The motivation to use drugs: a psychobiological analysis of urges. *The Nebraska Symposium on Motivation: alcohol use and abuse.* (pp. 257-323). Lincoln, NE: University of Nebraska Press. ISBN 9780803228801.

Blum, K., Braverman, E.R., Holder, J.M., Lubar, J.F., Monastra, V.J., Miller, D., Lubar, J.O., Chen, T.J., & Comings, D.E. (2000). Reward deficiency syndrome: a biogenetic model for the diagnosis and treatment of impulsive, addictive, and compulsive behaviors. *Journal of Psychoactive Drugs, 32,* Suppl:i-iv, 1-112. ISSN 0279-1072.

Cavallo, D.A. & Pinto, A. (2001). Effects of mood induction on eating behavior and cigarette craving in dietary restrainers. *Eating Behaviors, 2,* 113-127. ISSN 471-0153.

Cepeda-Benito, A. & Gleaves, D.H. (2001). A critique of food cravings research: Theory, measurement, food intake. In M.M. Hetherington (ed.), *Food cravings and addiction* (pp. 1-12). Surrey, U.K.: Leatherhead. ISBN 9780905748184.

Davis, M. (1992). The role of the amygdala in conditioned fear. In J. P. Aggleton (Ed.), *The amigdala: Neurobiological aspects of emotion, memory, and mental disfunction* (pp. 255-305). New York: Wiley-Liss. ISBN 9780471561293.

Drobes, D.J., Miller, E.J., Hillman, C.H., Bradley, M.M., Cuthbert, B.N., & Lang, P.J. (2001). Food deprivation and emotional reactions to food cues: Implications for eating disorders. *Biological Psychology, 57,* 153-177. ISSN 0301-0511.

Franken, I.H. (2003). Drug craving and addiction: integrating psychological and neuropsychopharmacological approaches. *Progress in Neuropsychopharmacology & Biological Psychiatry, 27,* 563-379. ISSN 0278-5846.

Garavan, H., Pankiewicz, J., Bloom, A., Cho, J.K., Sperry, L., Ross, T.J., Salmeron, B.J., Risinger, R., Kelley, D., & Stein, E.A. (2000). Cue-induced cocaine craving: neuroanatomical specificity for drug users and drug stimuli. *American Journal of Psychiatry, 157,* 1789-1798. ISSN 0002-953X.

Gendall, K.A. & Joyce, P.R. (2001). Characteristics of food cravers who binge eat. In M.M. Hetherington (Ed.), *Food Cravings and addiction* (pp. 88-101). Surrey, UK: Leatherhead Publishing. ISBN 9780905748184.

Green, M. (2001). Dietary restraint and craving. En M.M. Hetherington (Ed.), *Food Cravings and addiction* (pp.171-186). Surrey, UK: Leatherhead Publishing. ISBN 9780905748184.

Hetherington, M.M. & Macdiarmid, J.I. (1993). "Chocolate addiction": A preliminary srtudy of its description and its relationship to problem eating. *Appetite, 21,* 233-246. ISSN 0195-6663.

Jansen, A. (2001). Craving and binge eating. En M.M. Hetherington (Ed.), *Food cravings and addiction.* Surrey, UK: Leatherhead Publishing. ISBN 9780905748184.

Koob, G.F. & Le Moal, M. (2008). Addiction and the brain antireward system. *Annual Review of Psychology, 59,* 29-53. ISSN 0066-4308.

Laberg, J.C., Wilson, G.T., Eldredge, K., & Nordby, H. (1991). Effects of mood on heart rate reactivity in bulimia nervosa. *International Journal of Eating Disorders, 10* (2), 169-178. ISSN 0276-3478.

Lang, P.J., Davis, M., & Öhman, A. (2000). Fear and anxiety: Animals models and human cognitive psychophysiology. *Journal of Affective Disorders, 61,* 137-159. ISSN 0165-0327.

Lang, P.J., Greenwald, M.K., Bradley M.M., & Hamm, A.O. (1993). Looking at pictures: Affective, facial, visceral, and behavioral reactions. *Psychophysiology, 30,* 261-273. ISSN 0048-5772.

Le Moal, M. & Koob, G.F. (2007). Drug addiction: pathways to the disease and pathophysiological perspectives. *European Neuropsychopharmacology, 17,* 377-393. ISSN 0924-977X.

Legenbauer, T., Vögele, C., & Rüddel, H. (2004). Anticipatory effects of food exposure in women diagnosed with bulimia nervosa. *Appetite, 42,* 33-40. ISSN 0195-6663.

Moreno, S. (2003). *Ansia por la comida y Trastornos de la conducta alimentaria.* Tesis Doctoral. Universidad de Granada. Unpublished doctoral dissertation, University of Granada.

Obrist, P.A., Webb, R.A., Sutterer, J.R., & Howard, J.L. (1970). The cardiac-somatic relationship: some reformulations. *Psychophysiology, 6,* 569-587. ISSN 0048-5772.

Overduin, J., Jansen, A., & Eilkes, H. (1997). Cue reactivity to food- and body-related stimuli in restrained and unrestrained eaters. *Addictive Behaviors, 22* (3), 395-404. ISSN 0306-4603.

Pelchat, M.L., Johnson, A., Chan, R., Valdez, J., & Ragland, J.D. (2004). Images of desire: food-craving activation during fMRI. *Neuroimage, 23,* 1486-1493. ISSN 1053-8119.

Polivy, J. & Herman, P. (2002). Causes of eating disorders. *Annual Review Psychology, 53,* 187-213. ISSN 0066-4308.

Robinson, T.E. & Berridge, K.C. (1993). The neural basis of drug craving: an incentive-sensitization theory of addiction. *Brain Research. Brain Research Reviews, 18,* 247-291. ISSN 0165-0173.

Robinson, T.E. & Berridge, K.C. (2003). Addiction. *Annual Review of Psychology, 54,* 25-53. ISSN 0066-4308.

Schachter, S. (1968). Obesity and eating: internal and external cues differentially affect the eating behavior of obese and normal subjects. *Science, 161,* 751-756. ISSN 0036-8075.

Schachter, S. (1971). Some extraordinary facts about obese humans and rats. *American Psychologist, 26,* 129-144. ISSN 0003-066X.

Staiger, P.K., Greeley, J.D., & Wallace, S.D. (1999). Alcohol exposure therapy: Generalisation and changes in responsivity. *Drug and Alcohol Dependence, 57,* 29-40. ISSN 0376-8716.

Stice, E. (2001). A prospective test of the dual pathway model of bulimia pathology: mediating effects of dieting and negative affect. *Journal of Abnormal Psychology, 30,* 1089-1098. ISSN 0021-843X.

Stice, E. & Fairburn, C.G. (2003). Dietary and dietary-depressive subtypes of bulimia nervosa show differential symptom presentation, social impairment, comorbidity, and course of illness. *Journal of Consulting and Clinical Psychology, 71* (6), 1090-1094. ISSN 0022-006X.

Stormark, K.M., Laberg, J.C., Bjerland, T., & Hugdahl, K. (1993). Habituation of electrodermal reactivity to visual alcohol stimuli in alcoholics. *Addictive Behaviors,* 18, 437-443. ISSN 0306-4603.

Tiffany, S.T. (1990). A cognitive model of drug urges an drug use behaviour: Role of automatic and non-automatic processes. *Psychological Review, 97,* 147-168. ISSN 0033-295X.

Tiffany, S.T. (1995). The role of cognitive factors in reactivity to drug use. In D.C. Drummond, S.T. Tiffany, S. Glauter, & B. Remington (Eds.), *Addictive behavior: Cue exposure theory and practice* (pp. 145-162). New York: John Wiley & Sons. ISBN 0-471-94454-8.

Wang, G.J., Volkow, N.D., Thanos, P.K., & Fowler, J.S. (2004). Similarity between obesity and drug addiction as assessed by neurofunctional imaging: a concept review. *Journal of Addictive Diseases, 23,* 39-53. ISSN 1055-0887.

Waters, A., Hill, A., & Waller, G. (2001). Bulimics' response to food cravings: Is binge-eating a product of hunger or emotional state?. *Behaviour Research and Therapy, 39,* 877-886. 0005-7967.

Wexler, B.E., Gottschalk, C.H., Fulbright, R.K., Prohovnik, I., Lacadie, C.M., Rounsaville, B.J., & Gore, J.C. (2011). Functional magnetic resonance imaging of cocaine craving. *American Journal of Psychiatry, 158,* 86-95. ISSN 0002-953X.

Wilson, J.F. & Mercer, J.C. (1990). An electrophysiological correlate of Eating Attitudes Test scores in female college students. *Psychological Medicine, 20,* 973-975. ISSN 0033-2917.

Chapter 3

Screening of High-Risk Pregnant Women for Thyroid Dysfunctions in a Moderately Mild Iodine-Deficient Area

Imre Zoltán Kun, Zsuzsanna Szántó, Ildikó Kun and Béla Szabó

Additional information is available at the end of the chapter

http://dx.doi.org/10.5772/49971

1. Introduction

Pregnancy is a high risk condition for developing iodine-deficient disorders (IDD), mainly in circumstances of reduced iodine supply, due to the fact that during this physiological period of life the requirement of thyroid hormones increases with 30-50% (Alexander et al., 2012, Leung et al. 2011). Besides goiter, thyroid dysfunctions may develop. When the compensatory mechanisms become insufficient subclinical or overt hypothyroidism occur. Hypothyroidism may cause maternal and fetal complications: miscarriage, abortion, premature delivery, birth complications, neonatal respiratory distress syndrome, intellectual disabilities in offsprings including cretinism, growth retardation (Boyages, 1993; Pharoah et al., 1971, de Escobar et al., 2007; Cao et al., 1994). Thus hypothyroidism must be recognized and treated as early as possible, which would be before pregnancy, to avoid the above mentioned complications. Screening of pregnant women and of those who intend to become pregnant would be an adequate method for this purpose.

However, the screening for thyroid diseases in pregnant and lactating women is still an issue under debate. The inclusion criteria of the screening process are mostly disputed. Some authors consider the screening of high-risk pregnant women for thyroid disorders sufficient, others suggest universal screening program (the assessment of all women during pregnancy for thyroid conditions), mostly in iodine deficient areas. Iodine and thyroid hormones are essential for normal fetal and neonatal development, and their increased requirement in pregnancy rises the frequency of goiter and thyroid dysfunctions. These diseases are often oligosymptomatic and can easily remain undiagnosed, consequently fetal developmental impairments of different severity (even mental retardation, endemic cretinism) can appear in the circumstances of iodine and thyroid hormone deficiency.

Universal screening in pregnancy may be indicated in iodine deficient regions, but it represents a serious financial effort which was not considered justified by the evidences until 2007. Therefore, targeted case finding during early pregnancy, i.e. screening for thyroid diseases in high-risk pregnant women was recommended. This high-risk population group comprises pregnant women with history of hyper-/hypothyroidism, postpartum thyroiditis, thyroid surgery, previous head or neck radiation therapy, and miscarriage or preterm delivery, family history of thyroid disease, presence of goiter and/or thyroid antibodies, symptoms/clinical sings suggesting hyper-/hypothyroidism (including anemia, hypercholesterolemia, hyponatremia), type I diabetes and other autoimmune diseases (Endocrine Society's Clinical Guideline, 2007).

Iodine deficiency in Romania was confirmed by Milcu about 50-60 years ago (Milcu, 1956). The use of iodized alimentary salt has been introduced as a prophylactic method in our country since 1948 (15-25mg potassium iodide or 10mg potassium iodate per kg salt). From 1956 a supplementary iodine prophylaxis was started by administration of potassium iodide tablets (1mg KI/tb.) to school-age children and pregnant women.

The iodine status of our region, Mureş County, has been periodically assessed by a team of endocrinologists from the Endocrinology Clinic Târgu Mureş since 1960-70. From the geographic and epidemiologic point of view Mureş County is a 6,700 square km large hilly-mountainous region in the Transylvanian Basin, located in the centre of Romania, crossed by the river Mureş. Its estimated population is about 600,000, with a light variation in the last decades: the number of inhabitants was 614,000 in 1984, with a mild increase to 620,500 until 1990, followed by a slow decrease to 579,000 in 2007. These data are provided by the epidemiologic registers of National Institute of Statistics based on the censuses of population and housing realized in Romania (Romanian National Institute of Statistics, 2012).

In 2000 Balázs et al. reported in a study the assessment of iodine deficiency in the hydrographic basin of the superior and middle part of river Mureş, including the collected data of 508 children in their work: 26.97% (137) from urban and 73.03% (371) from rural localities. The thyroid volume was evaluated clinically and ultrasonographically. The majority of rural localities presented mild and the others moderate iodine-deficiency. The county town, Târgu Mureş was found iodine-sufficient. The mean urinary iodine excretion was 100.22μg/L, but with large inter-individual variations (SD: ± 73.37). This study emphasized the great frequency of small goiters in rural localities compared to their more reduced frequency in cities (Balázs et al., 2000/a).

Our studies performed during 2001-2004 (by the examination of urinary iodine content, thyroid ultrasound in school-age children and pregnant women, neonatal TSH screening) have confirmed that Mureş County was constantly a mild/moderate iodine deficient geographic area (Kun et al., 2003). During 2001-2003 we observed elevated serum TSH-values (above 10mIU/L, according to the criterion of WHO) in 8.23% out of 2,454 studied newborns, with a mean TSH-level of 19.81 ± 12.63mIU/L (Szántó et al., 2007).

According to these data is obvious that Mureş County, during the last decades of 20th century and beginning of the 21st century was characterized as a moderate/mild iodine deficient area, thus an extensive screening of thyroid disturbances in pregnant women could be indicated, but it was not performed for financial reasons. In these circumstances we started a targeted screening in pregnant women with history of thyroid diseases and gestational complications (previous miscarriage, preterm or post-term delivery, postpartum anemia), as well as suggestive clinical signs/symptoms for thyroid dysfunctions.

Extended studies realized during 2002-2004 have shown a moderate iodine deficiency in the majority (80%) of Romanian counties (mainly in rural areas), the prevalence of endemic goiter being between 0-40% and low urinary iodine excretion at 2/3 in the examined persons (Simescu et al., 2006).

In order to ameliorate this national endemic problem a Romanian governmental decision (no. 568/5 June 2002) regarding the universal alimentary salt-iodization decided the release of alimentary salt with increased iodine-content on the market (34 ± 8.5mg KIO_3/kg). This Decision was implemented into practice in December 2003, and in 2004 the mandatory use of iodized salt in baking industry was disposed in all 41 counties, both in households and bakeries (Second National Conference for the Elimination of Iodine Deficiency Disorders, 2005; Kun, 2006). Consequently, iodized salt was used in 96% of households in 2004, according to some authors (Simescu et al., 2006). At the same time, starting from 2002 a national program has begun in order to estimate the iodine status of the Romanian population by promulgating IDD screening programs in high risk population groups (newborns, school-children, pregnant women). After the implementation of universal salt-iodization the incidence of IDD has decreased considerably in school-children in several counties (Simescu et al., 2006).

After these legislative changes, during 2004-2006 we restarted neonatal screening for thyroid dysfunctions. Comparing screening data obtained before and after universal salt iodization (2001-2003 vs. 2004-2006) we did not find significant differences regarding the incidence of elevated TSH levels, but an important reduction of mean values was observed in the second period (15.63 ± 7.35mIU/L) compared to the first one (19.81 ± 12.63mIU/L, i.e. a decrease with 4.2mIU/L, p=0.02), pleading for the amelioration of iodine deficiency (Kun, 2006; Kun et al., 2007).

In 2005-2006 the assessment of iodine status in three mountain villages showed a significant improvement of urinary iodine excretion (UIE) compared to data published by Balázs et al. (2000/b): in 1999 UIE was 56.00 ± 38.07µg/L, being normal only in 6% of the investigated children, mild (50-99µg/L) and moderately low (20-49µg/L) each in 44%, and under 20µg/L (very low) in 6%. Our results in October 2006 were improved, but still subnormal: the mean UIE increased to 85.37 ± 60.05µg/L, 30.8% of the children had normal values, and iodine-deficiency related hypothyroidism had an incidence of 15% in the investigated school-children. Thyroid ultrasound performed in these children showed diffuse goiter in 27% of the cases. Rural mountain areas of Mureş County known before as moderate/mild iodine deficient zones have become mild-deficient ones, due to the new measures of iodine prophylaxis (Kun et al., 2007).

According to our previous studies Mureş County was considered a moderate/mild iodine-deficient area before 2003, and based on our new results this area still may be considered a mild iodine-deficient region, mainly in mountainous rural localities (Kun, 2006; Kun et al., 2007; Balázs et al., 2000/b; Szántó et al., 2007), and thus iodine-prophylaxis has an important role in preventing IDD and its complications, including thyroid dysfunctions.

The main cause of iodine deficiency in most rural localities of Mureş County is their localization on hilly-mountainous geographical regions, composition of the land and water (Mureş river and its affluents) having low iodine content. The geographical isolation of mountainous places could be involved to some extent, the more isolated a locality is the more severe the iodine deficiency is. Larger localities and cities, such as Târgu Mureş were iodine sufficient places.

The evaluation of thyroid status in pregnant women living in Mureş County has not been reported yet, although our targeted screening started in 2001. We consider targeted screening for thyroid dysfunctions in pregnant women the thyroid assessment of those subjects who had thyroid disease or gestational complications in the past or who recently have developed signs/symptoms of thyroid dysfunction or goiter during pregnancy – so we consider these pregnant women of high risk.

2. Objectives

We proposed to perform the screening of thyroid dysfunctions in pregnant women residents of Mureş County, being at high risk for these diseases, by determining the frequency and severity of hypo-/hyperthyroidism and the possible related gestational complications.

We also wanted to assess the influence of universal salt iodization on thyroid status of this population group by comparing the results of targeted screening of high-risk pregnant women realized before (2001-2003) and after (2004-2006) taking effect the governmental Decision 568/2002, starting from December 2003.

3. Material and methods

Material. During November 2001 – February 2003 we performed a targeted screening of thyroid dysfunctions in 321 pregnant women living in Mureş County. This screening meant that TSH- and FT_4-levels were measured in pregnant women with history of thyroid disease, clinical signs or symptoms suggestive for thyroid dysfunction or goiter, history of gestational complications (threatened abortion, abortion, imminent preterm birth, preterm delivery, miscarriage) or complications during current pregnancy. These inclusion criteria implied that subjects with history of thyroid condition and gestational complications firstly underwent endocrinological evaluation mainly in the first trimester, but others were screened when one of the mentioned criteria appeared, which could happen in any trimester, even in the third one.

These pregnant women were registered in endocrine out-patient units from Târgu Mureş, Sighişoara, Reghin and Târnăveni (all four cities of our county), as well as in the Obstetrics & Gynecology Clinics in Târgu Mureş (the main city of Mureş County). In some cases we determined the titer of thyroid peroxidase antibodies (TPO-Ab) and urinary iodine excretion, too.

In order to evaluate the influence of universal iodization of alimentary salt on thyroid function in pregnancy, starting from 2004 we performed a second targeted screening based on the same inclusion criteria. Thus, during February 2004–September 2006 we screened 206 pregnant women, then we compared the results with those obtained during 2001-2003.

Gestational complications were assessed according to data provided by out-patient Endocrinology units, and medical records of pregnant women hospitalized for gestational complications or for delivery in the Obstetrics & Gynecology Clinics from Târgu Mureş, or obstetrical and neonatal sections of Hospitals from Sighişoara, Reghin and Târnăveni.

The state of health of newborns to hypothyroid mothers was evaluated in the first 5 days of their life, and the distribution of neonatal complications were assessed. These data were compared to a group of neonates born from apparently healthy mothers: normal TSH-level (between 1.5-2.5mIU/L), absence of thyroid diseases and other gestational risk factors (Rh-incompatibility, twin pregnancy, smoking etc.).

Since 2007 a new large systematized screening of pregnant women has not been performed yet, further investigations being necessary depending on financial possibilities.

Methods. Serum thyrotropin (TSH) and free-thyroxine (FT_4) levels were measured from venous blood during the morning in all women included in the study. Third generation immunometric assay (ECLIA – electrochemiluminescence immunoassay) was applied at the Central Laboratory of Emergency Clinical Hospital Mureş County.

Until 2006 we considered the reference range for TSH-level 0.2-3.5mIU/L in the first and 0.4-4.0mIU/L in the second and third trimesters and in case of pathological levels we started specific treatment, but in 2006-2007 new normal TSH-values for pregnant women were adopted (Endocrine Society's Clinical Guideline, 2007) and according to these we have re-evaluated our data base.

Reference ranges for serum TSH-levels were adjusted for pregnant women according to the gestational trimester: between 0.03–2.5mIU/L during the I., between 0.1–3.1mIU/L in the II. and between 0.1–3.5mIU/L in the III. trimester.

FT_4 reference range is 0.86–1.86ng/dL in the first and 0.64–1.92ng/dL in the II.–III. trimesters.

We also assessed isolated maternal hypothyroxinaemia, which was considered by us as a reduced FT_4 along a normal TSH level. This definition is not well delineated in the literature, because the reference range of TSH-level varies between large limits according to different authors and the gestational trimester (Vaidya et al., 2012; Glinoer & Abalovich, 2007; Burman, 2009). We have evaluated the TSH- and FT_4-values based on the above mentioned normal intervals.

The titer of TPO-Ab was considered normal under 35IU/mL. We could measure this parameter randomly in a total of 46 pregnant women from the whole casuistry: 24 cases during 2001-2003 and 22 during 2004-2006.

Urinary iodine excretion (UIE) measured with a semiquantitative rapid test was included into three ranges: <10µg%, between 10–30µg% and >30µg%, values <30µg% are considered low. This was determined in 69 randomized cases: 34 pregnant women included in the first and 35 in the second period.

The obtained data were statistically evaluated by Students' „t" test and χ^2 test. The difference between parameters of two groups was considered significant, if P-value <0.05.

Ethical considerations: Every pregnant woman was informed about screening procedures, the benefit of hormonal assessment, possible side effects and than the hormonal results. In case of thyroid dysfunction specific endocrine treatment was performed. The Research Ethics Committee of the University of Medicine and Pharmacy Târgu Mureş has approved the outline of the research process and the obtained results for publication, as all ethical rules were respected.

4. Results

During *November 2001–February 2003*, before the implementation of the presented governmental decision about universal alimentary salt-iodization we screened 321 high-risk pregnant women: 263 (81.9%) were euthyroid, 51 (15.88%) hypothyroid and 7 (2.18%) hyperthyroid. Two third (34 cases) out of the investigated hypothyroid women had subclinical and one third (17 cases) overt form. Among the 7 hyperthyroid pregnant women 4 suffered of subclinical and 3 of overt form.

Trimester	Total cases	Hypothyroidism	Goiter*	Hyperthyroidism
I.	102	23 (22.5%)	41 (40.2%)	2 (1.96%)
II.	126	15 (11.9%)	53 (42.0%)	1 (0.79%)
III.	93	13 (13.9%)	48 (51.6%)	4 (4.3%)
Total	321	51 (15.88%)	142 (44.23%)	7 (2.18%)

Table 1. Thyroid state of pregnant women being in different gestational trimesters (2001-2003)
* I. grade diffuse goiter in >80%, II. grade goiter in 14.4%, III. grade goiter in 0.6% of women.

Only 31.8% of the subjects were screened in the first trimester, the others were detected later (39.2% in the II. and 29% in the III. trimester).

We could follow-up 28 hypothyroid pregnant women having thyroid hypofunction from the inclusion in the screening until delivery. Half of them presented gestational complications: 2 threatened abortions, one imminent preterm delivery, 5 preterm births, 2 prolonged deliveries, 2 caesarean sections for fearing fetal asphyxia, one miscarriage (hypertension, edema) and one pre-eclampsia. In four patients other gestational risk factors could contribute to the development of these complications (Rh-incompatibility, twin pregnancy, smoking).

We excluded these cases, so the rate of gestational complications in hypothyroid pregnant women without other apparent risk factors decreased to 45.8% (11/24).

<table>
<tr><th>Gestational age at delivery</th><th colspan="2">Newborns of hypothyroid mothers</th><th colspan="2">Newborns of apparently healthy mothers</th></tr>
<tr><td rowspan="4">preterm</td><td rowspan="4">5</td><td>2 clinically healthy</td><td rowspan="4">2</td><td rowspan="2">1 clinically healthy</td></tr>
<tr><td>1 preterm – premature grade II.</td></tr>
<tr><td>1 preterm – premature grade I., A= 7/1′</td><td rowspan="2">1 asphyxia, A=7/1′</td></tr>
<tr><td>1 death by severe asphyxia*</td></tr>
<tr><td rowspan="2">post-term</td><td rowspan="2">2</td><td>1 clinically healthy</td><td colspan="2" rowspan="2">–</td></tr>
<tr><td>1 asphyxia, A=8/1′</td></tr>
<tr><td rowspan="2">born at term</td><td rowspan="2">21</td><td>20 clinically healthy</td><td rowspan="2">24</td><td>23 clinically healthy</td></tr>
<tr><td>1 asphyxia, A=8/1′(thyroidectomized mother, subclinical hypothyroidism)</td><td>1 asphyxia, A=7/1′</td></tr>
<tr><td>Total</td><td>28</td><td></td><td>26</td><td></td></tr>
</table>

Table 2. Newborns' health status at delivery and on the first 5 days of life
A: Apgar score; case marked with * is presented in the text

Seven (25%) out of the 28 neonates from hypothyroid mothers were born preterm or post-term, while 2 (7.7%) out of 26 apparently healthy women gave birth to preterm newborn. We observed preterm or post-term delivery in hypothyroid pregnant women significantly more often than in apparently healthy women (P-value: 0.07, OR: 3.7, 95%CI: 0.86–5.91), although these cases of hypothyroidism were mainly subclinical forms.

In one woman diagnosed with Hashimoto's thyroiditis in the third trimester multiple complications have developed: late miscarriage, severe pre-eclampsia, grade II. utero-placental apoplexia, which needed caesarean section at the 32-33. gestational week. The newborn (case marked with * in Table 2.) presented acute fetal suffering (Apgar score 1/1′, 2/5′, 3/10′). The newborn died on the 14th day of life due to severe asphyxia during birth, hyaline membrane disease, persistent pulmonary hypertension and pneumonia.

One pregnant woman with overt hyperthyroidism out of the total 7 hyperthyroid cases during 2001-2003 developed imminent premature birth.

TPO-Ab determined in 24 randomized cases was elevated in 3 patients (12.5%).

During November 2001 – February 2002 urinary iodine excretion measured with semi-quantitative method in 35 pregnant women showed values above 30µg% in 11.4%, between 10-30µg% in 20% and <10µg% in 68.6% out of the total investigated women. Thus, UIE was subnormal in 88.6% of the cases.

During *February 2004–September 2006*, after the legislative changes regarding universal iodine prophylaxis took effect we screened 206 pregnant women, their hormone status being presented in Table 3.

Thyroid function	No. cases	%	Trimester		
			I.	II.	III.
hypothyroidism	20	9.7	13.8%	8.1 %	11.9%
hyperthyroidism	6	2.9	5.8 %	4.3 %	0 %
euthyroid state	180	87.4			
Total	206				

Table 3. Thyroid function of 206 high-risk pregnant women screened during 2004-2006

Out of the 20 hypothyroid pregnant women 12 (60%) had subclinical and 8 (40%) overt hypofunction. Out of the 6 thyrotoxic pregnant women 4 had overt and the other 2 subclinical disease.

The titer of TPO-Abs determined only in 22 women was normal in all cases. Urinary iodine excretion measured in 34 pregnant women detected iodine deficiency in 84.2% of these cases.

Half of the pregnant women with hypothyroidism detected by targeted screening during 2004-2006 suffered from gestational complications: 5 imminent abortions, 2 imminent premature births, 3 miscarriages. One woman with thyroid cancer treated before pregnancy by thyroidectomy and insufficient substitutive-suppressive T_4-therapy presented imminent abortion (the case was included into the previously mentioned complications).

Three pregnant women out of the 6 hyperthyroid cases developed imminent abortion, hyperemesis gravidarum and imminent premature birth. All 3 had overt thyrotoxicosis (the majority of overt forms).

Thyroid dysfunction	2001-2003	2004-2006	P-value
Hypothyroidism	51 cases – 15.88% (3 post-thyroidectomy)	20 cases – 9.7% (1 PTC, thyroidectomy)	0.049
Overt/Subclinical hypothyroidism	17:34 (=1:2)	8:12 (=2:3)	0.081
Hyperthyroidism	7 cases – 2.18%	6 cases – 2.91%	0.44
Overt/Subclinical hyperthyroidism	3:4	2:1	

Table 4. Comparison of data obtained during 2001-2003 and 2004-2006
PTC: papillary thyroid carcinoma

During 2004-2006 the frequency of hypothyroidism in pregnant women has decreased significantly (with about 40%) compared to the previous period (2001-2003), but the ratio of overt/subclinical forms remained almost the same. The proportion of complications in hypothyroid women was similar in the two studied periods, but the total number of cases decreased in the second interval so the absolute number of gestational complications among pregnant women was reduced in the second period. Targeted case finding screening could identify high-risk pregnant women in the first trimester only in 1/3 of the cases, the others being detected later.

The rate of hyperthyroidism showed mild increase, which proved to be non-significant compared to 2001-2003. All hyperthyroid pregnant women with gestational complications suffered from overt hyperthyroidism.

Finally we evaluated a very controversial problem: the *isolated maternal hypothyroxinaemia*. This means a low free-T_4 concentration along a normal TSH-level. In our group we observed a few women suffering from such condition, and we considered them patients who need thyroid hormone replacement therapy.

During 2001-2003 a number of 8 (2.96%) cases had isolated hypothyroxinaemia among the 270 pregnant women with normal TSH-value: 2 in the first trimester (mean TSH: 1.10 ± 0.66mIU/L, mean FT4: 0.69 ± 0.08ng/dL), 3 in the second (mean TSH: 1.39 ± 0.41mIU/L, mean FT_4: 0.61 ± 0.02ng/dL), and 3 in the third trimester (mean TSH: 2.8 ± 0.34mIU/L, mean FT_4: 0.58 ± 0.06ng/dL).

During 2004-2006 only two (1.1%) pregnant women in the third trimester presented low FT_4 among the 182 subjects with normal thyrotropin (mean TSH: 1.68mIU/L, mean FT_4: 0.63ng/dL).

Thus, among the total number of 527 pregnant women 1.89% had isolated hypothyroxinaemia, mainly in the third trimester (half of the cases), when the upper normal limit of TSH-level is extended to 3.5mIU/L. In these latter cases the TSH-levels were situated mainly between 2.8-3.2 approaching to the upper normal limit in the III. trimester.

5. Discussion

During pregnancy the iodine requirement is increased by different mechanisms. One of these is the increase of maternal thyroxine secretion to maintain euthyroidism: the elevated TBG-level due to hyperestrogenism binds T_4 in higher amounts as in non-pregnant conditions and must be saturated to obtain normal free thyroid hormone levels. At the same time, a part of iodine and maternal thyroid hormones are transferred to the fetus, particularly in later gestation. The other cause is the secretion of placental hCG (human chorionic gonadotropin), which stimulates thyroid hormone secretion (similarly with TSH) mainly near the end of the first trimester, and thus it can be associated with a transient lowering in serum TSH (Glinoer, 1999). Finally, a presumed cause of increased iodine requirement is the augmented renal iodine clearance in pregnancy (see Tabel 5).

The iodine and the thyroid hormones are essential for the normal general development of offspring, especially for the differentiation of CNS, being indispensable for neuronal migration, arborization of dendrites, myelination of axons, normal synaptogenesis, synaptic transmission and plasticity during fetal and early postnatal life. The increased iodine and thyroid hormone requirement during pregnancy favours the development of *iodine-deficiency disorders (IDD)* and of subsequent hypothyroidism, having serious consequences on both maternal and fetal organisms, especially in conditions of reduced iodine supply in endemic regions.

Causes	Consequences
Hyperestrogenism	elevated TBG-level and increased binding of thyroid hormones: for maintenance of euthyroidism maternal thyroxine secretion must be augmented
Placental hCG	stimulates the thyroid hormone secretion
Transplacental transfer	primarily in the first trimester and in fetal hypothyroidism
Increased renal iodine clearance	urinary iodine losing

Table 5. The causes of increased iodine requirement in pregnancy

Iodine deficiency is still a health problem, not only worldwide but also in Europe. Recent French data show that in Northern Paris area the mean UIE was low (49.8µg/L), far under 100µg/L, the formerly considered normal value (Luton et al., 2011). Taking into account that WHO currently recommends a median UIE in pregnant women of 150-249 µg/L, this result is still more alarming. Similarly, in the Lyon metropolitan area Raverot et al. (2012) found that pregnant women are iodine-deficient, 77% of them having a median UIE under 150µg/L.

In countries or regions where under 90% of households are using iodized salt and the median UIE in school-age children is under 100µg/L, WHO recommends iodine supplementation during pregnancy and infancy. Recently, WHO/UNICEF/ICCIDD increased the Recommended Nutrient Intake for iodine during *pregnancy* from *200 to 250µg/day* and considered that the adequate iodine intake is reflected by a median *UIE* of *150-249µg/L* (Zimmermann, 2009). In *lactating women and children under the age of 2 years* a median *UIE of 100µg/L* can be used to define adequate iodine intake; although lactating women have the same requirement as pregnant women, the median urinary iodine is lower because iodine is also excreted in breast milk (WHO, 2007, see Table 6).

Iodine dose (µg/day)	Organization and date	Median urinary iodine excretion (median UIE µg/L)
200	World Health Organization 1994; WHO/NUT/94.6,Geneva	100
250	WHO/UNICEF/ICCIDD 2007	150-249

Table 6. The evolution of recommended iodine intake during pregnancy

WHO: World Health Organization; UNICEF: United Nations Children's Fund; ICCIDD: International Council for the Control of Iodine Deficiency Disorders

In *lactating women and children under the age of 2 years* a median *UIE of 100µg/L* indicates adequate iodine intake; although lactating and pregnant women have the same iodine requirement, in formers the median UIE is lower due to iodine excretion in breast milk (WHO, 1994; 2007).

It is well known, that in severe iodine deficient regions maternal and fetal hypothyroidism can cause classic or masked cretinism or reduces cognitive development in children; to prevent fetal damage, iodine should be given before or in early pregnancy. During the 1st trimester, the fetus is completely dependent upon the thyroxine produced by the mother (Springer et al., 2011).

A new USA trial has shown that when a hypothyroid woman becomes pregnant, she should immediately increase her levothyroxine dose by two tablets per week in order to remain biochemically euthyroid. This protocol significantly reduces the risk of maternal hypothyroidism during the first trimester and mimics normal physiology (Alexander et al., 2004; Reuters Health Information 2010). It was previously reported that T_4 requirement may rise as early as the fifth week of gestation (Alexander et al., 2004). In general, pregnant women started this protocol at a median of 5.5 weeks of pregnancy. Other authors recommended for women who became pregnant to increase the dose of levothyroxine by 30-50%. Several authors would first check thyroid function tests before adjusting the dose (Vaidya et al., 2012). Thyroid hormone levels must be monitored at least every 4 week until 20th weeks, because the required doses of T_4 increase during pregnancy. The recommended control of thyroid hormone levels only at the 30th weeks of pregnancy may be considered insufficient, because in 92% of the cases were detected abnormal TSH values (Alexander et al., 2004; Reuters Health Information 2010).

Our study shows that the targeted screening of high-risk pregnant women for thyroid dysfunctions according to the before mentioned inclusion criteria resulted the inclusion into the screening of only about 1/3 of pregnant women in the first gestational trimester (31.8% – 102 subjects from the 321 cases during 2001-2003), the others being detected only in the second or third trimester (39.2% in the II. and 29% in the III. trimester) according to symptoms, signs and/or gestational complications developed later during pregnancy.

Early maternal iodine deficiency and hypothyroidism may cause developmental impairments in the fetal nervous system, but evidences about the consequences of later (after the first trimester) initiated thyroid hormone replacement therapy and of mild-to-moderate iodine deficient maternal status are still limited. It is not clarified whether this mild maternal iodine deficiency can influence, and if so in what extent the cognitive function of offsprings. Studies showed impaired intellectual and motor development in children from endemic areas, but presumably other factors could affect mental development, too (Zimmermann, 2009).

Taking into account that under the circumstances of targeted screening in high-risk pregnant women a large number of subjects are screened later, after the first gestational trimester, it is recommended to start thyroid hormone replacement as soon as possible. Thus the tendency to perform universal screening in early pregnancy for thyroid conditions, first of all in iodine deficient regions is justifiable.

Aggressive thyroid hormone replacement before or in early pregnancy is justified, but to recommend or discuss the possibility of therapeutic abortion in case of initiation the substitutive hormone therapy after the first trimester, because of fearing evident cognitive delay in offsprings, is not warranted (Downing et al., 2012). A quarter of the European thyroidologists recently responding to the electronic questionnaire survey of Vaidya et al. proved to have this opinion. In case of fetal hypothyroxinaemia it must be taken into account that there are also compensatory mechanisms that favour the transfer of thyroid hormones through placenta into the fetus. In this respect, it can be mentioned that according to a study the IQ of children born from mothers diagnosed with hypothyroidism during early pregnancy was normal, similarly to children born from mothers without thyroid hypofunction (Liu et al., 1994).

The iodine state of a geographical area can be quantified by more indicators. Besides the screening of pregnant women using TSH and/or FT_4, TPO-Ab assays, the serum TSH concentration in neonates measured in blood collected between the 3rd and 7th days of life is another indirect indicator. The incidence of cases with neonatal serum TSH>10mIU/L reflects the grade of iodine deficiency: between 3-19.9% indicates moderate, between 20-39.9% severe and >40% very serious iodine deficiency (WHO, 1994; Delange, 1998). A frequency under 3% of TSH > 5mIU/L indicates iodine sufficiency.

We obtained in the studied periods TSH>10mIU/L in 8-9% of newborns, indicating moderate iodine deficiency in Mureş County (Szántó et al., 2007).

Other laboratory and imagistic parameters are urinary iodine excretion and thyroid ultrasound effectuated in school-children and pregnant women.

The increased iodine and thyroid hormone requirement during pregnancy favours the development of *hypothyroidism* with consequences on both maternal and fetal organisms, and this may be aggravated in iodine deficient endemic regions. Since iodine deficiency is a continuous health problem worldwide, and knowing our region as a hilly-mountainous one, we have started to evaluate the iodine status of our county in the mirror of the criteria for iodine deficiency estimation (WHO, 1994). The studies realized on neonates and school-aged children cohorts have demonstrated that during 1990-2003 Mureş County was a moderately mild iodine deficient area (Kun et al., 2003; 2007; Kun, 2006) in the condition of relatively systematic iodine prophylaxis, but not rigorously controlled by legislative means. In that period of time iodized alimentary salt contained about 16mg KI per kg, and it was not mandatory to sell on market exclusively iodized alimentary salt. Simultaneously we started to evaluate pregnant women known with previous or present thyroid conditions and gestational complications, without the possibility of screening all pregnant women. Although, in recent recommendations living in an area with iodine insufficiency represents a risk factor for thyroid disorders in pregnant women (Stagnaro-Green et al., 2011), so our endemic region represents increased risk factor during pregnancy.

In our study the rate of hypothyroidism in pregnant women with history of thyroid conditions or gestational complications, as well as signs/symptoms of thyroid dysfunction was 15.88% during 2001–2003, subclinical forms being diagnosed in 2/3 of cases. Gestational goiter was present in average 44.2% of the cohort and the randomly measured UIE showed reduced values in the majority of cases (88.6%), that suggest the insufficient prophylactic effect of the used iodized alimentary salt at that time (mean 16mg KI/kg salt). A proportion of 2.18% of high-risk pregnant women had hyperthyroidism. According to reported data thyroid dysfunction is observed in about 10% (0.4-25%) of pregnant women, its frequency being dependent on the severity of iodine-deficiency and the presence of thyroid antibodies.

Our targeted screening of high-risk pregnant women has detected mainly subclinical hypothyroidism in the circumstances of moderately mild iodine deficiency before 2003. This mild form of thyroid dysfunction develops due to increased requirement of iodine and thyroid hormones during pregnancy and/or due to iodine deficiency and autoimmune lymphocytic thyroiditis (Badenhoop, 2000; Hehrmann, 2002). Anyway, the prevalence of Hashimoto's thyroiditis in pregnancy is low, about 0.8–1% (Badenhoop, 2000), but it can increase during iodine prophylaxis, and this disease can also provoke gestational complications without any thyroid dysfunction (Negro et al., 2007; Thangaratinam et al., 2011). In our cohort severe maternal and fetal complications developed in one case of chronic autoimmune thyroiditis and mild hypothyroidism, but we suppose that other factors might also contribute to this severe case of miscarriage (e.g. immunologic ones), taking into account that the grade of maternal hypothyroidism was mild.

Neonates born to hypothyroid mothers presented almost significantly higher frequency of pre- or post-term delivery in comparison with the control group (newborns of apparently healthy mothers) – 25% vs. 7.7%.

The screening and treatment of subclinical hypothyroidism in pregnancy have been recommended since 2001-2002 (Mann, 2001; Hehrmann, 2002), after the recognition of its role in development of maternal and fetal complications. Although subclinical hypothyroidism is a very mild thyroid dysfunction, it can favour both gestational/delivery and fetal complications (delay of central nervous system development and consecutive mental retardation). According to data reported by Abalovich in 2002 the frequency of both abortion and premature birth in inadequately treated pregnant woman with overt hypothyroidism was high (60% and 20%, respectively), but, surprisingly, the frequency of abortion in subclinical forms was much higher (above 70%). The rate of premature birth was 7% in case of subclinical hypothyroidism. Under the condition of adequate T_4-substitution of overt hypothyroidism 100%, but in state of subclinical form about 90% of pregnant women had normal termed delivery (Abalovich et al., 2002). Several studies showed that pregnancy was more likely to be complicated if subclinical hypothyroidism was present (Casey et al., 2005; Pop et al., 2003).

Other studies showed, that in course of pregnancy, the outcome of delivery and postpartum period, the neuromuscular development of newborns is mainly dependent on TPO-Ab level.

In pregnant women the frequency of increased TPO antibodies is about 9% (Hehrmann, 2002). During 2001–2003 we could determine in our targeted screening the TPO-Ab-level in only 24 pregnant women, and we obtained elevated levels in 3 women. One of these three cases was diagnosed with Hashimoto-thyroiditis in the III. trimester, she developed high blood pressure, oedema, pre-eclampsia and premature birth, the new-born presenting severe asphyxia and died after birth. Data in the literature showed that from the second trimester onward, the major adverse obstetrical outcome associated with raised TSH was the increased rate of fetal death (Allan et al., 2000). The reduced number of TPO-Ab-positive cases in our cohort may be explained by immunsuppression during pregnancy: in the first trimester the level of antithyroid antibodies can increase, but after that TPO-Ab-level may decrease to the normal level until delivery.

Iodine and thyroid hormone deficiency in the first trimester inhibits the development of the nervous system in the fetus, because the fetal organism is unable to produce sufficient amounts of thyroid hormones. Iodine deficiency in the precocious period of pregnancy conducts to the most severe neural impairments (mental retardation, dwarfism, neuromuscular complications, as spastic paresis of the limbs). These complications are irreversible, thus their prevention is indispensable. Later (II.-III. trimesters) may appear growth disturbances, but these are not irreversible.

As our results show, during 2001-2003 the frequency of goiter increased gradually with gestational trimester. In the I. and II. trimester 40.2% and 42.1% of pregnant women had goiter, respectively, and this rate increased to 51.6% in the III. trimester. These results show indirectly the endemic character of our geographical area.

After 2002, when the government decree took effect, universal iodine prophylaxis was applied with an increased iodine content alimentary salt (34±5mg/kg) and a more stable iodine salt (KIO_3). Our targeted screening to detect thyroid dysfunction in pregnant women showed a decreasing tendency in the frequency of hypothyroidism (9.7%, P:0.049), being significantly reduced compared to the first period (15.88%), although, the distribution according to severity remained practically identical (subclinical forms in 50% vs. 40% in the first and second studied period of time). The ratio of overt:subclinical hypothyroidism remains almost unchanged during the two studied periods (1:2 vs. 2:3). The values of urinary iodine excretion of the two intervals did not differ significantly, in concordance with the similar data obtained in the whole country in 2004.

Conversely, the frequency of hyperthyroidism had a slightly increasing tendency after universal iodine prophylaxis, but this change was not significant (2.18% in 2001-2003 vs. 2.91% in 2004-2006). According to the literature the prevalence of hyperthyroidism in the United States is about 1%. The distribution of clinical and subclinical forms is almost equal: 0.4% overt and 0.6% subclinical forms. The activity level of autoimmune thyroid diseases may fluctuate during gestation, with exacerbation during the first trimester and gradual improvement during the later gestational period (The Endocrine Society's

Clinical Guideline, 2007). Graves' disease accounts for about 85% of hyperthyroidism during pregnancy. In autoimmune thyroiditis a hyperthyroid phase of Hashimoto's thyroiditis and silent thyroiditis may occur. The risk of complications for both mother and fetus is related to the duration and control of maternal hyperthyroidism. Inadequately treated maternal thyrotoxicosis is associated with increased risk of preterm delivery, which can occur in up to 88% of these pregnant women (The Endocrine Society's Clinical Guideline, 2007).

Iodine prophylaxis is needed in all pregnant women, not only for those living in endemic regions. In euthyroid (normal TSH-level), TPO-Ab-negative pregnant women without goiter, iodine usually must be applied in doses of *200-260µg/day.* The use of iodine supplementation is also indicated in cases of elevated TPO-Ab-level, primarily for the fetus. We should also inform pregnant women that iodine overdose can induce hypothyroidism, so for detection repeated laboratory investigations may be necessary. This statement is also valid for the lactation period.

In the treatment of endemic goiter, the increased need for iodine and thyroid hormones for both pregnant and fetus requires iodine administration (in the before mentioned doses) with or without association of T_4-treatment (e.g. in doses of 50-75µg/day), the later alone being not sufficient during pregnancy.

We must emphasize that in the II. trimester, the T_4-level decreases and the TSH and the T_3/T_4 ratio increase in one third of pregnant women. In this situation we must increase the T_4 dose individually (but avoid the suppression of TSH). Generally, an adequate treatment of hypothyroidism needs increasing T_4 doses as pregnancy progress. Thus, in early pregnancy we must monitor the thyroid hormone and TSH-levels frequently (e.g. on 10 days interval at the beginning, after that every 3-4 weeks during the first half of pregnancy, and monthly or every 6 weeks during the second half), to administer T_4-preparations properly, in increasing doses.

At the same time during pregnancy and lactation smoking and all medications with inhibitory effect on the thyroid function must be avoided. Among these iodine excess (iodinated contrast materials, amiodarone) must be emphasized. Iodine excess can induce not only hypothyroidism (through Wolff-Chaikoff effect), but also thyrotoxicosis (hyperthyroidism or subacute thyroiditis). These dysfunctions may appear both in mother and offspring (fetuses and neonates). The appearance of these adverse reactions depend on several factors, among them the iodine dose is very important. In this respect Kochi et al. (2012) show that there was no significant adverse clinical reaction of thyroid function abnormalities in the fetus after administering iv. iodinated contrast material to the mothers for computed tomography scan. In contrast, radioiodine administration is strictly contraindicated for both diagnostic and therapeutic purposes in pregnant women, because it can destroy the offspring's thyroid function. This rule is also valid in case of the thyroid cancer. When thyroid cancer is diagnosed during pregnancy, a decision must be taken regarding performing thyroidectomy during the pregnancy or postponing surgical resection until the postpartum period. Radioactive iodine is absolutely contraindicated during pregnancy and lactation (Yazbeck & Sullivan, 2012).

Isolated maternal hypothyroxinemia may have negative effects on motor, cognitive and neurobehavioural performance of the offspring, taking into account that maternal thyroxine plays a pivote role upon the normal nervous system development of the fetus. Screening of pregnant women for thyroid dysfunctions firstly measures TSH-levels, while free-T_4 assays have limitations in clinical use. In these situations isolated maternal hypothyroxinemia may not be detected.

The *frequency* of isolated maternal hypothyroxinemia and its impact on maternal/fetal complications, as well as therapeutical recommendations are not clarified entirely, yet. The incidence of this special hormonal state during pregnancy varies among wide intervals, depending on the iodine status of the geographical area, the trimester-specific hormonal assays and the used normal ranges, thus according to these influencing factors published data showed an incidence ranging between 1.3-26.5% (Casey et al., 2007; Vaidya et al., 2007; Clear-Goldman et al., 2008; Berbel et al., 2009; Moleti et al., 2009; Shan et al. 2009; Hendrichs et al., 2010). The prevalence is the lowest in the first gestational trimester (1.2-3.2%) but than it starts to increase gradually during the II. and III. trimesters reaching values as high as 26.5% (Berbel et al., 2009). The true incidence of isolated maternal hypothyroxinemia is not known, yet.

The influence of this state on *pregnancy outcome* and on *fetal development* is a question under debate. Some researchers have stated that isolated maternal hypothyroxinemia has no influence on obstetrical adverse outcomes (Casey et al., 2007), but further investigations in this respect are needed. It was reported, that isolated maternal hypothyroxinemia is associated with impaired neurodevelopment of offsprings (Pop et al., 1999), but this must also be confirmed by further surveys.

The *etiology* of this state is also not known exactly. It was reported that in the circumstances of short-term iodine prophylaxis the prevalence of isolated hypothyroxinemia is 5-fold higher than in pregnant women who had regularly used iodized salt for at least 2 years before pregnancy occurred (36.8% versus 6.4%) (Moleti et al., 2011). It was suggested, that the cause of isolated hypothyroxinemia is iodine deficiency instead of autoimmune thyroid processes, such as among 56/220 (25.4%) pregnant women with isolated hypothyroxinemia TPO-Ab were detectable in only 7.1% of them (Moleti et al., 2009). Data published so far are not sufficient to recommend thyroxine replacement therapy in this case in pregnancy, although a study analysing questionnaires about the treatment of hypothyroidism during pregnancy filled in by over 600 members of the European Thyroid Society (ETA) showed that 38% of the responders would treat isolated maternal hypothyroxinemia, but the responders' definition of this disorder was not consistent (Vaidya et al., 2012), which reflects the lack of clear definition and management of this state.

6. Conclusions

During 2001-2003 the frequency of hypothyroidism in high-risk pregnant women was 15.88% in Mureş County, a region with moderately mild iodine deficiency, the subclinical forms predominate versus overt hypothyroidism. During 2004-2006, after the implementation in practice of universal salt-iodization and more rigorous follow-up of thyroid dysfunctions the frequency of hypothyroidism in pregnancy decreased significantly (to 9.7%). Complications (imminent abortion, premature birth, gestational hypertension, pre-eclampsia) appeared with high frequency (in 50%) among hypothyroid pregnant women in the two periods of time. Special measures of iodine-prophylaxis are necessary in case of every pregnant woman, mainly for those living in endemic regions, because the universal salt-iodization (in our region iodized alimentary salt with 34 ± 8.5mg/kg KIO_3) is not sufficient in all cases. Targeted screening could identify high-risk pregnant women in the first trimester only in 1/3 of cases, the others being detected later. Thus, our results plead for the necessity of *universal screening of pregnant women* for thyroid dysfunctions and their regular follow-up even in a mild iodine deficient area, taking into account that iodine deficiency, primarily through inducing hypothyroidism, can have detrimental effects on fetal brain development even from the first gestational trimester. Similarly, the early recognition and adequate treatment of thyroid disorders can contribute substantially to decrease of frequency and severity of other maternal and fetal complications related to these dysfunctions.

Author details

Imre Zoltán Kun and Ildikó Kun
University of Medicine and Pharmacy, Târgu Mureş,
Mureş County Clinical Hospital, Endocrinology Clinic, Târgu Mureş,
Romania

Zsuzsanna Szántó
University of Medicine and Pharmacy, Târgu Mureş,
Romania

Béla Szabó
University of Medicine and Pharmacy, Târgu Mureş,
Clinic of Obstetrics & Gynecology No. 1., Târgu Mureş,
Romania

Acknowledgement

The authors are grateful to the Sapientia Foundation from Cluj-Napoca, Romania for its financial contribution in supporting the costs of hormonal measurements. The authors express their gratitude to Győrfi Annamária for her collaboration in the translating process of this text.

7. References

Abalovich M, Gutierrez S, Alcaraz G, Maccallini G, Garcia A, Levalle O (2002) Overt and subclinical hypothyroidism complicating pregnancy. Thyroid 12/1: 63-68.

Alexander EK, Marqusee E, Lawrence J, Jarolim P, Fischer GA, Larsen PR (2004) Timing and magnitude of increases in levothyroxine requirements during pregnancy in women with hypothyroidism. New Engl J Med 351: 241-249. (doi:10.1056/NEJMoa 040079).

Allan WC, Haddow JE, Palomaki GE, Williams JR, Mitchell ML, Hermos RJ, Faix JD, Klein RZ (2000) Maternal thyroid deficiency and pregnancy complications: implications for population screening. J Med Screen 7: 127-130.

Badenhoop K (2000) Hashimoto-Thyreoiditis in der Schwangerschaft. In: Derwahl, K.M.–Heufelder, AE editors. Endokrine Erkrankungen während der Schwangerschaft und Postpartalphase. Berlin, Blackwell Wissenschafts Verlag. Pp. 68-72.

Balázs J, Kun IZ, Buksa C, Coroş L, Vasilescu G, Năsălean A (2000/a) Study of endemic goiter, chronic thyroiditis, thyroid function in corelation with iodine intake at school-children living in the superior and middle hydrographic basin of the river Mureş [in Romanian] Revista de Medicină şi Farmacie Targu Mureş 46: 240-244.

Balázs J, Pintea A, Buksa C, Vasilescu G (2000/b) The thyroid volume and the iodine intake in school-children from Târgu-Mureş [in Romanian]. Revista de Medicină şi Farmacie Targu Mureş 46: 60-63.

Berbel P, Mestre JL, Santamaria A, Palazon I, Franco A, Graells M, Gonzales-Torga A, de Escobar GM (2009) Delayed neurobehavioral development in children born to pregnant women with mild hypothyroxinemia during the first month of gestation: the importance of early iodine supplementaion. Thyroid 19/5: 511-519.

Boyages SC (1993) Clinical review: iodine deficiency disorders. J Clin Endocrinol Metab. 1993; 77/3: 587-591

Burman KD (2009) Controversies surrounding pregnancy, maternal thyroid status, and fetal outcome. Thyroid 19: 323-326.

Cao XY, Jiang XM, Dou ZH, Rakeman MA, Zhang ML, O'Donnell K, Ma T, Amette K, DeLong N, DeLong GR (1994) Timing of vulnerability of the brain to iodine deficiency in endemic cretenism. N Eng J Med 331/26: 1739-1744.

Casey B, Dashe JS, Wells CE, McIntire DD, Byrd W, Leveno KJ, Cunningham FG (2005) Subclinical hypothyroidism and pregnancy outcome. Ostet Gynecol 105: 239-245.

Casey BM, Dashe JS, Spong CY, McIntire DD, Leveno KJ, Cunningham GF (2007) Perinatal significance of isolated maternal hypothyroxinemia identified in the first half of pregnancy. Obstet Gynecol 109(5): 1129-1135.

Cleary-Goldman J, Malone FD, Lambert-Messerlian G, Sullivan L, Canick J, Porter TF, Luthy D, Gross S, Bianchi DW, D'Alton ME (2008) Maternal thyroid hypofunction and pregnancy outcome. Obstet Gynecol 112/1: 85-92.

de Escobar GM, Obregon MJ, del Rey FE (2007) Iodine deficiency and brain development in the first half of pregnancy. Public Health Nutr 10/12A: 1554-1570

Delange F (1998) Screening for congenital hypothyroidism used as an indicator of IDD control. In: Pinchera A, Mann K, Hostalek U editors. The Thyroid and Age, Merck European Thyroid Symposium Italy, April 30–May 2, 1998. Stuttgart: Schattauer Verlagsgesellschaft mbH. pp. 121-134.

Downing SD, Halpern L, Carswell J, Brown RS (2012) Severe Early Maternal Hypothyroidism Corrected Prior to the Third Trimester Associated with Normal Cognitive Outcome in the Offspring. Thyroid, 2012 Mar 7.

Glinoer D (1999) What happens to the normal thyroid during pregnancy? Thyroid 9(7): 631-635.

Glinoer D, Abalovich M (2007) Unresolved questions in managing hypothyroidism during pregnancy. BMJ 335: 300-302.

Henrichs J, Bongers-Schokking JJ, Schenk JJ, Ghassabian A, Schmidt HG, Visser TJ, Hooijkaas H, de Muinck Keizer-Schrama SM,Hofman A, Jaddoe VV, Visser W, Steegers EA, Verhulst FC, de Rijke YB, Tiemeier H (2010) Maternal thyroid function during early pregnancy and cognitive functioning in early childhood: the generation R study. J Clin Endocr Metab 95/9: 4227-4234.

Hehrmann R (2002) Immunthyreopathien in der Schwangerschaft – Auswirkungen auf den Fetus. In: Mann K, Weinheimer B, Janßen OE editor. Schilddrüse und Autoimmunität. Berlin, Walter de Gruyter GmbH & Co. KG. pp. 284-294.

Kochi MH, Kaloudis EV, Ahmed W, Moore WH (2012) Effect of in utero exposure of iodinated intravenous contrast on neonatal thyroid function. J Comput Assist Tomogr 36/2:165-169.

Kun I (2006) Hypothyroidism in Mureş County – Doctoral thesis. [in Romanian: Insuficienţa tirodiană în judeţul Mureş], University of Medicine and Pharmacy Târgu Mureş.

Kun IZ, Szántó Zs (2003) The frequency and complications of hypothyroidism in Mureş County - [in Hungarian: A pajzsmirigyelégtelenség és szövődményeinek gyakorisága Maros megye területén]. In: Brassai A editor. Orvostudományi Tanulmányok – Sapientia Könyvek. Scientia Cluj-Napoca, pp. 131-206.

Kun IZ, Balázs J, Năsălean A, Gliga C, Deteşan G, Simescu M, Coroş L, Ionescu A, Madaras G, Szántó Zs, Macarie C (2007) Iodine deficiency detected through urinary iodine excretion in school-children living in goiter prevalent regions of County Mureş (2005–2006). 9th European Congress of Endocrinology Budapest, 28 April – 2 May 2007, Budapest. Endocrine Abstracts. 14: P353.

Leung AM, Pearce EN, Braverman LE (2011) Iodine nutrition in pregnancy and lactation. Endocrinol Metab Clin North Am 40/4: 765-777.

Liu H, Momotani N, Noh JY, Ishikawa N, Takebe K, Ito K (1994) Maternal hypothyroidism during early pregnancy and intellectual development of the progeny. Arch Intern Med 154: 785–787. (doi:10.1001/archinte.154.7.785)

Luton D, C Alberti, E Vuillard, G Ducarme, JF Oury, J Guibourdenche (2011) Iodine Deficiency in Northern Paris Area: Impact on Fetal Thyroid Mensuration. PLoS ONE 6(2): e14707, doi:10.1371/journal.pone.0014707.

Mann K (2001) Latente Schilddrüsenfunktionsstörungen – Welche Diagnostik, welche Therapie? In: Hensen J, Allolio B, Grußendorf M et alii editors. VI. Intensivkurs für Klinische Endokrinologie, 24.–27. Oktober 2001, Hannover. pp. 209-218.

Milcu SM (1956) Guşa endemică [in Romanian] - Editura Academiei Republicii Populare Române, Bucharest.

Moleti M, Lo Presti VP, Mattina F, Mancuso A, De Vivo A, Giorgianni G, Di Bella B, Trimarchi F, Vermiqlio F (2009) Gestational thyroid function abnormalities in conditions of mild iodine deficiency: early screening versus continuous monitoring of maternal thyroid status. Eur J Endocrinol 160/4: 611-617.

Moleti M, Di Bella B, Giorgianni G, Mancuso A, De Vivo A, Alibrandi A, Trimarchi F, Vermiglio F (2011) Maternal thyroid function in different conditions of iodine nutrition in pregnant women exposed to mild-moderate iodine deficiency: An observational study. Clin Endocrinol 74/6: 762-768.

Negro R, Formoso G, Coppola L, Presicce G, Mangieri T, Pezzarossa A, Dazzi D (2007) Euthyroid women with autoimmune disease undergoing assisted reproduction technologies: the role of autoimmunity and thyroid function. J Endocrinol Invest 30(1): 3-8.

Pharoah PO, Butterfield IH, Hetzel BS (1971) Neurological damage to the fetus resulting from severe iodine deficiency during pregnancy. Lancet 1:308-310.

Pop VJ, Kuijpens JL, van Baar AL, Verkerk G, van Son MM, de Vijlder JJ, Vulsma T, Wiersinga WM, Drexhage HA. Vader HL (1999) Low maternal free thyroxine concentrations during early pregnancy are associated with impaired psychomotor development in infancy. Clin Endocrinol 50: 149-155.

Pop V, Brouwers EP, Vader HL, Vulsma T, Van Baar AL, De Vijlder JJ. (2003) Maternal hypothyroximaemia during early pregnancy and subsequent child development: a 3-year follow-up study. Clin Endocrinol (Oxf) 59: 282-288.

Raverot V, Bournaud C, Sassolas G, Orgiazzi JJ, Claustrat F, Gaucherand P, Mellier G, Claustrat B, Borson-Chazot F, Zimmermann M (2012) French pregnant women in the Lyon area are iodine deficient and have elevated serum thyroglobulin concentrations. Thyroid 2012 Feb 23.

Shan ZY, Chen YY, Teng WP, Yu XH, Li CY, Zhou WW, Gao B, Zhou JR, Ding B, Ma Y, Wu Y, Liu Q, Xu H, Liu W, Li J, Wang WW, Li YB,Fan CL, Wang H, Guo R, Zhang HM (2009) A study for maternal thyroid hormone deficiency during the first half of pregnancy in China. Eur J Clin Invest 39/1: 37-42.

Simescu M, Dimitriu L, Sava M, Chiovernache D, Colda A, Balmes E, Ursu H, Bistriceanu M, Zosin I, Duncea I, Balazs J, Kun IZ, Dragatoiu G, Hazi G, Coamesu I, Harsan T, Stamoran L, Florescu E, Vitiuc M, Varciu M, Budura I, Fugaciu A, Hutanu T, Lepadatu D, Sulac H, Munteanu M, Parlog L, Podia Igna C, Sirbu A (2006) Urinary iodine levels in schoolchildren and pregnant women after the legislative changes in the salt iodization. Acta Endocrinol (Buc) 2(1): 33-44.

Springer D, Limanova Z, Zima T (2011) Thyroid in Pregnancy. In: Fulya Akin editor. Basic and Clinical Endocrinology Up-to-Date. Rijeka: Intech. pp. 37-50.

Stagnaro-Green A, Abalovich M, Alexander E, Azizi F, Mestman J, Negro R, Nixon A, Pearce EN, Soldin OP, Sullivan S, Wiersinga W (2011) Guidelines of the American Thyroid Association for the diagnosis and management of thyroid disease during pregnancy and postpartum. Thyroid 21: 1081-1125

Szántó Zs, Kun I, Kun IZ, Coroş L, Cucerea M (2007) The influence of universal salt iodization on the iodine status reflected by TSH serum levels of newborns, in Mureş County, between years 2001-2006. Acta Endocrinol (Buc) III(3): 291-301.

Thangaratinam S, Tan A, Knox E, Kilby MD, Franklyn J, Coomarasamy A. (2011) Association between thyroid autoantibodies and miscarriage and preterm birth: meta-analysis of evidence. BMJ 9: 42: d2616. doi: 10.1136/bmj.d2616.

Vaidya B, Anthony S, Bilous M, Shields B, Drury J, Hutchison S, Bilous R (2007) Brief report: detection of thyroid dysfunction in early pregnancy: universal screening or targeted high-risk case finding?" J Clin Endocrinol Metab 92/1: 203-207.

Vaidya B, Hubalewska-Dydejczyk A, Laurberg P, Negro R, Vermiglio F, Poppe K (2012) Treatment and screening of hypothyroidism in pregnancy: results of a European survey. Eur J Endocrinol 166(1): 49-54.

Yazbeck CF, Sullivan SD (2012) Thyroid disorders during pregnancy. Med Clin North Am 96(2): 235-256.

Zimmermann MB (2009) Iodine deficiency in pregnancy and the effects of maternal iodine supplementation on the offspring: a review. Am J Clin Nutr 89(2): 668S-72S.

The Endocrine Society's Clinical Guideline (2007) Management of Thyroid Dysfunction during Pregnancy and Postpartum: An Endocrine Society Clinical Practice Guideline. J Clin Endocrinol Metab 92/8: 12-31.

The Second National Conference for the elimination of Iodine Deficiency Disorders (IDD) (2005) The National Strategy to eliminate the iodine deficiency disturbances by the universal salt iodization in alimentary and bakery industry 2004-2012. Bucharest, 14 November 2005:3-12. Abstracts on CD.

Reuters Health Information (2010) Hypothyroid Women in 1st Trimester Need 2 Extra Levothyroxine Pills/week. J Clin Endocrinol Metab http://jcem.endojournals.org/cgi/ cn tent/abstract/jc.2010-0013v1

Romanian National Institute of Statistics. Censuses of Population and Housing, http://www.recensamantromania.ro

World Health Organization, United Nations Children's Fund, International Council for Control of Iodine Deficiency Disorders (1994) Indicators for assessing Iodine Deficiency Disorders and their control through salt iodization. WHO/NUT/94.6,Geneva: World Health Organization 1994 pp. 1-55.

World Health Organization. United Nations Children's Fund & International Council for the Control of Iodine Deficiency Disorders (2007) Assessment of iodine deficiency disorders and monitoring their elimination. 2nd ed. Geneva, Switzerland: WHO.

Chapter 4

Behavioral and Somatic Disorders in Children Exposed in Utero to Synthetic Hormones: A Testimony-Case Study in a French Family Troop

Marie-Odile Soyer-Gobillard and Charles Sultan

Additional information is available at the end of the chapter

http://dx.doi.org/10.5772/48637

1. Introduction

Development and maturation of the human brain especially genesis of neurones and synaptogenesis are under the genetic control of neurohormones secreted by hypothalamus during fetal and early postnatal life. So the lesser modification in the hormonal status might influence either the neurodevelopment course or the sexual differentiation. This study shows that there are serious effects on the psychological and physical health of the descendants of women treated with synthetic hormones during their pregnancy. Preliminary results by a group in Paris have recently been published [1], based on observations and diagnoses of psychiatric disorders in a small sample of children from the HHORAGES families. As synthesized by Dodds in 1938, but not patented, diethylstilbestrol (DES), a synthetic non-steroid estrogen, given among others to pregnant women, was considered at the time as "an indisputable progress in the therapeutics of ovarian deficiency", and was described in such terms as early as May 1939 in an advertisement shown in *"Le Progrès Médical"*, a French journal. Despite various alerts which were published as early as 1940, and after research work was conducted on animals proving carcinogenic effects, and despite Dieckmann et al. [2], which demonstrated the ineffectiveness of DES to prevent miscarriages or premature births in a large cohort of DES-treated women versus placebo-treated women, the product has been much used worldwide, and has caused a long list of damaging effects in the past, the present and very likely in the future [3-5]. The discovery of vaginal clear cell adenocarcinomas in "DES daughters" [6] led to DES being banned for pregnant women in 1971 in the US, but it was only in 1977 that it was banned in France, where this particular use of DES was removed from the Vidal pharmaceutical handbook. However, DES was still sporadically prescribed until 1981. Meanwhile, another steroid estrogen, also synthesized in 1938 by H. Herloff Inhoffen and W.

Hohlweg, 17-alpha-ethinylestradiol, was often added to DES in cocktails, or at a later stage was used as a replacement, sometimes with synthetic delayed progestin. An example of prescription, time and doses is shown in **Table 1**.

History: Miscarriage, two years before, at 6 weeks amenorrhea.
1st pregnancy: 1966-67. At 7 weeks amenorrhea: Ethinylestradiol (EE) 100mg/d. From 10th to 20th week: Distilbene 25mg/d + EE 100mg/d. From 20th to 37th week: Distilbene 15mg/d + EE 250mg/d+ Delay Progestin 500mg/week. Full term delivery: girl, 3,870kg weight, Apgar score 10/10. No problem during pregnancy and delivery.
2nd pregnancy: 1970-71. At 6 weeks amenorrhea: EE 500mg/d. From 8th to 37th week: EE 500mg/j + Distilbène 25 mg+ Delay Progesterone 500mg/d. Full term delivery, boy, 3,900 kg weight, Apgar Score 10/10. No problem during pregnancy and delivery.
Twenty years after: 1stchild (girl): Recurrent depressions and eating disorders, 14 suicide attempts, then suicide in 1995 (28 years old). 2ndchild (boy): Borderline Schizophrenia. Suicide in 1998 (27 years old).

Table 1. An example of synthetic hormone prescription during two successive pregnancies (dose and exposure periods), confirmed by medical file and its "20 years after" consequences (MOSG personal data).

As visible in Table 1 the doses/kg/day prescribed to this pregnant woman for her first pregnancy were: ethinyl-estradiol (EE): 19μg/kg^{-1}/d; DES: 28.8μg/kg^{-1}/d; Progestin delay: 1,37 mg/kg/d. For the second pregnancy, prescribed doses were slightly higher except for synthetic progestin delay prescribed at identical dose. Similar doses were administered to other pregnant French women and in the whole world, not only to women who had miscarriages (as the prevalent idea at the time was that they suffered from a hormonal deficiency which caused the miscarriage, whilst it is well known nowadays that the deficiency is caused by the miscarriage itself), but also to other women as a pain-relieving medicine, or even as a morning-after pill or for comfort.

Although DES and 17-alpha-ethinylestradiol belong to different estrogenic categories (non-steroid and steroid) and degrade in different ways, they do bind to the same ER-beta-estrogen receptors. The (natural) 17-beta-estradiol belongs to the family of steroid estrogens, which are lipophilic compounds. So it should bind to lipids, but thanks to the metabolization enzymes Cytochromes P-450 [7] it will be disposed of in the form of hydrosoluble products such as estriol, which can be found in the urine in the sulphate form. The (synthetic) 17-alpha-ethinylestradiol undergoes different metabolization pathways relative to its acetylenic function. These pathways deactivate the metabolization enzymes Cytochromes P-450, unlike the hydrosoluble natural estradiol, estrogen, which degrades in estriol. Hence the 17-ethinylestradiol remains bound to the lipids. Diethylstilbestrol, a non-steroid oestrogen, is a very lipophilic synthetic diphenol. Its metabolization is also different from natural estradiol; it is a molecular degradation by means of a very harmful oxidation reaction, as it will release toxic "quinone"-type structures, which are highly reactive to proteins and to DNA in particular **(Table 2)**.

Up to now, many research studies have been carried out on animals (mice and rats), showing the toxicity of such synthetic oestrogens upon the descendants, and inducing in particular behavioral disorders – along with other effects such as cancers [8,5] with multigenerational carcinogenesis effects on mice (9). Prenatal exposure to three different synthetic chemicals, DES and two pesticides (DDT and its chemical analogue, methoxychlor), was studied [10]: it affects the behavior of young mice, showing increased aggressiveness in males (increase of the number of attacks and decrease in reaction time before the attack). However, the DES doses were 1000 times smaller (0.02 and 0.2 µg/kg) than the DDT ones (and analogue) (20 and 200µg/kg), while the subsequent aggressive reactions were far more severe, showing the tremendous impact of DES, even at low doses. The treatment period of the mothers from the 11th to the 17th day of the gestation also played a key role, as it represents a crucial period in the differentiation of the reproductive system and in the development of the brain in the rodents studied [11]. Newbold [4] unambiguously demonstrated the validity of the "rodent model" transposed to humans. Injection of 17-alpha-ethinylestradiol (EE) in pregnant rats not only induces many abortions, but also anxiety and depression-type disorders in pups (strain Dark Agouti) [12, 13] (15µg/kg^{-1}/d). In terms of brain cytology, an alteration of the frontal part of the hippocampus in young rats (Long Evans strain) which were EE-treated *in utero* was also demonstrated [14] at the same doses which were calculated to be relatively comparable to the doses prescribed to pregnant women (see Table 1).

The (natural) 17-beta-estradiol belongs to the family of steroid estrogens, which are lipophilic compounds. So it should bind to lipids, but thanks to the metabolization enzymes of the Cytochromes P-450 type, it will be disposed of in the form of hydrosoluble products such as Estriol, which will be found in the urine in the sulphate form.
The (synthetic) 17-alpha-ethinylestradiol undergoes different metabolization pathways relative to its acetylenic function. These pathways induce the inactivation of the Cytochromes P-450. Hence the 17-Ethinyl-Estradiol will remain bound to the lipids.
The diethylstilbestrol, a non-steroid estrogen, is a very lipophilic synthetic diphenol. Its metabolization is also different from natural Estradiol; it is a molecular degradation by means of a very harmful oxidation reaction, as it will release toxic "quinone"-type structures, which are highly reactive to proteins and to DNA in particular.

Table 2. Difference between natural sexual hormone, the 17-beta-estradiol type, and the synthetic hormones of the 17-alpha-ethinylestradiol or diethylstilbestrol type.

In humans, research work on the effects of synthetic hormones on women is scarce, but as early as 1977, June Reinisch [15] published a paper in Nature showing that the personality of the children whose mothers had been treated with synthetic oestrogens and progestin could be affected. Behavioral disorders starting in post-adolescence have since been reported in the children exposed *in utero* to the two mentioned estrogens: depression [16, 17], anxiety [17- 19], schizophrenia [20, 21], anorexia and bulimia [22]. These observations were summarized by Pillard et al [17] and Verdoux [21]. As early as 1987, was described [20] the case of 4 male adults prenatally exposed to DES and showing psychotic disorders. It is only during late adolescence that psychotic disorders develop, which often requires a neuroleptic treatment, even in the absence of family history of same. They hypothesized then that there could be a causal relationships between disruptions in the neuro-development linked to DES, and the subsequent appearance of psychotic disorders. Pillard et al. [17] showed that the frequency of major recurrent depressive episodes was significantly higher in DES sons than in their unexposed brothers, which was recently confirmed in 2010 [23] in DES daughters from a cohort of 74,628 women (known as "Nurses Health Cohort"), 1,612 of whom were exposed to DES. In critical literature reviews Kébir and Krebs [24, 25] analyse in particular the results of the only three epidemiological large cohort studies, as well as smaller cohorts in relation to the effects of DES on the onset of psychiatric disorders. Out of the three epidemiological studies on large cohorts, two favour the hypothesis of an existing causal link [18, 23], and one reaches a different conclusion (study based on 1,352 mothers) [26].

The mothers' exposure to synthetic hormones, and in particular to DES and 17-alpha-ethinylestradiol, during pregnancy, and the study of its impact on exposed children, represents an almost experimental model to evaluate the toxicity of these products: the French HHORAGES troop, the results of which are presented in this work, is a "real-world" experimental group, in real-life conditions.

2. Materials and methods: Gathering questionnaires and the evidence

This study is not epidemiological. Its purpose is to put together a database that will enable HHORAGES-France to advance the evidence of serious effects on the psychological and physical health of the descendants of women treated with synthetic hormones during their pregnancy. This study has been carried out based on spontaneous testimonies from families affected. Families were alerted to this initiative either by TV, by radio, or by direct confidential communication. After an initial contact with the association (by phone, post, or via e-mail), a detailed questionnaire **(Table 3)**, prepared by researchers and doctors, was sent without consideration of race only to the families affected by psychiatric disorders in one or more of their children with or without somatic problems. More often mothers answered but also daughters or sons if the mother was deceased or too old or ill or in denial of the effects. Concerning the age of the children, psychiatric diseases appearing generally at the post adolescence after 18 years or later, testimonies concern people born between 1946 to 2000. In order to avoid some deviations in the sample, other factors as contamination with pesticides or other chemicals were questioned in the paragraph "professional exposure".

An authorization request about such questionnaires and files was sent to the CNIL (French "*Commission Nationale de l'Informatique et des Libertés*") and obtained. Subsequently the data were synthesized in the form of synoptic data for further studies. In 2006 a first detailed analysis of 2002-2004 and 2005 data was carried out in the *Laboratoire d'Endocrinologie-Pédiatrique* of the Montpellier University Hospital (CHU Lapeyronie), and was conducted according to specific descriptive criteria: exposed and unexposed children, daughters and sons, ranking in the sibling order, treatment by synthetics (oestrogens, oestrogen-progestin, or progestin), and pathologies, malformations and other disorders. In May 2009, all files with prescriptions attached were validated in psychiatric terms by representatives of the CERC (*Centre d'Etude et de Recherche Clinique*, Hôpital Sainte-Anne, Paris, run by Professor M.O. Krebs), a research laboratory with which HHORAGES established a partnership from 2007 via a PICRI project (*Partenariat Institution Citoyen pour la Recherche et l'Innovation*) subsidized by the Île-de-France region, and for the benefit of said Laboratory.

Mother's Situation: Surname, First Name, Date of Birth, Address, Home phone number, Professional phone number, Mobile number, E-mail address
Family Situation, Number of children, children's first names and dates of birth. Professional Situation.
Pill taken: before first pregnancy, and between pregnancies
Hormonal treatment before pregnancy (or pregnancies). (If a treatment was prescribed, please indicate the nature of the treatment and the time elapsed between the end of treatment and the beginning of the pregnancy)
Miscarriage(s): Indicate the time when it occurred, in relation to the other full term pregnancies, if any (*before the first one, or between two full term pregnancies?*)
Professional Exposure to hormones, to chemicals (pesticides, etc...)
Psychiatric or psychopathological family history (father, mother, ...)
Health problems after first child birth
Pregnancy and childbirth (For more than 2 children, T.O.P.)
1st child 2nd child
Treatment during pregnancy: *(Yes/No)* - Nature of medicines - Doses – What time during pregnancy (first and last day of treatment, expressed in weeks from the beginning of pregnancy)?
What medical reason was put forward (possible miscarriage, comfort, etc...)?
At what month did the delivery occur, from the start of the pregnancy?
General condition of the child, Sex, Weight, Health problems at birth *(mother and child)*
Existing documents (prescriptions, medical files, etc...) and testimonies
Would you be so kind as to send us the copies of the files and documents? If yes, in order to save time, please attach the copies of all relative documents in your possession.
Health problems of your children (For more than 2 children, T.OP)
1st child, 2nd child First name, Sex, Birth Date, Rank in the sibling order
Physical disorders: Which ones? What age? Sterility treatment? Surgery?
Psychological disorders: Nature of first symptoms? What age? Subsequent aggravation? And at what age?
Other data: Hospitalization, Violence, Suicide attempt(s), Medical Treatments, Diagnosis, AAH, Disability?
Relational difficulties: in married life, in professional life?
Children, grandchildren: How many? Full term? Health condition? Malformations or observed disorders?

Table 3. Questionnaire sent to families.

3. Results

3.1. Data analysis

Chronological evolution of number of cases issued from the HHORAGES-France association was studied from testimonies collected from 2002 to 2007 (**Figures 1-4**). From 2002 (foundation of the HHORAGES association) to 2004 our first crude analysis was based on the testimonies of 297 mothers with a total number of 511 children, the birth years ranging from 1946 to 1994 **(Figure 1)**. 161 unexposed children had no disorder ("control"), 35 children exposed *in utero* had no disorder, 297 children exposed *in utero* showed various psychiatric pathologies, while 18 unexposed children also showed psychiatric disorders. It must be noted that in most families without any psychiatric antecedent and having several children, only the exposed child showed psychiatric disorders.

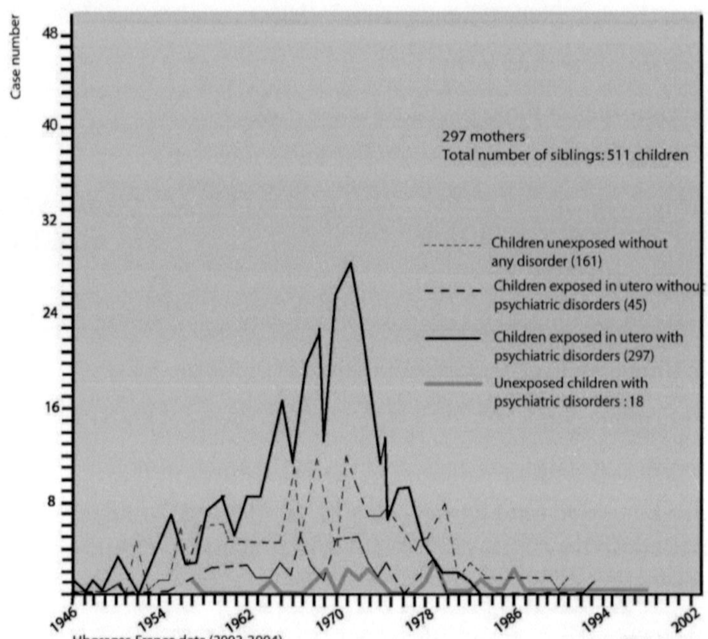

Figure 1. Representation of case numbers as a function of administered or not synthetic hormonal treatments during pregnancies (children born between 1946 and 1996), in a cohort of 511 children born from 297 mothers. The x-axis shows the birth years and the y-axis the number of cases. A prescription peak can be observed in the seventies. Black line: children exposed *in utero* with psychiatric disorders; dotted line: children unexposed without any disorders; dash line: children exposed *in utero* without psychiatric disorders; thick grey line: unexposed children with psychiatric disorders (HHORAGES-FRANCE data 2002-2004).

In 2005, a larger overall analysis based the testimony of 470 mothers **(Figure 2)** with a total number of 967 siblings: 381 of whom were not exposed, 345 exhibited no disorder, and 18 of whom showed psychiatric disorders. Interestingly, 9 of those unexposed with psychiatric disorders were born after their mother had been treated with synthetic hormones during a previous pregnancy. 586 children were exposed, during their mother's pregnancy, to DES only or to DES in association with synthetic ethinylestradiol, and sometimes with synthetic delayed progestin, 538 children displayed psychiatric disorders and 35 were without any psychiatric disorders nor any malformation whatsoever and 13 were stillborn.

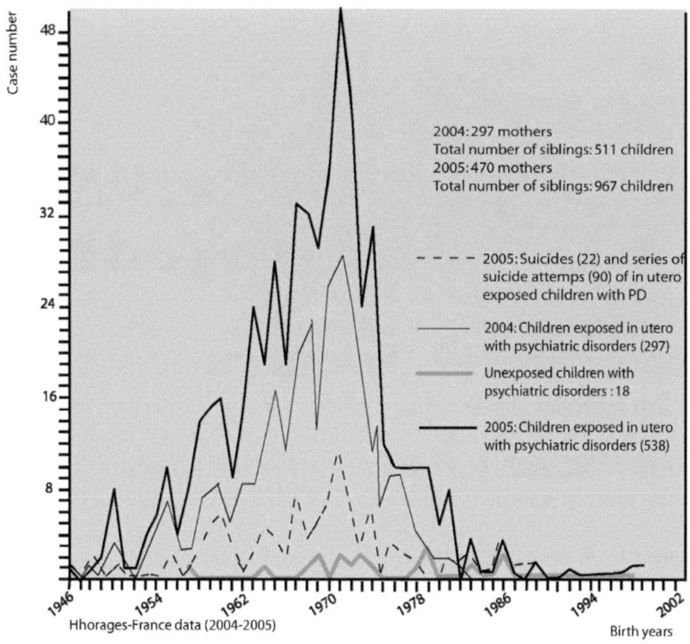

Figure 2. A detailed representation of case numbers in a group of 967 children born from 470 mothers. 363 unexposed children do not present any disorder. 586 children were exposed *in utero,* 48 of whom without disorders and 538 with psychiatric disorders (PD). 18 unexposed children showed PD, 9 of whom after their mother was treated in a previous pregnancy. Thin grey line: children exposed *in utero* with psychiatric disorders collected in 2004; black line: children exposed *in utero* with psychiatric disorders (2005). Thick grey line: unexposed children with psychiatric disorders. Dash line: Suicides and series of suicide attempts of *in utero* exposed children with psychiatric disorders. Comparison between 2004 and 2005 curves and suicide curve show the same prescription peak than in Fig.1 as observed in the seventies (1971) (HHORAGES-France data 2005).

By refining these observations, it appeared that out of the 538 children exhibiting psychiatric disorders, 200 suffered also from genital malformations. However, 74 presented genital malformations or other somatic disorders only, whereas 126 exhibited somatic and psychiatric disorders. In total, 538 children had psychiatric disorders. There were 18 non-exposed children who presented psychiatric disorders, 9 of which after their mothers had been exposed in a previous pregnancy. Among the children showing psychiatric disorders, it must be stressed that a significant number of suicides (22 S) and 90 series of suicide attempts were observed (dash line curve). The comparison between the 2004 and 2005 curves represented on Figure 2 shows a homothety, the peak of children suffering psychiatric disorders being for children born on the 1971-1972 years as well as the peak of suicide and suicide attempts.

In 2006-2007, a detailed analysis covered 529 testimonies, representing a total number of 1182 children as shown in the synthetic tree diagram of **Figures 3.**

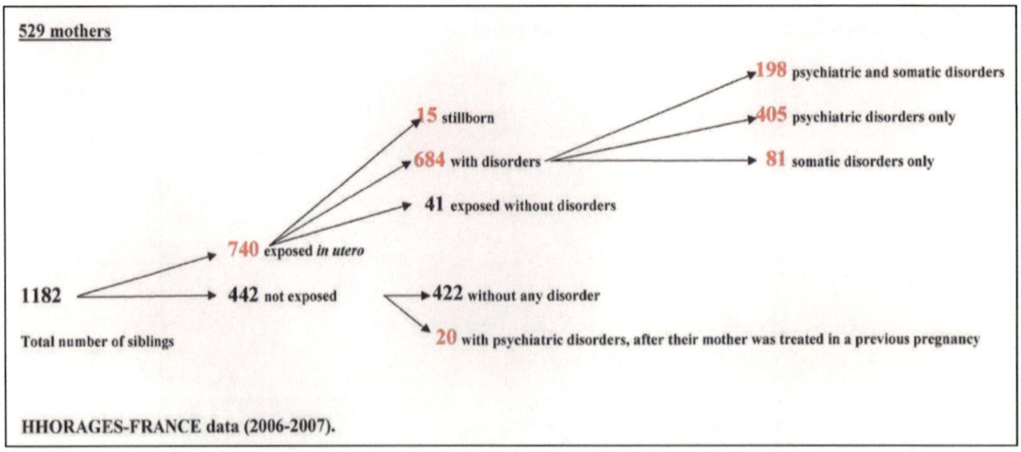

Figure 3. Tree diagram showing the distribution of a cohort of 1182 children born from 529 mothers, 740 of whom were exposed to synthetic hormones during their mothers' pregnancies. 41 exposed children did not show any disorder, 15 were stillborn and 684 were affected either by psychiatric disorders only, or by somatic disorders only, or by both (HHORAGES-France data 2006-2007).

442 children were not exposed, of which 422 did not exhibit any disorder or malformation; while 20 whose mothers had been exposed in a previous pregnancy exhibited psychiatric disorders. Among the 740 who were exposed *in utero*, 15 were stillborn (10 boys and 5 girls), 41 were not affected (25 boys and 16 girls) and 684 were affected, 405 of which with psychiatric disorders only, 198 psychiatric disorders associated with genital malformations and other somatic disorders, and 81 were affected only physically.

In **Figure 4** is shown the ratio of Boys/Girls, as well as their numbers. Thus 740 children were exposed and 684 were affected either by psychiatric disorders only, or by somatic ones, or by both. 65 girls and 16 boys were affected by somatic disorders only, while 134 girls and 64 boys were affected by psychiatric and somatic disorders. 219 girls and 186 boys are affected by psychiatric diseases only. Our group of 1182 total children is composed of 630 girls and 552 boys, so the gender ratio is 1.14. For children suffering from psychiatric diseases only, gender ratio is 1.17, psychiatric and somatic disorders 2.09, and somatic disorders only, 4.06.

Among the 442 "non-exposed" pregnancies, 422 children were not affected and 20 (mothers previously treated) were affected presenting psychiatric and/or somatic disorders. Among the 422 not affected 182 are free from all exposure (104 boys and 78 girls) and 240 were born after their mother was treated in a previous pregnancy (123 boys and 117 girls); so we observed a majority of unaffected boys. Among the 20 affected are 14 girls and 6 boys. Of these 14 girls, 7 suffered psychiatric disorders only, 3 presented psychiatric and somatic disorders, 4 somatic disorders only. Of the 6 boys, 4 presented psychiatric disorders, 2 psychiatric and somatic, and none with somatic disorder only. It is clear overall that disorders in girls are more numerous than in boys.

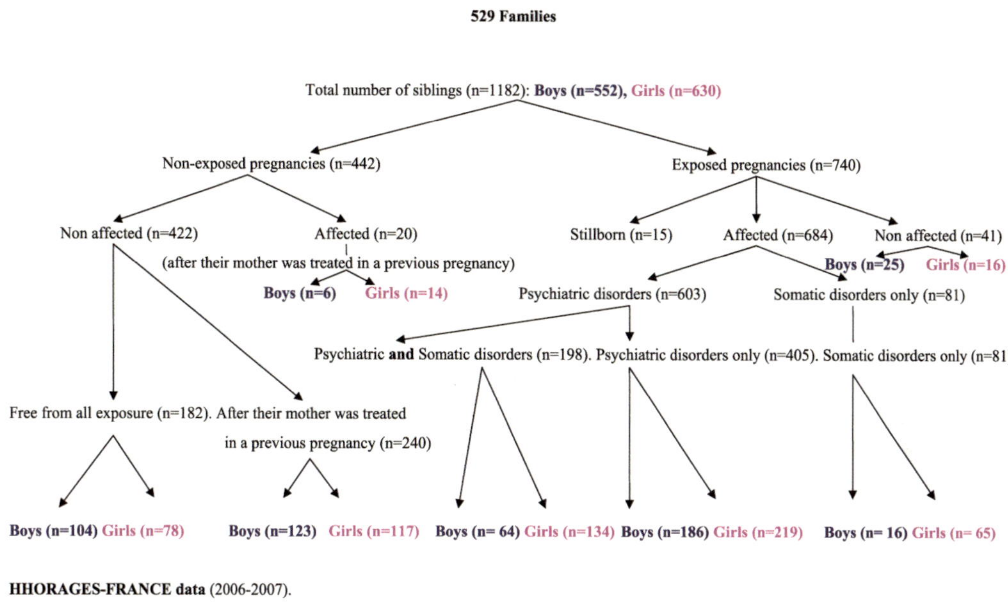

Figure 4. Detailed testimony group included in the study showing the distribution of girls and boys of second generation in a cohort of 1,182 children born from 529 mothers: 740 of whom were exposed to synthetic hormones during their mothers' pregnancies collected from 2002 to 2007. 15 were stillborn and 684 were affected either by psychiatric disorders only, or by somatic malformations only, or by both (HHORAGES-FRANCE data 2006-2007). In all cases girls suffered more than boys either from psychiatric, and/or somatic disorders, while boys are more likely than girls to be unaffected even after exposure: 41 exposed children did not show any disorder (25 boys versus 16 girls) (HHORAGES-France data 2006-2007).

For boys among somatic disorders associated or not with psychiatric disorders (on a total of 80 boys), we have counted 28 cryptorchidia, 22 hypospadias, 14 sterility, azoospermia or semen abnormalities, 12 cancers or others, 4 micropenis. (**Figure 5**).

Among a total of 210 girls, somatic disorders associated or not with psychiatric disorders are: 70 womb malformations, 50 sterility, 31 difficulty to procreate (primary and secondary infertility), miscarriage, extra uterine pregnancies, 31 cancers (often of breast) or others, 21 ovarian cysts, 8 endometriosis. (**Figure 6**).

As of today (April 2012), we are receiving an ever-increasing number of testimonies, the total number of testimonies collected by HHORAGES is 1,223, which represents 2,674 children from them 409 unexposed, 1,676 children exposed to synthetic hormones after medical prescriptions and 589 (post-DES) born after a previous exposure from which 20 presented psychiatric and/or somatic disorders. Amongst this total amount of 1,676 exposed children, 1,549 children are affected: 916 present psychiatric disorders, 418 somatic plus psychiatric disorders, 183 somatic disorders, 126 exposed are non affected. In addition, we numbered 48 suicides and 128 series of suicide attempts. Many HHORAGES families collaborated in genetic and epigenetic studies, as carried out in the Inserm U796 Laboratory in St-Anne Hospital, Paris, in order to understand the cellular and molecular mechanisms disrupted by these xenooestrogens [1] in the cadre of the PICRI (*Partenariat Institution Citoyens pour la Recherche et l'Innovation*) project. In addition, the HHORAGES families participate to a vast study on the origin of schizophrenia, this study, granted by the French National Research Agency (ANR), is larger than the PICRI one and also developed in the St Anne Hospital, Paris, by the Professor M.O. Krebs team.

Somatic disorders :boys	Impregnation:Synthetic hormones (DES, EE..)
Hypospads	22
Cryptorchidia	28
Micropenis	4
Sterility, Azoospermia, Abnomal.spz.	14
Cancers, others	12
Total	80

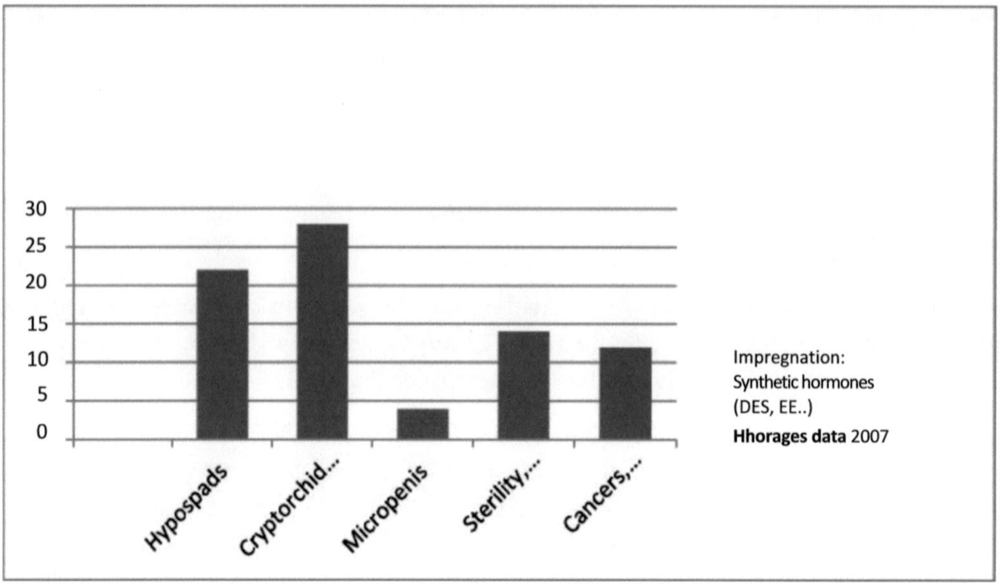

Figure 5. Somatic disorders in boys after exposition to synthetic hormones (DES, EE,.). Cryptorchidia and hypospadias are the most numerous disorders. These disorders are whether or not associated with the psychiatric ones (HHORAGES-France data 2007).

Somatic disorders : girls (associated or not to psychiatric disorders)	Impregnation: synthetic hormones (DES, EE..)
Uterine malformations	70
Sterility	50
Difficulty procreating, miscarriages, extra-uterinepregnancies	31
Ovarian cyst	21
Endometriosis	8
Cancers, others	31
Total	210

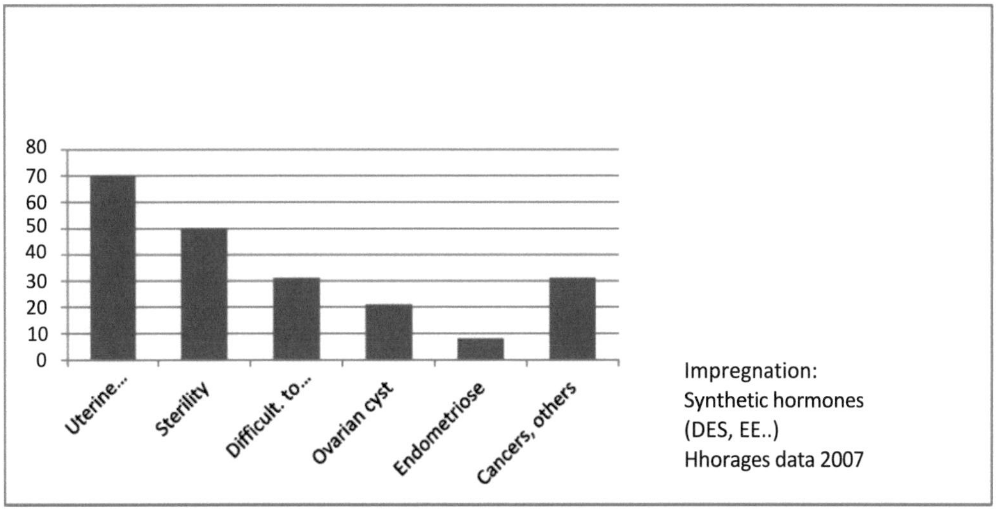

Figure 6. Somatic disorders in girls after exposure to synthetic hormones (DES, EE,). Womb malformations and sterility are the most numerous disorders. These disorders are whether or not associated with psychiatric ones (HHORAGES-France data 2007).

4. Discussion

1. Research work on behavioral disorders in humans after prenatal exposure to synthetic hormones is scarce, as people affected by severe psychotic disorders and their families are not usually very inclined to answer epidemiological inquiries. Similarly, as suggested in a preliminary work [27] the number of families who spontaneously gave their testimony to HHORAGES (more than 1220 to date) is rather low in comparison to the total number of pregnancies effectively treated with these products, about 160,000 in France according to [28,29]. Nevertheless, in our results presented in Figure 2, we observe in addition to the fact that curves deducted from successive year data are homothetic and that the peak of the curve representing children suffering psychiatric disorders as well as the peak of suicide and suicide attempts correspond to the years 1971-72. This could be put in parallel to the curve published in Figure 1 in [28] and calculated from the DES plaques sold in our country (EE sold plaques not estimated).

   But some testimonies remained anonymous, or some families were not properly informed, or failed to answer the questionnaires, in these cases, certain factors should be taken into account: -The fact that psychiatric disorders appear during post-adolescence implies on average a twenty-year gap between the time when the mothers were treated and the appearance of the disorder, hence the difficulty finding the prescriptions and the medical files.– Psychiatric disorders are often treated with denial and shame, which presents problems connecting families with HHORAGES, or in their answering any inquiry whatsoever; and the children (DES sons and daughters for instance), if and when they are informed (often very late) about their family (mother) history, they first try to find a cure, as psychotic disorders can often be very incapacitating, especially if these disorders are in addition to genital malformations, sterility, semen abnormalities or total azoospermy.

2. Somatic disorders of boys and girls as genital malformations (see Figures 5 and 6), sterility, azoospermie, endometriosis, cancers, are now completely recognized as being a consequence of DES or EE *in utero* exposure. In our troop, they are found associated with psychiatric disorders for 198 children, while 81 were only somatically affected. The total amount of 279 children represent more than 1/3 of the 684 affected children exposed to synthetic estrogens that demonstrate the DES and EE signature.

   A preliminary result concerning a small part of the total number of children linked to the HHORAGES families was published in 2009 in a congress communication [1] (**Table 4**). A series of cases were studied, consisting of 31 files about 31 mothers and 72 children born alive. Among the 72 children, the following were found: 43 children exposed and affected, 4 exposed, but not affected, 23 non-exposed and not affected, 1 non-exposed but affected. The involved hormones were DES and 17-alpha-ethinylestradiol and synthetic progestin. The psychiatric disorders found were: Alcohol addiction: 3, Learning disorders: 3, Eating disorders: 9, Behavioral disorders (aggressiveness, impulsivity): 5, Sleeping disorders: 3, Anxiety disorders: 7, Mood swings: 12, Major depressive episodes: 2, Bipolar disorders, Personality disorders: 3, Schizophrenia: 10, Acute psychotic episodes: 4, Series of suicide attempts: 9, and Suicides: 5. As concluded in this communication "The clinical pictures relative to the children studied are quite complex and involve some atypical associations, for instance mood swings associated with psychotic features." A larger study pertaining to this cohort is under way.

   It is known that psychosis as schizophrenia for example affects about 1% of the world population, a few part being of genetic familial origin. Neuro developmental and environmental causal factors of schizophrenia (or of other psychoses as bipolar diseases) are yet badly known, the epigenetic track and the conjunction gene X environment theory being the best hypothesis from several years [24, 25, 30]. So the HHORAGES family group participates also to a study largest than PICRI on the origin of schizophrenia also developed in the St Anne Hospital by Professor M.O. Krebs team.

3. In this study, we observed that girls seem more vulnerable to synthetic estrogens than boys either for somatic and psychiatric disorders (see **Figure 4**). The preferential effects of DES on female *versus* male are not fully understood. It is likely that prenatal DES exposure affected behavior through its action on estrogen receptor alpha or beta of the

hypothalamic area which concentration may be higher in female fetus as shown in [30]. A sex difference in DNA methylation and gene regulation after prenatal DES exposure cannot be excluded [31] and last, hypomethylation of COMT promotor, a major risk factor for schizophrenia and bipolar disorder, may be different between male and female fetus and infant [32]. Our observations are reinforced by these of Braun et al [33] about BPA exposure and cognitive disorders or hyperactivity observations in *in utero* exposed children. In their study authors observed this BPA exposure affected behavioral and emotional regulation domains from 3 years of age, especially among girls which present aggressiveness and impulsivity. Authors suggest that girls would be more sensitive than boys *in utero* to BPA, which acts as mimetic of natural estrogen hormones, and in surplus to them.

Among the 72 children born alive, 40 exposed children were affected, 7 exposed were not affected, 1 exposed but deceased by the age of 10 months, 23 children were not exposed and not affected, et 1 unexposed child was affected. The psychiatric disorders are as follows :
Alcohol addiction: 3; Learning disorders: 3; Eating disorders : 9
Behavioral disorders (aggressiveness, impulsivity): 5
Sleeping disorders: 3; Anxiety disorders: 7
Mood swings: 12; Major depressive episodes, 2
Bipolar disorders, Personality disorders: 3
Schizophrenia: 10; Acute psychotic episodes: 4
Series of suicide attempts: 9 and Suicides: 5.

Table 4. Analysis of the psychiatric cases of 72 children from 31 testimonies [1]. From this observation, authors suggest that the vulnerability toward psychiatric disorders could be enhanced after impregnation with diethylstilbestrol (DES), ethinyl estradiol and/or synthetic delay progestin during the mother's pregnancy.

Concerning the manifestation of psychiatric disorders in boys and girls, appearing often post adolescence, Verdoux [21] had suggested that these diseases could be due to the exposed status of the children after being informed of it by the mother: In our cohort, during our contacts with families, we carefully questioned them about this point: most of children had never been previously informed of the exposure, or were never informed at all.

Concerning the 41 children exposed and not affected (25 boys/16 girls) and the 422 children unaffected (226 boys/196 girls) of which 242 mothers had been treated in a previous pregnancy, a majority of boys is observable: we think that this fact could be linked to the specific and unequal detoxification potential of each individual, and could concern either the treated mother or/and the fetus in correlation with Cytochromes P450 gene activity and their regulation, as well analysed in the recent work of the Seralini group [34].

Concerning the 20 boys and girls (14 girls and 6 boys) "post DES" (whose mothers were only exposed during a previous pregnancy) and suffering psychiatric and somatic disorders, this could be linked with the lipophily (see Table 2) of the synthetic estrogens (DES and/or EE) administrated to mothers during a previous pregnancy, due to their likely residuum (remanence) in the maternal tissues.

4. There is a large amount of convincing research on animals (rodents) showing an indisputable link between synthetic estrogen exposition during gestation of the females and various disorders in exposed pups. Newbold et al [35] did not hesitate to extrapolate from rodents to humans where anatomical disorders observed in older mice are concerned after they were prenatally exposed to DES (cancers, lesions of the male as cryptorchidism, testicular hypoplasia, semen abnormalities [36] or female genital abnomalies, also of DNA and genetic lesions) as well as a function of the doses as of exposure time. She believes that the DES makes an excellent predictive model for other environmental estrogens. Indeed, O'Reilly *et al.* [23], in their epidemiological work on the depression rates in DES daughters, suggest that studies on this pathology may be extrapolated to children exposed to BPA *in utero*. Endocrine disrupter Bis-Phenol A (BPA) was nearly chosen instead of DES, but ultimately was not. However, its action inside plastic materials is even more insidious, as it is present in a large number of materials and consumer goods and as it contaminates therefore the whole population, including fetuses and infants via their breast feeding mothers. Among the many research works carried out on animals (rats, mice, monkeys) showing that there is a detectable effect for doses lower than the ADI (Acceptable Daily Intake) of 50μg/kg, one is specially interesting: it has been demonstrated in mice, that a prenatal exposure to the low dose of 10μg/kg (from the 11th day of gestation) unambiguously triggers behavioral disorders, besides other effects [37]. As recently published [38] the effects of low dose cannot be predicted by the effects observed at high doses. And as far as some organophosphate pesticides that mimic oestrogens are concerned, it has been recently shown that residues of such chemicals in urine samples of 1139 children aged 8-15 came from the family food (based on garden fruits and vegetables), and that their presence was strongly correlated to behavioral disorders of hyperactivity type and cognitive disorders (attention deficit disorder) type [39].

5. A multi-generational effect? By what mechanism?

Multi-generational carcinogenesis studies were realized on mice after diethylstilbestrol impregnation with impressive and undisputable results [8, 9]. Our observations presented in this present work from the French HHORAGES troop raises the question of the mechanism through with synthetic hormones as DES cause either psychiatric disorders in exposed children and/or adverse effects in subsequent generations. Since Abdomaleky et al

[40,41,30] concluded that modulation of gene-environment interactions may be trough DNA methylation, in [42] and [24, 25] authors put forward hypothesis that DES-induced changes in epigenetic background and alteration of DNA methylations could be significant factors. The pregnant mother's exposure to DES at very early neurodevelopment time and/or at time of sex determination would appear to be sufficient to alter the remethylation of neuron precursors and/or of the fetus germ line. Only a few third-generation children suffering psychiatric illness are mentioned in testimonies. This is understandable because third generation exposed children are still too young (excepted in some cases) to present psychiatric disorders as schizophrenia which is not the case for hypospads that are detectable from birth in male children and grand-children [42]. Work is already under way concerning the gene X environment DES impact hypothesis by comparing DES and EE exposed children, various genetic and epigenetic factors to those of mother and unexposed children of the same family as studied by the INSERM team U796 in collaboration with the HHORAGES families.

6. Conclusions

In the present familial case control study, we have shown that there are serious effects on the psychological and physical health of the descendants of women treated with synthetic hormones during their pregnancy: psychiatric illnesses are often found associated with somatic disorders which are well known to be the DES and EE signature. Synthetic hormones, acting as endocrine disturbers, are toxic for humans, especially for pregnant women and their children, probably partly in relation with their toxic degradation status. In all cases girls suffered more than boys either of somatic and/or psychiatric disorders due to the estrogen receptor alpha or beta concentration higher in female fetus than in male. It is also clear that in all the families most of the exposed children are ill while quite the unexposed are not.

So what now? As the precautionary principle was not applied in the past, and still is not in force today, and since the lessons of recent history were never taken into account [33], it is our common duty to repair the damage by supporting the devastated families, and by pursuing research work on the observation of trans-generational effects. Such effects are already highlighted by the demonstration that cancers are observed even in the fourth generation in mice [9]. According to the Skinner's mini review [43] "the ability of an environmental compound (as DES or EE) to promote the reprogramming of the germ-line appears to be the causal factor in the epigenetic transgenerational phenotype," we observed an increase of the genital malformations in the third generation in male infants whose mothers were treated with xenoestrogens [42]. In the HHORAGES troop, DES and EE-exposed infants are already pointed out as bodily and/or psychologically impaired after their mothers were treated with clomifene citrate (an ovulation stimulator previously used for IVF-type medically assisted procreation). Another concern is the putative future effect of ethinylestradiol containing oral estrogenic contraception on future generations due to its lipophily after its metabolization and its future release in fetus through the placenta. As for the demonstration of the causality link within the HHORAGES troop, will we have to wait for a large-scale epidemiological study, or are we allowed to think that the impressive figures that we are publishing in this work are not merely random? The only way now is to respect absolutely the precautionary principle and to delete completely or to give the less possible toxic (synthetic) hormone medication: for example Clavel Chapelon and her Endogenous Hormones and Breast Cancer Collaborative Group in Villejuif [44] informed that natural hormone as micronized (natural) progestin associated with estrogens (synthetic alas!) is more often ordered for SHT (Substitutive Hormonal Treatment) in order to avoid breast cancer. Unfortunately, she said also that in the contrary the same SHT is not recommended to avoid the endometrium cancer [45]…

As Newbold et al [35] said after they reviewed the damages caused by DES [4], "only new advances in the knowledge of genetic and epigenetic mechanisms of the disruptions of fetal development will enable us to be aware of the risks entailed by the other estrogenic disruptors which are present around us and in ourselves, even at very low doses", whilst Theo Colborn [46] insists on the fact that the foetus cannot be protected against endocrine disruptors, whatever they may be, except at zero level.

Author details

Marie-Odile Soyer-Gobillard
Centre National de la Recherche Scientifique, Unité Mixte de Recherche 7628 Université P. et M. Curie (Paris6) Laboratoire Arago, F-66650 Banyuls sur mer and Association HHORAGES, (Halte aux HORmones Artificielles pour les GrossessES), Le Prieuré de Baillon, Asnières sur Oise, France

Charles Sultan
Service d'Hormonologie (Développement et Reproduction), Hôpital Lapeyronie, CHU de Montpellier, Montpellier, France et Institut de Génétique Humaine, CNRS UPR 1142, Montpellier, France
Service de Pédiatrie I, Unité d'endocrinologie et gynécologie pédiatrique, Hôpital Arnaud-de-Villeneuve, CHU de Montpellier, Montpellier Cedex 5, France

Disclaimer

The authors declare they have no competitive financial interests; the financing of HHORAGES-France association comes exclusively from the donations of families and of sympathetic individuals.

Acknowledgement

Mr René Alexandre, Dr Henri Pézerat and Pfr Jean Caston worked tirelessly to demonstrate the harmful role of the endocrine disruptors, and in particular of synthetic hormones, before passing away: we shall never forget their efficient help. This work could not continue without the daily ongoing support of the HHORAGES board especially Mrs Geneviève

Alchourroun, Mauricette Puillandre, Denise Hemmerdinger, Michel Datry and Yette Blanchet. We are very grateful to Mr André Cicolella, President of the French RES (Réseau Environnement Santé) for his constant support. We thank particularly Henri Diaz, Herrade Hemmerdinger, and James di Properzio (USA) for their help and critical reading in the preparation of the manuscript.

7. References

[1] Roblin J, Chayet M, Bon Saint Come M, Kebir O, Bannour S, Guedj F (2009) Troubles psychiatriques et exposition *in utero* aux hormones de synthèse: Etude d'une série de cas. 7ème Congrès de l'Encéphale, Paris, 22-24-01, PO 010.

[2] Dieckman WJ, Davis ME, Rynkiewicz LM, Pottinger RE (1953) Does the administration of diethylstilbestrol during pregnancy have therapeutic value? American Journal of Obstetrics and Gynaecology 66: 1062-1081.

[3] Giusti RM, Iwamoto K, Hatch E (1995) Diethylstilbestrol revisited: A review of the long term health effects. Annals of Internal Medicine 122: 778-788.

[4] Newbold RR (2004) Lessons learned from perinatal exposure to diethylstilbestrol. Toxicology and Applied Pharmacology 199: 142-150.

[5] Hoover RN, Hyer M, Pfeiffer RM, Adam E, Bond B, Cheville AL, Colton T, Hartge P, Hatch EE, Herbst AL, Karlan BY, Kaufman R, Noller KL, Palmer JR, Robboy SJ, Saal RC, Strohsnitter W, Titus-Ernstoff L, Troisi R (2011) Adverse health outcomes in women exposed *in utero* to Diethylstilbestrol. New England Journal of Medicine: 1304-1314.

[6] Herbst AL, Ulfelder H, Poskanzer DC (1971) Adenocarcinoma of the vagina. Association of maternal stilbestrol therapy with tumor appearance in young women. New England Journal of Medicine 284 (15): 878-881.

[7] Gueguen Y, Mouzat K, Ferrari L, Tissandie E, Lobaccaro JM, Batt AM, et al (2006) Cytochromes P450: xenobiotic metabolism, regulation and clinical importance. Ann Biol Clin (Paris) 64(6) : 535-548.

[8] Turusov VS, Trukhanova LS, Parfenov Yu D, Tomatis L (1992) Occurrence of tumors in the descendants of CBA male mice prenatally treated with diethylstilbestrol. International Journal of Cancer 50: 131-135.

[9] Walker BE, Haven MI (1997) Intensity of multigenerational carcinogenesis from diethylstilbestrol in mice. Carcinogenesis 18, 791-793.

[10] Palanza P, Gioiosa L, Vom Saal F, Parmigiani S (2008) Effects on developmental exposure to bisphenol A on brain and behavior in mice. Environmental Research 108: 150-157.

[11] Vom Saal FS, Montano MM, Wang HS (1992) Sexual differentiation in mammals. In Colborn T, Clement C, editors. Chemically induced alterations in sexual and functional development: the wildlife/human connection. Princeton, NJ: Princeton Specific 17-83.

[12] Dugard ML, Tremblay-Leveau H, Mellier D, Caston J (2001) Prenatal exposure to ethinylestradiol elicits behavioural abnormalities in the rat. Developmental Brain Research 129: 189-199.

[13] Arabo A, Lefebvre M, Fermanel M, Caston J (2005) Administration of 17-alpha-ethinylestradiol during pregnancy elicits modifications of maternal behaviour and emotional alteration of the offspring in the rat. Developmental Brain Research 156: 93-103.

[14] Sandner G, Barbosa Silva MJ, Angst J, Knobloch JM, Danion JM (2004) Prenatal exposure of Long-Evans rats to 17alpha-ethinylestradiol modifies neither latent inhibition nor prepulse inhibition of the statle reflex but elicits minor deficiency in exploratory behaviour. Developmental Brain Research 152: 177-187.

[15] Reinisch JM (1977) Prenatal exposure of human foetuses to synthetic progestin and oestrogen affects personality. Nature 266: 561-562.

[16] Ehrhardt AA, Feldman JF, Rosen LR, Meyer-Bhalburg R, Gruen NP, Veridiano NP (1987) Psychopathology in prenatally DES-exposed females: current and lifetime adjustement. Psychosomatic Medicine 49: 183-196.

[17] Pillard RC, Rosen H, Meyer-Bahlburg JD, Weinrich JF, Feldman, JF, Gruen R, Ehrhard AA (1993) Psychopathology and social functioning in men prenatally exposed to diethylstilbestrol (DES). Psychosomatic medicine 55: 485-491.

[18] Vessey MP, Faiweather DV, Norman-Smith B, Buckley J (1983) A randomized double-blind controlled trial of the value of stilboestrol therapy in pregnancy: long term follow-up of mothers and their offspring. British Journal of Obstetrics and Gynaecology 90:1007-1017.

[19] Saunders G (1988) Physical and psychological problems associated with exposure to diethylstilbestrol (DES). Hospital and Community Psychiatry 39: 73-77.

[20] Katz DL, Frankenburg FR, Frances R, Benowitz LI, Gilbert JM (1987) Psychosis and prenatal exposure to diethylstilbestrol. The Journal of Nervous and Mental Disease 175: 306-308.

[21] Verdoux H (2000) Quelles sont les conséquences psychiatriques de l'exposition intra-utérine au diethylstilbestrol (DES)? Annales médico-psychologiques 158: 105-117.

[22] Geary N (1998) The effect of estrogen on appetite. Medscape Women's Health 3: 3 (10).

[23] O'Reilly EJ, Mirzaei F, Forman MR, Ascherio A (2010) Diethylstilbestrol exposure *in utero* and depression in women. American Journal of Epidemiology 171: 876-882.

[24] Kebir O, Krebs, MO (2011) Perturbateurs endocriniens et troubles du comportement: Endocrine disruptors and behavioural anomalies. Médecine et Longévité 3: 94-98.

[25] Kebir O, Krebs, MO (2012) Diethylstilbestrol and risk of psychiatric disorders: A critical review and new insights. The World Journal of Biological Psychiatry, 13(2): 84-95.

[26] Verdoux H, Ropers J, Costagliola D, Clavel-Chapelon F, Paoletti X (2007) Serious psychiatric outcome of subjects prenatally exposed to diethylstilbestrol in the E3N cohort study. Psychological Medicine 37: 1315-1322.

[27] Soyer-Gobillard MO (2011). Perturbateurs endocriniens et troubles du comportement: Non, nous n'avons pas encore tiré toutes les leçons de l'histoire du DES. Médecine et Longévité 3: 67-74.

[28] Palmlund I, Apfel R, Buitendijk S, Cabau A, Forsberg JG (1993) Effects of diethylstilbestrol (DES) medication during pregnancy: report from a symposium at the

10th International Congress of ISPOG. Journal of Psychosomatic Obstetrical Gynaecology 14:71-89.

[29] Palmlund I (1996) Exposure to xenooestrogen before birth: the diethylstilbestrol experience. Journal of Psychosomatic Obstetrical Gynaecology 17: 71-84.

[30] Abdomaleky HM, Cheng K, Faraone SV, Wilcox M, Glatt SJ, Gao F, Smith CL, Shafa R, Aeali B, Carnevale J, Pan H, Papageorgis P, Ponte JF, Sivaraman V, Tsuang MT, and Thiagalingam S (2006) Hypomethylation of MB-COMT promoter is a major risk factor for schizophrenia and bipolar disorder. Human Molecular Genetics 15(21): 3132-3145.

[31] Tanaka M, Ohtani-Kaneko R, Yokosuka M, Watanabe C (2004) Low-dose perinatal diethylstilbestrol exposure affected behaviors and hypothalamic estrogen receptor-alpha-positive cells in the mouse. Neurotoxicology and Teratology 26 : 261-269.

[32] Li S, Hursting, Davis BJ., McLachlan JA., Barrett JC (2003) Environmental exposure, DNA methylation, and gene regulation: lessons from diethylstilbestrol-induced cancers. Ann N Y Acad Sci, 983: 161-169.

[33] Braun J M, Kalkbrenner AE,. Calafat AM, Yolton K, Ye X, Dietrich KN, Lanphear BP (2011) Impact of early life Bisphenol A Exposure on behavior and executive function in children. Pediatrics 128: 873-882.

[34] Benachour N, Clair E, Mesnage R, Seralini GE (2012) Endocrine disruptors: New Discoveries and possible Progress of Evaluation. In: Advances in Medicine and Biology. Volume 29 ISBN 978-1-61324-361-9 Leon V. Berhardt: Nova Science Publishers Inc. pp 1-58.

[35] Newbold RR, Padilla-Banks E, Jefferson WN (2006) Adverse effects of the model environmental Estrogen Diethylstilbestrol are transmitted to subsequent generations. Endocrinology 147: 11-17.

[36] Gill WB, Schumacher GF, Bibbo M, Straus FH 2nd, Schoenberg HW (1979) Association of diethylstilbestrol exposure *in utero* with cryptorchidism, testicular hypoplasia and semen abnormalities. Journal of Urology 22(1): 36-39.

[37] Palanza P, Gioiosa L, Vom Saal F, Parmigiani S (2008) Effects on developmental exposure to bisphenol A on brain and behavior in mice. Environmental Research 108: 150-157.

[38] Vandenberg LN, Colborn Th, Hayes TB, Heindel JJ, Jacobs DR, Lee DH, Shioda T, Soto AM, Vom Saal FS, Welshons Wv, Zoeller RT, Myers JP. (2012) Hormones and endocrine-disrupting chemicals: Low-dose effects and nonmonotonic dose responses.Endocrine Reviews. 33 (3): 0000-0000. Available: edrv.endojournals.org. Accessed 2012 March 14.

[39] Bouchard MF, Bellinger DC, Wright RO, Weisskopf MG (2010) Organophosphate Pesticides Attention-Deficit/Hyperactivity Disorder and Urinary Metabolites of Organophosphate Pesticides. Pediatrics 125: 1270-1277.

[40] Abdolmaleky HM, Smith, CL, Faraone SV, Shafa R, StoneW, Glatt, SJ and Tsuang MT (2004) Methylomics in psychiatry: modulation of gene–environment interactions may be through DNA methylation. American Journal of Medicine Genetics B Neuropsychiatric Genetics, 127, 51–59.

[41] Abdolmaleky H.M., Thiagalingam S, and Wilcox M (2005) Genetics and epigenetics in major psychiatric disorders: Dilemmas, achievements, applications, and future scope. American Journal of Pharmaco genomics 5: 149–160.

[42] Kalfa N, Paris F, Soyer-Gobillard MO, Daures JP, Sultan Ch (2011) Incidence of hypospadias in grandsons of DES-exposed women during pregnancy: a multigenerational national cohort study. Fertility and Sterility 95 (8): 2574-2577.

[43] Skinner MK (2008) What is an epigenetic transgenerational phenotype? F3 or F2 Reproduction Toxicology 25(1): 1-8.

[44] Endogenous Hormones and Breast Cancer Collaborative Group (2011) Circulating sex hormones and breast cancer risk factors in postmenopausal women: reanalysis of 13 studies. British Journal of Cancer 105 (5): 709-722.

[45] Interview of Dr F. Clavel Chapelon published on internet 23/11/2011: "E3N Study has clarified several problems of public health, especially links between SHT and breast cancer".

[46] Colborn T (2004) Neurodevelopment and endocrine disruption. Environmental Health Perspectives 112: 944-949.

Chapter 5

Role of Corticosteroids in Oral Lesions

Masoumeh Mehdipour and Ali Taghavi Zenouz

Additional information is available at the end of the chapter

http://dx. doi. org/10. 5772/50287

1. Introduction

Glucocorticoids were first introduced in the 1940s and have become a widely prescribed class of drugs. Corticosteroids are a class of chemicals that includes steroid hormones naturally produced in the adrenal cortex of vertebrates and analogues of these hormones that are synthesized in laboratories. Corticosteroids are involved in a wide range of physiologic processes, including stress response, immune response, and regulation of inflammation, carbohydrate metabolism, protein catabolism, blood electrolyte levels, and behavior. They are some of the most common drugs for management of patients undergoing stressful situations such as surgery and dentstry (Gibson 2004).

It has thus become common for standard textbooks in dentistry to recommend the administration of oral or intravenous steroids in the management of oral lesions.

Steroids have different effects on different tissues, which are dose dependent. The reason for varied effect of steroids lies in its mechanism of action (Grover 2007).

Glucocorticoids have potent anti-inflammatory actions, including the reduction in the number and function of various immune cells, such as T and B lymphocytes, monocytes, neutrophils, and eosinophils, at sites of inflammation. Glucocorticoids decrease the production of cytokines, chemokines, and eicosanoids and enhances the production of macrophage migration inhibitory factor (Gibson 2004).

Corticosteroid drugs are widely used in oral medicine such as in vesiculobullous diseases, orofacial granulomatosis, temporal arteritis and other oral mucosal disorders. Topical corticosteroids should be considered the treatment of choice unless the disease is very extensive. Systemic therapy is reserved for those with severe, refractory disease.

2. Mucosal ulceration and inflammation

2.1. Recurrent Aphthous Stomatitis

Recurrent Aphthous Stomatitis (RAS) are among the most common oral lesions in the general population, with a frequency of 5–25% and three month recurrence rates as high as 50%. Aphthous ulcers are often quite painful; may lead to difficulty in speaking, eating, and swallowing; and may negatively affect patients' quality of life (Ship 1996).

RAS is classified as minor, major, and herpetiform. Minor RAS involves the presence of one to five ulcers at a time, with each ulcer less than 1 cm in diameter.

Major aphthae are a cause of significant dysphagia and often result in extensive scarring. In herpetiform RAU there are 10–100 ulcers at a time, ulcer size is usually 1–3 cm, and the ulcers form clustersthat coalesce into widespread areas of ulceration lasting 7–10 days (Rees, Woo 1996).

The use of topical and systemic steroids in an attempt to manage apthous stomatitis is based on the presumption that the aphthae are the result of a noninfectious inflammatory process. Corticosteroids may act directly on T lymphocytes or alter the response of effect or cells to precipitants of immunopathogenesis (Vincent 1992).

2.1.1. Topical corticosteroids

Topical corticosteroid use in patients with RAS is intended to limit the inflammatory process associated with the formation of aphthae.

There are two double-blind, placebo-controlled trials have evaluated the efficacy of topical corticosteroids for RAS (Merchant 1978; Thompson 1989). The patients enrolled in one trial had minor RAS. Classification of ulcers was not available for the other trial. Both trials assessed patients for immuno -competence through laboratory studies. One trial excluded other medications used in RAS (Thompson 1989). In both trials there were significant reductions, compared with placebo, in ulcer duration and pain severity and no changes in the frequency of RAS in patients who applied betamethasone gel or beclomethasone aerosol spray to ulcers four times daily for six days to four weeks (Vincent 1992; Thompson 1989).

Two non-placebo controlled trials found no significant differences between triamcinolone ointment or betamethasone tablets and adhesive vehicles and Orabase in the frequency and duration of severe RAS. Subjective improvement tended to be greater with corticosteroids than with adhesive vehicle (Orabase), although the difference was not statistically significant (MacPhee 1968). A single blind, placebo-controlled trial involving fluocinonide ointment was performed in patients with minor and major RAS. Fluocinonide ointment significantly reduced ulcer duration, but ulcer frequency and subjective improvement were the same as for adhesive vehicle (Orabase). In the latter three trials, study design, ulcer severity, and vehicle activity may have contributed to findings inconsistent with those in the doubleblind, placebo-controlled studies (Pimlott 1983).

The drugs most commonly adopted for local oral application in RAS are hydrocortisone hemisuccinate (as pellets of 2. 5 mg) and triamcinolone acetonide (in an adhesive paste containing 0. 1% of the steroid). There is little risk of adrenal suppression provided that the recommended dose (fourtimes daily) is adhered to (Field 2003).

In severe RAS may be necessary to use a more potent steroid preparation. High potency topical steroid preparation such as fluocinonide, betamethasone or clobetasol placed directly on the lesions shortens healing time and reduces the size of lesion. The gel can be carefully applied directly to the lesion after meals and at bedtime 2-3 times a day or mixed with an adhesive such as orabase prior to application. Recently, Lo Muzio et al. treated oral aphthous lesions by applying clobetasol propionate with a bioadhesive system, which resulted insurprisingly good outcomes (Lo Muzio 2001).

Larger lesions can be treated by placing a gauge sponge containing the topical steroid on the ulcer and leaving it in place for 15-30 min to allow for longer contact of the medication. Ulcerations located in the areas that make them difficult to see or reach can be controlled by topical dexamethasone elixir, 0. 5 mg / 5 ml held over the area or applied with a saturated gauge pad to the ulcers, four times per day for 15 min (Lo Muzio 2001) and betamethasone sodium phosphate rinse (dissolve 0. 5 mg in 5 mL of water and rinse for 2–3 min), steroid aerosol (e. g. beclometasone diproprionate, 100 lg/puff) , or a high-potency topical corticosteroid, such as clobetasol 0. 05% in orabase or fluocinonide 0. 05% in orabase (Natah 2004).

2.1.2. *Systemic corticosteroids*

Major apthous ulcers often require systemic treatment as an initial approach. Therapy with prednisone 40 mg/day for one week is usually adequate to control the presenting outbreak. Systemically, oral prednisone is most commonly employed. Systemic prednisone therapy should be started at 1. 0 mg/kg a day as a single dose in patients with severe RAS and should be tapered after 1-2 weeks. Intralesional steroids can be used to treat large indolent major RAS lesions (Field 2003).

2.2. Behcet's disease

Behcet's disease is a multisystem, chronic relapsing inflammatory disease of unknown cause, which is characterized by recurrent oral (aphthous) ulcers, genital ulcers, uveitis and skin lesions. There maybe a variety of other manifestations including joint, central nervous system, vascular and intestinal lesions of variable severity (Lai 1995).

Patients with Behcet's disease usually have repeated exacerbations and remission of their clinical symptoms, and in these individuals treatment is essentially symptomatic. The choice of therapy depends on whether the clinical manifestations of the disease are local or systemic.

Local treatment with corticosteroids often controls oral and genital ulcers, and immunosuppressive therapy is reserved for severe cases of mucocutaneous involvement (Yazici 1991).

Immunosuppressive therapy is the mainstay of treatment for Behcet's disease. Successful treatment consists of anti-inflammatory agents that modify neutrophil activity. In the acute phase, prednisone, at doses of 40-60 mg/day, may be helpful, used alone or in combination with other immunosuppressive agents (Reich 1998).

Systemic corticosteroids continue to be used extensively, and may be administered as intravenous pulse therapy.

2.3. Oral Lichen Planus (OLP)

Lichen Planus (LP) is an unique inflammatory disorder that affects the skin, mucous membranes, nails and hair was first described and named by Erasmus Wilson in 1869 (Oztas 2003). The pathogenesis of LP is not entirely understood. It is a disorder of altered cell mediated immunity with exogenous antigens targeting the epidermis.

Various medical therapies are used for the treatment of Phototherapy has been used in the treatment of LP for many years. The therapeutic properties of corticosteroids were first demonstrated by Edward Kendall and Philip Hench in 1948 (Hench 1949).

Corticosteroids may be applied topically as ointments, pastes, lozenges or mouthwashes or through an inhaler with a special adapter.

The best treatment for OLP includes the use of high-potency topical corticosteroids (Setterfield 2000, Bruce 2007).

It has been reported that topical corticosteroids, which have fewer side effects, are equally or even more effective than systemic corticosteroids (Lodi 2005).

2.3.1. Topical corticosteroids

Topical corticosteroids are the main stay in treating mild to moderately symptomatic lesions. They are widely used in the treatment of OLP to reduce pain and inflammation. Options (presented in terms of decreasing potency) include 0. 05% clobetasol proprionate gel, 0. 1-0. 05% betamethasone valerate gel, 0. 05% fluocinonide gel, 0. 05% clobetasol ointment or cream and 0. 1% triamcinolone acetonide ointment (Levin 2002).

Triamcinolone acetonide is commonly used either in orabase or lozenge (Thongprasom 1992, Zegarelli 1969). A number of investigations have determined the efficacy of triamcinolone acetonide 0. 1% suspension in the treatment of OLP. This drug is available over the counter and is useful in the treatment of OLP (Rabiyi 2003).

An aqueous suspension of triamcinolone acetonide 0. 1% was used as an oral rinse in the treatment of 46 patients with symptomatic oral lichen planus (Vincent 1990). This method proved to be effective, resulting in "complete relief " in 27 patients. Although these results most likely refer to improvement in patients' symptoms, no specific information is provided regarding the clinical improvement with this therapy.

Betamethasone valerate, an even more potent anti-inflammatory agent, produced dramatic results in a number of controlled studies in patients with oral lichen planus. In a double-blind study, Cawson treated 30 patients with symptomatic oral lichen planus with betamethasone (0.1 mg) pellets. In 8 patients, all lesions virtually disappeared within 1 month, and during the same period, 20 of 30 patients showed substantial improvement. Only two patients failed to respond to this therapy (Cawson 1968).

Similarly, Tyldesley and Harding showed betamethasone valerate aerosol fitted with a special intraoral adaptor was an excellent treatment in the majority of 23 patients tested in a double-blind study (Tyldesley 1977). Greenspan et al. confirmed the efficacy of both betamethasone valerate aerosol and pellets in a double-blind study, noting improvement in 17 of 19 patients (Greenspan 1978).

High-potency steroid mouthwashes such as disodium betamethasone phosphate or clobetasol propionate, can be used in widespread oral LP but these may cause a significative systemic absorption leading to a pituitary- adrenal axis suppression (Gonzalez-Moles 2002).

Fluocinolone is another steroid, which has been used for treatment of OLP. Compared with the placebo, this drug has been found to be more effective (Voute 1993).

Recently, fluticasone propionate spray has been used effectively in the short-term management of symptomatic OLP, but 10% of the patients did not tolerate such treatment for more than 3 weeks (Hegarty 2002). The more potent fluorinated steroids can be very effective and include fluocinonide 0. 05% (Silverman 1991; Lozada 1980) and fluocinolone acetonide 0. 1%. (Thongprasom 1992) Fluocinonide 0. 05% and fluocinolone acetonide 0. 1% have been found to be effective in the treatment of severe oral LP that has failed to respond to other medications (Thongprasom 1992; Voute 1993).

A study evaluated fluocinolone acetonide 0. 1% in three groups: solution (FAS), Orabase (FAO), and both. The best results achieved with FAO (complete remission of 77. 3% of patients). This study had a long-term follow-up, without having a control group (Thongprasom 2003).

A study confirmed the efficacy of topical fluocinolone acetonide gel 0. 025 %, along with the topical antimicrobial drug chlorhexidine, in treatment of erosive OLP (Thongprasom 2003).

Another study showed no difference between the fluticasone propionate (FP) spray and betamethasone sodium phosphate (BSP) mouth rinse. But FP was found to be more acceptable to patients than BSP, because of the convenience of the spray form (Hegarty 2002).

The application of fluocinonide ointment (0. 05%) compounded with orabase 6 times per day or clobetasol propionate ointment (0. 05%) with orabase 3 times per day can control erosive lichen planus effectively in most patients (Edwards 2002).

Fluocinolone acetonide 0. 1% in orabase has been shown to be more effective than a similar triamcinolone acetonide 0. 1% preparation with no serious side effects (Thongprasom 1992).

Clobetasol propionate in aqueous solution, ointment, or orabase has also been shown to be effective in OLP. Clobetasol can be more effective than fluocinonide in improving lesions and the long-term use of clobetasol (6 months) may help to control the disease, offering substantial disease-free periods in 65% of the patients after 6 months of follow-up (Carbone1999).

Clobetasol propionate, a very potent corticosteroid in the Miller and Munro classification, was used in a 4% hydroxy ethylcellulose bioadhesive gel (Carbone1997). Clobetasol propionate 0. 05% ointment has been shown to heal OLP, but this study had a small sample group, without any control group or follow-up (Roed-Petersen 1992). Among the three preparations of clobetasol propionate 0. 05% (ointment, Orabase, and the adhesive denture paste) the best results have been achieved with clobetasol propionate in an adhesive denture paste (Lo Muzio 2001).

Although there are some reports of systemic absorption and adrenal suppression from super-potent topical steroids in the treatment of chronic skin disorders, adrenal suppression has not been found in long-term oral application of topical corticosteroids such as fluocinonide 0. 05%, fluocinolone acetonide 0. 1%, and clobetasol 0. 05% (Carbone1999).

Acute pseudomembranous candidiasis is the only common side effect from topical corticosteroid therapy (Thongprasom 1992). This can be prevented with antifungal (miconazole gel) alone or with chlorhexidine mouthwashes (Carbone1999).

2.3.2. *Intralesional corticosteroids*

Intralesional injection of corticosteroid for recalcitrant or extensive lesions involves the subcutaneous injection of 0. 2–0. 4 mL of a 10 mg/mL solution of triamcinolone acetonide by means of a 1. 0-mL 23 or 25 gauge tuberculin syringe (Edwards 2002).

Intralesional injections of hydrocortisone, dexamethasone, triamcinolone acetonide and methylprednisolone have been used in the treatment of OLP (Zegarelli 1980). However, the injections can be painful, are not invariably effective, and have a localized effect such as mucosal atrophy. Three to four or twice weekly treatments of intralesional triamcinolone acetonide in doses of 0. 5–1 ml of a 1-mg/ml suspension seem to be a practical supplement for the treatment of erosions (Edwards 2002).

Zegarelli combined the use of topical and weekly intralesional corticosteroids in seven patients. After 3 weeks, five patients were graded as having 100% clinical improvement. Furthermore, in most cases, a remission of several months was noted; recurrences were milder than the original disease state and were managed with topical agents alone (Zegarelli 1983). It is unclear why the response to topical corticosteroid therapy is so variable. Undoubtedly, the frequency of application of topical corticosteroids makes compliance difficult because optimal effects are not achieved unless they are applied between five and ten times daily (Zegarelli 1980).

2.3.3. *Systemic corticosteroids*

Systemic corticosteroids are reserved for recalcitrant erosive or erythematous LP where topical approaches have failed. Systemic prednisolone is the drug of choice, but should be used at the lowest possible dosage for the shortest duration (40-80 mg for 5-7 days) (Eisen 2005).

Systemic prednisone can be used to control the ulcers and erythema in OLP. Systemic corticosteroids may be indicated in patients whose condition is unresponsive to topical steroids or in patients with mucocutaneous disease and in high doses (1. 5-2 mg/kg/daily), but adverse effects are possible even with short courses (Zegarelli 1980; Chainani-Wu 2001).

The oral dose of prednisone for a 70-kg adult ranges from 10–20 mg/day for moderately severe cases to as high as 35 mg/day (0. 5 mg/kg daily) for severe cases (Zegarelli 1983). Prednisone should be taken as a single morning dose to reduce the potential for insomnia and should be taken with food to avoid nausea and peptic ulceration. Significant response should be observed within one to 2 weeks.

When systemic corticosteroids are prescribed for periods of longer than 2 weeks, the dosage of steroid must be gradually tapered to avoid precipitating an adrenal crisis. Tapering can be accomplished by decreasing the daily dose of prednisone by 5 mg per week (Edwards 2002).

Some studies have compared the efficacy of corticosteroids with some other drugs. For example in a double-blind randomized controlled study, compared the efficacy of topical zinc sulfate in combination with 0. 05% fluocinolone ointment in the treatment of OLP after 2 weeks of treatment, was founded that topical zinc sulfate in combination with 0. 05% fluocinolone ointment reduced the severity erosive OLP better than 0. 05% fluocinolone separately (Mehdipour & Taghavi 2010).

2.4. Erythema Multiforme (EM)

Erythema Multiforme is a skin condition considered to be hypersensitivity reaction to infections or drugs. It consists of a polymorphous eruption of macules, papules, and characteristic 'target' lesions that are symmetrically distributed with a propensity for the distal extremities. There is minimal mucosal involvement. Herpes simplex virus (HSV) is the most commonly identified etiology of this hypersensitivity reaction, accounting for more than 50 percent of cases. Although EM was first clinically recognized in the early 19th century and referred to by a variety of names, it was not until 1860 that Ferdin and von Hebra termed the disease "Erythema Multiforme (Forman 2002).

Erythema multiforme (EM) was once thought to be the early presentation of a continuum of diseases related to Stevens-Johnson syndrome (SJS), with toxic epidermal necrolysis (TEN) believed to be a distinct entity. It is now generally accepted that a separation exists between EM and SJS. Currently, two different classifications exist: first, an erythema multiforme spectrum (minor and major) and second, an SJS and TEN spectrum (Lamoreux 2006; French 2008).

SJS and its more severe progression, TEN, are both rare mucocutaneous diseases that can be life-threatening and almost always caused by drugs (49). SJS was first described in 1922 by two physicians, Stevens and Johnson, who described a skin eruption similar to EM that also included purulent conjunctivitis, stomatitis,, and fever (Forman 2002).

Management of erythema multiforme involves determining the etiology when possible. The first step is to treat the suspected infectious disease or to discontinue the causal drug.

2.4.1. Topical steroid therapy

Mild cases of Erythema Multiforme do not require treatment. Oral topical steroids may be used to provide symptom relief (Shin 2001).

Lozada-Nur and Zhong Huang reported that an adhesive paste (Orabase) form of clobetasol propionate, the most potent topical corticosteroidis a safe and efficacious alternative to systemic therapy in erosive oral lesions (Lozada-Nur F 1994).

Mouthwashes of clobetasol propionate in aqueous solution may offer an alternative topical approach to this patient population. The mouthwash solution provides ready access to all lesional areas, and there is excellent control over the contact time between drug and lesion (Jacobson 1986).

2.4.2. Systemic steroid therapy

The role of systemic corticosteroids in Erythema Multiforme Major (EMM) and SJS is controversial. There is no literature to date based on a large, prospective, randomized, or double-blind study evaluating use of systemic corticosteroids in EMM/SJS.

Moderate to severe oral Erythema Multiforme may be treated with a short course of systemic glucocorticosteroid in patients without significant contraindications to their use. Prednisone may be used in patients with many lesions at dosages of 40 to 80 mg per day for one to two weeks then tapered rapidly (Lamoreux 2006). There have been no controlled studies of prednisone's effectiveness, and its use in patients with herpes-associated Erythema Multiforme may lower the patient's resistance to HSV and promote recurrent HSV infection followed by recurrent Erythema Multiforme (Volcheck 2004).

The dosing and route of administration that provides the most benefit for EMM and SJS patients is in question. Early therapy with systemic prednisone (0. 5 to 1. 0mg/kg/day) or pulse methylprednisolone (1mg/kg/day for 3 days) has been shown to be effective (Scully 2008). One author suggests tapering the oral prednisolone over 7 to 10 days, while Patterson et al. suggests a high dose of corticosteroids for EMM patients followed by a four-week tapering course (Chrousos 2004). Still another suggests a bolus infusion for 3 to 7 days of coricosteroids, which showed no relapses after treatment was discontinued (Kakourou1997). Intravenous (IV) pulsed dose methylprednisolone (3 consecutive daily infusions of 20–30mg/kg to a maximum of 500 mg given over 2 to 3 hours) has also been reported, with the suggestion that this approach is superior to oral prednisone because the greatest benefit is seen when treatment is administered as early as possible in the progression of the cutaneous insult (Martinez 2000).

Kardaun and Jonkman recently proposed dexamethasone pulse therapy (1. 5mg/kg IV over 30 to 60 minutes on 3 consecutive days) to avoid long-term use of systemic corticosteroids (Kardaun 2007). The authors described the pleomorphic effects of dexamethasone on the immune system, including inhibition of epidermal apoptosis by several mechanisms. These mechanisms include suppression of various cytokines, such as TNF-alpha; inhibition of interferon-gamma-induced apoptosis; and inhibition of Fas-mediated keratinocyte apoptosis (Yeung 2005).

When treating TEN, it is generally agreed that after widespread sloughing occurs, any risk of infection outweighs the potential benefits of systemic corticosteroid therapy (Wolverton 2007).

Recurrent Erythema Multiforme often is secondary to HSV-1 and -2 reactivation, although the HSV may be clinically silent (Huff 1992).

2.5. Pemphigus

Pemphigus refers to a group of rare chronic mucocutaneous diseases characterized by painful lesions caused by intraepidermal antholytic structures in the skin and mucous membrane (Sirois 2000).

Oral mucosal lesions in Pemphigus are common (50%-70%) and predominantly appear as buccal erosions in the occlusal line, which is most exposed to trauma and also on the palate, gingival and tongue (Sirois 2000).

The exact nature of the disease remains unknown. Pemphigus is characterized by intra-epithelial bulla formation, due to autoantibodies directed against proteins of the desmosome-tonofilament complex between keratinocytes (Sirois 2000).

Pemphigus vulgaris (PV) has a high morbidity and mortality rate without treatment. Because of the rarity of the disease, there is not yet a standard treatment regimen (Cotell 2000).

The aim of treatment in pemphigus vulgaris is the same as in other autoimmune bullous diseases, which is to decrease blister formation, promote healing of blisters and erosions, and determine the minimal dose of medication necessary to control the disease process (Knudson 2010).

Until now, treatment consists mostly of the use of corticosteroid and immunosuppressive drugs. The use of corticosteroids in the 1950s had reduced mortality from 60% to 90% to about 30%. The current mortality was about 6. 2% (range 0 to 10%) and did not show further significant reduction (Bystryn 1996).

The treatment depends on the prognostic elements of the condition, such as the extent of the lesions and antibody levels. Treatment is administered in 2 phases: a loading phase, to control the disease, and a maintenance phase, which is further divided into consolidation and treatment tapering. The basic treatment for pemphigus consists of either local or systemic corticosteroid therapy (Fellner 2001).

2.5.1. *Topical corticosteroids*

Local corticosteroid therapy is used in cases where the PV is not extensive and lesions are limited to the oral cavity. Corticosteroids can be prescribed in the form of a paste, an ointment or a mouthwash administered as monotherapy or as adjunctive therapy with a systemic treatment (Fellner; Ruocco 2001).

In patients with no progressing oral lesions, moderate to high potency topical corticosteroids are recommended, applied 2-3 times a day, such as 0. 05% fluocinolone acetonide or 0. 05% clobetasol propionate (Hashimoto; Prajapati 2008).

Dumas et al. described 7 pemphigus patients, 3 of whom were treated with clobetasol propionate 0. 05% cream as monotherapy for their mild PV. PV was defined as "mild" if fewer than 10 new bullae appeared per week and if the circulating pemphigus antibody titer was 1:320. The cream was applied twice a day for at least 15 days, and then tapered. Lesions were controlled in only 1 of the 3 PV patients (Dumas 1999).

2.5.2. *Systemic corticosteroid therapy*

In patients with severe disease and spreading of the lesions to skin surfaces, systemic corticosteroids are the treatment of choice (Knudson 2010).

The dosing schedule of systemic corticosteroids in pemphigus is largely empirical (Ratnam 1990). Prednisolone was the first drug used to treat this disease and almost in all situations, is the first line of treatment (Camisa 1998).

The starting dose is high; a total oral dose of 100–200 mg Prednison is administered daily until subsidence of clinical signs. This dose can gradually be decreased to a maintenance level of 40 to 50 mg daily. Topical application of corticoids is effective if small, isolated areas of the oral mucosa are involved. The acute phase of pemphigus is associated with changes in gastric mucosa and this condition is further aggravated by ingestion of corticosteroids (Fassmann 2003).

Corticosteroids taken by mouth have many long-term harmful effects, including adrenal atrophy, abnormal sensitivity to infection, high blood pressure, hypertriglyceridemia, hyperglycemia, cortisone myopathy, erosive duodenitis and stress fracture, as in the case presented here. To minimize iatrogenic effects, Lever and Schaumburg recommended a treatment called the "high Lever scheme" with very high loading doses (100–175 mg taken twice daily for 5–10 weeks) , followed by the "low Lever scheme," which includes a rapid reduction in dosage over a few weeks, with a maintenance dose of 40 mg every 2 days accompanied by local adjuvant treatment (Lever 1984).

The British Association of Dermatologists recommends patients with mild disease to receive an initial prednisolone dose of 40-60 mg daily and in more severe cases, 60-100 mg daily. If there is no response within a week, the dose is increased by 50-100% until disease control. There is no unitized handling considering the tapering of corticosteroids. A 25% dose reduction may be performed biweekly with slower decrease after a dose of 20 mg/day has been reached (Harman 2003).

Two prospective controlled trials explored the effect of i. v. corticosteroid pulses in addition to oral prednisolone but did not observe statistical differences between treatment groups (Femiano 2002; Mentink 2006).

In one controlled trial, patients randomized to treatment with either low-dose oral prednisolone (45-60mg/day) or high-dose oral prednisolone (120-150mg/day) showed no significant difference in the time to achieve remission and in relapse rates at 5 years (Ratnam 1990).

A nonrandomized retrospective controlled trial of 71 pemphigus patients assigned participants to cohorts receiving prednisone 1 mg/kg/day or 2 mg/kg/day. No statistical difference was observed between cohorts in terms of response to treatment; however, there was a significantly higher frequency of adverse events, particularly infection, in the 2 mg/kg/day cohort. Despite the retrospective, nonrandomized nature of the study, the results indicate that higher doses of corticosteroid are no more effective than lower doses, and are associated with higher rates of complications. Overall, the limited evidence indicates that lower steroid dose regimens (=1 mg/kg/day) have equivalent efficacy in controlling disease as higher dose regimens, and may have decreased associated morbidity (Fernandes 2001).

Another nonrandomized, controlled trial of 20 PV patients studied participants receiving either a 125 mg/day tapering schedule of prednisone or a 50 mg/day tapering schedule of prednisone plus intravenous betamethasone 20 mg/day. In this study, the cohort receiving the pulse therapy was found to have faster clinical resolution of symptoms, with statistically significant difference (Femiano 2002).

Pulse corticosteroid usually seems to result only in short-term relief from the disease and most likely needs continued administration of oral corticosteroids (Funauchi 1997).

Werth has compared these two therapeutic protocols. It was only a retrospective study that included two heterogeneous groups of patients with completely different therapeutic regimens for each patient. It included nine patients who had received pulse therapy and six patients who had received conventional treatment. Some received only one course of pulse therapy, while others received two courses. This study showed the superiority of pulse therapy over conventional treatment (Werth 1996).

2.5.3. Intralesional corticosteroid therapy

Intralesional corticosteroid therapy accelerates the scarring process of a lesion or is used to treat persistent lesions. This treatment, which gives inconsistent results, involves sublesional injections given every 7 to 15 days; treatment is stopped after 3 injections if there is no improvement. Scarring is accompanied by cutaneous or mucosal atrophy the major drawback of this treatment (Fellner; Ruocco 2001). If the patient has extraoral lesions or if the oral damage is extensive, systemic corticosteroid therapy is initiated immediately. The initial dose depends on the chronicity of the lesions and the severity of the disease. A daily application of prednisone 0. 5–2 mg/kg is recommended (Fellner; Toth 2001). Depending on the response, the dose is gradually decreased to the minimum therapeutic dose, taken once a day in the morning to minimize side effects.

The lack of randomized controlled trials precludes any conclusions as to whether these protocols are superior to those using higher loading doses. An adjuvant drug is prescribed for most patients with severe PV, with the objectives of reducing the cortisone dose and ensuring stable remission. However, the use of adjuvant therapy remains controversial (Mutasim 2004).

2.6. Mucous Membrane Pemphigoid (MMP)

Mucous Membrane Pemphigoid (MMP) or Cicatricial pemphigoid is a rare autoimmune blistering disorder that affects the mucous membranes and skin. It was first described by Thost in 1911 (Thost 1911).

This disease is extremely difficult to treat despite the use of aggressive combination immunosuppressive regimens. Cicatricial pemphigoid with multiple mucosal site involvement has the worst prognosis due to its high resistance to medical therapy resulting in loss of function through scarring (Tht Yu 2007).

During the past 50 years, the mainstay of treatment for MMP has been systemic glucocorticoids. However, the high doses needed to obtain clinical response are generally poorly tolerated, especially in young patients, and are associated with many adverse effects (Borradori 2004).

2.6.1. Topical steroid therapy

Mild localized lesions usually respond to topical steroids, including triamcinolone, fluocinonide and clobetasol propionate. Patients with mild oral disease should be treated with topical and intralesional steroids.

Desquamative gingivitis can often be managed with topical steroids in soft dental splint that covers the gingiva, although the clinician using topical steroids over large areas of mucosa must closely monitor the patient for side effects such as candidiasis and effects of systemic absorption (Reich 1998).

Lozada -Nur and Zhong Huang treated patients with severe erosive disease, using clobetasol propionate mixed in an adhesive paste. They reported a complete response in 62. 5% of the series (15 patients), an excellent response in 29. 7% (7 patients), and a failed response in 8. 3% (2 patients). They concluded that their treatment was efficacious and safe (Lozada-Nur 1991).

In low risk patients with lesions confined to the oral mucosa and/or skin, topical corticosteroids are advised, such as 0. 1% triamcinolone acetonide, 0. 05% fluocinoloneacetonide, or 0. 05% clobetasol propionate in orabase, applied 3-4 times a day during 9-24 weeks. In patients with isolated erosions, intralesional corticosteroid injections (triamcinolone in 5-10 mg/ml solution) can be used. In subjects presenting gingival lesions in the form of desquamative gingivitis, 0. 05% clobetasol propionate is recommended, with nystatin 100,000 IU to avoid candidiasis overinfection (Bagan 2005, Scully 2008). When MMP affects the palate, esophagus or nasal mucosa, beclomethasone dipropionate or budesonide (50-200 μg) can be prescribed (Bagan 2005).

2.6.2. *Systemic steroid therapy*

MMP can be rapidly progressive, and systemic steroids have been used as initial treatment for patients with extensive oral ulceration or as additional treatment on patients who did not respond to topical steroids. Systemic corticosteroids such as prednisolone at 1- 2 mg/kg/day are the first-line medications in CP because of their potent anti-inflammatory and immunosuppressive effects (Mondino 1981).

The serum autoantibody titers remain very high after the disappearance of clinical lesions. Therefore the benefit of steroids in benign mucous membrane pemphigoid might be due to anti-inflammatory actions, including lowered enzyme release, reduced cell migration and decreased leakage of humoral factors (Knudson 2010).

In high risk patients with multiple oral lesions, rapidly progressing spread of the disease to other mucosal membranes such as the eyes, genital, esophagus or nasopharyngeal zone, or recurrent lesions, the administration of prednisone 1-2 mg/kg/day, with gradual dose reduction, and immune suppressors such as cyclophosphamide (0. 5-2 mg/kg/day) , azathioprine 1-2 mg/ kg/day, or mycophenolate mofetil 2-2. 5 g/day has been described (Bagan 2005; Knudson 2010).

2.7. Bullous Pemphigoid (BP)

Bullous Pemphigoid (BP) is an autoimmune disease characterized by subepidermal blistering , which are often pruritic (Fitzpatrick 2008).

Bullous pemphigoid occurs most commonly in the elderly, with an onset between 65 and 75 years of age. Prognosis is influenced by age and general condition of the patient, not by extent of disease activity.

Treatment includes topical and systemic corticosteroids, steroid-sparing immunosuppressants, and tetracycline in combination with niacinamide (Joly 2005).

2.7.1. *Topical steroid therapy*

In a study of 10 patients with extensive and generalized BP, treatment with 0. 05% clobetasol propionate cream achieved complete healing in all patients within 17 days of treatment. Seven of the 10 patients remained in remission at the time of reporting (1–10 months) (Westerhof 1989).

Twenty patients with BP (involvement of less than 60% body surface) in a second study were treated with very potent topical corticosteroids: in seven patients BP was completely suppressed and the same number obtained remission with an 11-month follow-up. There were mild side-effects of cutaneous infection and skin atrophy. The use of topical corticosteroids has also been reported in a large number of case reports and smaller series of fewer than five patients (Zimmermann 1999).

Potent topical corticosteroids should be considered in patients with limited or moderate disease (Mutasim 2004).

In a large randomized controlled trial, initial disease control and 1-year survival were significantly better when treating extensive BP with clobetasol propionate cream 40 mg daily compared with oral prednisolone 1mg/kg/day while in moderate BP (< 10 blisters/day) outcomes using clobetasol cream and prednisolone 0. 5mg/kg were similar (Joly 2002).

Recently, lower doses of topical clobetasol propionate (10-30g daily) were shown to have similar short-term efficacy but reduced side-effects compared to the high dose topical regimen (40g daily clobetasol propionate) (Joly 2009).

2.7.2. Systemic steroid therapy

High-doses of systemic corticosteroids are the standard for initial treatment of BP to gain control over the eruptions, and prolonged high-doses are often used in severe cases. Adverse side effects from systemic corticosteroids seem to be the main cause of mortality in BP (Mamelak 2007).

Recommended initial doses of prednisolone are 20 mg/day or 0. 3 mg/kg/day in localised or mild disease, 40 mg/day or 0. 6 mg/kg/day in moderate disease, and 50-70 mg or 0. 75-1 mg/kg/day in severe disease (Wojnarowska 2002).

In patients with limited disease, clobetasol propionate cream alone is used; in patients with moderate disease, clobetasol propionate cream is combined with dapsone (1. 0-1. 5mg/kg/day) and in severe cases, oral prednisolone (0. 5mg/kg/day) is added. Instead of dapsone, doxycycline (200mg/day) may be given (Kasperkiewicz 2009).

2.7.3. Intralesional corticosteroid therapy

Intralesional triamcinolone acetonide 3-10 mg per ml can be administered to resistant lesions. Experience in injecting correctly is necessary to maximise efficacy and minimise atrophy. Where pemphigoid does not respond to steroids, or large maintenance doses are required, other 'steroid-sparing' agents can be used. However, the evidence for effectiveness of these drugs is limited and many have worrying side effect profiles. They should therefore be used cautiously by those with experience in their actions (Reich 1998).

2.8. Systemic Lupus Erythematosus

Lupus Erythematosus may run in one of the two well recognized forms. Systemic (acute) or Discoid (chronic). Both of them may have oral manifestations. Discoid Lupus Erythematosus (DLE) is a chronic skin condition of sores with inflammation and scarring favoring the face, ears and scalp. It probably occurs in genetically predisposed individuals (Khare 2011).

Systemic Lupus Erythematosus (SLE) is a chronic disease characterized by protean manifestations, often with a waxing and waning course. In the past, a diagnosis of SLE often implied a decreased life span caused by internal organ system involvement or the toxic effects of therapy, but recent improvements in care have dramatically enhanced the survival of SLE patients. Nonetheless, increased mortality remains a major concern and current treatments for SLE remain inadequate (Ippolito 2008).

Oral ulcerations of systemic lupus erythematosus are transient, occurring with acute lupus flares. Symptomatic lesions can be treated with high potency topical corticoids or intralesional steroid injections. Systemically low dose prednisone 10-20 mg /day or an alternate day dose of 20-40 mg may be needed (Pedersen 1984; Reich 1998).

Reducing corticosteroid use is an important goal in treatment of patients with SLE if it occurs in the context of a treatment that effectively controls disease activity. Therefore, for a medical product to be labeled as reducing corticosteroid usage, it should also demonstrate another clinical benefit, such as reduction in disease activity as the primary endpoint.

The evaluation of efficacy should be based on the proportion of patients in treatment and control groups that achieve a reduction in steroid dose to less than or equal to 10 mg per day of prednisone or equivalent, with quiescent disease and no flares for at least 3 consecutive months during a 1-year clinical trial. For a result to be clinically meaningful, the patient population should be on moderate to high doses of steroids at baseline. Trials should also assess the occurrence of clinically significant steroid toxicities (Ad Hoc Working Group on Steroid-Sparing Criteria in Lupus 2004).

In the localized variety of Discoid Lupus the lesions tend to be confined to the head and neck and in the generalized variety they occur both above and below the neck. The disease may occur at any age; with higher incidence between 20 to 40 years of age. It has a prolonged course and can have a considerable effect on quality of life. Potent topical steroids and antimalarials are the mainstay of treatment (Khare 2011).

Topical steroids are the mainstay of treatment of DLE. Patients usually start with a potent topical steroid (e. g., betamethasone or clobetasol) applied twice a day, then switch to a lower-potency steroid as soon as possible. The minimal use of steroids reduces the recognized side effects like atrophy, telengiaectasiae, striae, and purpura.

Intralesional injection of corticosteroids (typically, this author uses triamcinolone acetonide 3 mg/mL) is useful as adjunctive therapy for individual lesions. Potential for atrophy relates to the amount of corticosteroid injected in any area; therefore, dilute concentrations are preferred. In addition, the treating physician must take care to limit the total dose of the injections at any given office/clinic visit to avoid systemic toxicity from the steroids; eg, if a patient is given 10 mL of triamcinolone 3 mg/mL, this means that the patient has received a total of 30 mg, and toxicity is the same as if it had been delivered orally or by intramuscular injection (Panjwani 2009).

Oral steroids may be required for the control of systemic lupus but are not generally beneficial in DLE. For patients with progressive or disseminated disease or in those with localized disease that does not respond to topical measures, the addition of systemic agents should be considered.

3. Facial pain

3.1. Bell's palsy

Idiopathic facial palsy, also called Bell's palsy, is an acute disorder of the facial nerve, which may begin with symptoms of pain in the mastoid region and produce full or partial paralys is of movement of one side of the face (Valença 2001).

Facial nerve paralysis may be congenital or neoplastic or may result from infection, trauma, toxic exposures, or iatrogenic causes. Increasing evidence suggests that the main cause of Bell's palsy is reactivation of latent herpes simplex virus type 1 in the cranial nerve ganglia. How the virus damages the facial nerve is uncertain (Gilden 2004).

Treatment of Bell palsy should be conservative and guided by the severity and probable prognosis in each particular case. Studies have shown the benefit of high-dose corticosteroids for acute Bell palsy (Sullivan 2007; Engström 2008).

Taverner in 1954 was the first to design a controlled treatment trial of steroids but unfortunately the number of patients was too small to permit a signifcant statistical evaluation (Taverner 1954).

Attempts to treat Bell's palsy with steroids changed in the 1970s. After the initial publication of Adour et al. several series of treatments with prednisone for Bell'spalsy were designed, but almost all of them were of unsatisfactory quality (Adour 1972). Nevertheless, the majority of authors claimed that they had shown steroids to be benefcial to a statistically signifcant degree.

Two recent systematic reviews concluded that Bell's palsy could be effectively treated with corticosteroids in the first seven days, providing up to a further 17% of patients with a good outcome in addition to the 80% that spontaneously improve (Ramsey 2000; Grogan 2001).

Other studies have shown the benefits of treatment with steroids; in one, patients with severe facial palsy showed a significant improvement after treatment within 24 hours (Shafshak 1994; Williamson 1996).

Immunocompetent patients without specific contraindications are prescribed prednisone at 1 mg/kg/d (maximum 80 mg) for the first week, which is tapered over the second week. Around a fifth of patients will progress from partial palsy, so these patients should also be treated (Ramsey 2000).

However the Sullivan study with 496 participants compared different combinations of prednisolone, acyclovir and placebo. They found significant benefit from prednisolone but not acyclovir (Sullivan 2007).

Hato assessed the efficacy of valacyclovir with 296 participants divided into two groups (valacyclovir with prednisolone,and placebowith prednisolone) and found significant benefit from valacyclovir (Hato 2007).

3.2. Ramsay Hunt syndrome

Ramsay Hunt syndrome (RHS) is caused by the reactivation of a previous Varicella zoster virus (VZV) infection. RHS is a potentially serious viral infection that accounts for approximately 12% of all facial nerve palsies (Robillard 1986; Uri 2003).

VZV is also the cause of "shingles," which frequently presents with a classic painful dermatomal distribution of vesicles and crusted skin ulcerations. In addition to the alarming facial palsy, RHS may also be characterized by severe otalgia, sensorineural hearing loss, vertigo, painful skin vesicles and aguesia in the ipsilateral anterior tongue (Hiroshige 2002).

The treatment of Ramsay Hunt syndrome is not entirely agreed upon. Definitive treatment consists of antiviral therapy and sometimes includes steroids. Adjunctive steroid therapy can be helpful in the management of the facial paralysis of RHS (Kinishi 2001).

However, many authors caution against implementing steroid therapy, especially with periocular lesions, as they fear dissemination of the VZV infection (Van de Steene 2004; Hyvernat; Hill 2005).

The largest retrospective treatment study showed a statistically significant improvement in patients treated with acyclovir and prednisone within 3 days of onset. Complete recovery occurred in 75% of patients treated within the first 3 days, but in only 30% of those treated after 7 days. This suggests that prompt diagnosis and management improves outcome in Ramsay Hunt syndrome. Importantly, no statistically significant outcome differences were noted between patients treated with intravenous or oral acyclovir (Murakami 1997).

A large prospective study demonstrated that combination therapy with acyclovir and steroids led to better recovery of facial nerve function than steroids alone (Kinishi 2001). These findings were confirmed by responses to nerve excitability testing. Although there are no evidence-based dosing recommendations, published trials typically administered acyclovir at 800 mg by mouth 5 times/day for 7-10 days and prednisone at 1 mg/kg/day by mouth for 5 days followed by a taper (Murakami 1997).

RHS may present with a spectrum of clinical variations, including facial swellings that appear to be of odontogenic origin. As a result, dentists may be challenged to make the correct diagnosis of RHS versus an odontogenic infection in a timely manner. Appropriate supportive and prompt antiviral therapy combined with close follow-up is associated with significantly better functional recovery and outcomes (Kinishi 2001).

3.3. Postherpetic Neuralgia (PHN)

Postherpetic Neuralgia (PHN) continues to be a significant clinical problem, with an average of 25% of patients developing persistent neuropathic pain after acute herpes zoster (HZ) (Pavan-Langston; Schmader 2008).

This condition signals damage to the affected nerve. Patients may continue experiencing pain and discomfort even after blisters have already cleared. Usually, patients may feel a sharp or deep pain along the area were blisters first appeared. It is believed that repetitive painful stimuli that reach the central nervous system might lead to central sensitization of the nociceptive system, the most important mechanism underlying long-lasting chronic pain. Interventions that decrease the repetitive painful stimuli and inflammation during the acute phase of HZ may attenuate central sensitization and substantially reduce the incidence of chronic pain (Kelly 2001; Johnson 2002).

Treatment includes corticosteroids, which are used to treat pain, swelling and effectively reduces the risk of recurrence of post-herpetic neuralgia. Steroids were found to accelerate the resolution of acute neuritis and provide a clear improvement in quality-of-life measures in comparison to those patients treated with antivirals alone. The use of oral steroids had no effect on the development or duration of postherpetic neuralgia (Dworkin 2007).

Historically, epidural, intrathecal, and sympathetic nerve blocks have all been used in the treatment of pain caused by HZ and PHN. It was accepted by some investigators that nerve blocks do not provide lasting relief in established PHN, but injection of corticosteroids has been suggested to be of some benefit.

Prednisolone, a corticosteroid, is the most common drug administered in heavy doses to herpes patients. Moderate doses of prednisone 40 mg daily for 10 days, which is gradually tailed off over the following 3 weeks is an effective and safe regime which reduces the occurrence of postherpetic neuralgia.

The use of steroids in conjunction with an antiviral for uncomplicated herpes zoster is controversial. Steroids were found to accelerate the resolution of acute neuritis and provide a clear improvement in quality-of-life measures in comparison to those patients treated with antivirals alone. The use of oral steroids had no effect on the development or duration of postherpetic neuralgia. The optimal duration of steroid therapy is not known. If prescribed, it seems reasonable for steroids to be used concurrently with antiviral therapy. The duration of steroid use should not extend beyond the period of antiviral therapy. Steroids should not be given alone (without antiviral therapy) , owing to concern about the promotion of viral replication (Van Wijck 2006).

Intrathecal administration of corticosteroids has also been attempted. A trial involving a series of 4 intrathecal injections of methylprednisolone and lidocaine in patients with established postherpetic neuralgia demonstrated a significant and persistent reduction in pain among corticosteroid-treated patients when compared with untreated patients or those treated with intrathecal lidocaine alone. Kotani et al. published remarkable results after the intrathecal injection of methylprednisolone in patients with intractable PHN for at least 1 yr, which showed a 50% decrease in interleukin-8 concentrations, and this decrease correlated with the duration of neuralgia and with the extent of global pain relief (Kotani 2000).

The use of oral or epidural corticosteroids in conjunction with antiviral therapy has been found to be beneficial in treating moderate-to-severe acute zoster, but to have no effect on the development or duration of postherpetic neuralgia (Wood1994; Whitley 1996).

3.4. Temporomandibular joint disorders

Temporomandibular joint (TMJ) disorders are the main cause of chronic facial pain and a major cause of disability (Horten 1953).

Several decades ago, Toller suggested that intra-articular corticosteroid injections were only useful in adult patients with TMJ disorders; a single intra-articular injection resulted in resolution of TMJ pain and other symptoms in 62% of adult patients, compared to only 17% of pediatric patients (Toller 1977).

Intra-articular injection of steroids into the temporomandibular joint (TMJ) space is not a recent subject. Horten in 1953, was the first who reported this procedure which was based on the work of Hollander et al. in which they described the effect of intra-articular injection of hydrocortisone in various joint disorders. Since then, a number of papers have reported varying degrees of success (Wood1994; Hollander 1951).

A variety of methods are currently used for intra-articular corticosteroid injection to the TMJ, each with the goal of minimizing the potential for tissue damage. Intra-articular corticosteroid formulations are often diluted with a local anesthetic prior to injection into the TMJ (Kopp 1981; Alstergren 1996).

Numerous corticosteroid formulations are available for intra-articular injection, ranging from solutions of more soluble agents to suspensions of triamcinolone hexacetonide and other relatively insoluble steroids. Although the efficacy of various corticosteroids is presumed to differ, studies of this topic have been limited (Wise 2005; Gerwin 2006; Lavelle 2007).

Triamcinolone acetonide which has been used for intra-articular injection is very slowly absorbed from the injection sites. The dose ranges between 2 to 40 mg, depending upon the size of the joint injected (Hollander 1951; Silbermann1978). In cases of TMJ, the dose is usually 10 mg (Gray 1994). Triamcinolone acetonide is a safe drug, although anaphylactic shock following injection of triamcinolone acetonide has been reported. A repeat injection is occasionally used but the third injection should be used with caution as the expectation of further improvement decreases with successive injections (Larsson 1989).

In recent studies of juvenile idiopathic arthritis, intra-articular corticosteroid (triamcinolone) injections improved or even completely eliminated TMJ pain in 77-88% of children for several months (Arabshahi 2005; Cahill 2007; Ringold 2008).

In a controlled study of adults with TMJ arthritis, a single intra-articular injection of corticosteroid (methylprednisolone) diluted with lidocaine significantly reduced joint pain and other symptoms for 4-6 weeks. The pharmacologic effect of intra-articular methylprednisolone lasts 3-4 weeks, so these findings were consistent with the expected timeline of corticosteroid effect. No adverse events were reported (Alstergren 1996).

However, the efficacy may vary depending on the specific cause of TMJ degeneration.

3.5. Temporal arteritis (TA)

Temporal arteritis (TA) , also known as cranial arteritis or Giant Cell Arteritis (GCA) , was first clinically recognized in 1890 when Hutchinson described an 80-year-old man whose painful inflamed temporal arteries precluded his wearing a hat (Hutchinson 1890). In 1932, Horton et al. correlated the histopathologic features with the clinical features and applied the name arteritis temporalis. Other names include arteritis cranialis, Horton disease, granulomatous arteritis, and arteritis of the aged (Horton 1932).

There is universal agreement that glucocorticosteroids are the mainstay of treatment for GCA and should be initiated immediately and aggressively, with the goal of suppressing inflammation and preventing visual loss and ischemic stroke (Hayreh 2003; Rahman; Pipitone 2005).

Oral prednisone is first-line acute therapy for GCA. Although no consensus exists for initial dose of prednisone, the vast majority of patients respond to a dose of 1 mg/kg/d, or between 40 and 60 mg/d (Salvarani 2002; Weyand 2003). The dose of prednisone is lowered after 2–4 weeks, and slowly tapered over 9–12 months (Chan 2001).

Higher doses of 80 to 100 mg/d are suggested for patients with visual or neurological symptoms of GCA. IV pulse methylprednisolone has been proposed as an induction therapy, particularly in cases where vision is at risk (Rahman; Rahman 2005).

4. Medical emergencies in dental practice

4.1. Adrenal crisis prophylaxis

Patients with a history compatible with adrenal suppression and presenting with features of adrenal crisis should be treated urgently.

Acute adrenal crisis, with insufficiency of mineralocorticoids and glucocorticoids, is a medical emergency. The patient presents with abdominal pain, weakness, hypotension, dehydration, nausea and vomiting. Laboratory findings may include decreased sodium (hyponatraemia), elevated potassium (hyperkalaemia) , decreased blood glucose (hypoglycemia), acidosis and uraemia. Few patients have all these findings, with hypotension and nausea being most common.

Patients with secondary Addison's most typical presentation is of hypotension, and hyponatraemia without volume depletion. Additional symptoms may include fatigue, weakness, arthralgia, nausea, and orthostatic dizziness associated with hypotension.

Patients taking exogenous glucocorticoids. Exogenous glucocorticoids can cause adrenal gland suppression and resultant atrophy. With atrophy of the adrenal glands there is a decreased glucocorticoid response to stress, and this may precipitate an adrenal crisis (Edwards 1995).

4.1.1. Management

i. Intravenous fluids, in the form of 5% dextrose in normal saline, should be given to address the volume depletion that is often present.

ii. Primary adrenal insufficiency: start on 20–25 mg hydrocortisone per 24 h

iii. Secondary adrenal insufficiency: 15–20 mg hydrocortisone per 24 h; if borderline fail in cosyntropin test consider 10 mg or stress dose cover only

iv. Hydrocortisone should be given intravenously initially. If improvement has occurred within 24 hours, which is common, the hydrocortisone dose can be decreased. This can be changed to an oral formulation whenever the patient is stable. The dose can be decreased by one third to one half the dose daily until a maintenance dose of 20 mg in the morning and 10 mg in the afternoon or at night is attained. Some patients may need only a dose of 20 mg/day total (i.e., 20 mg every morning, or 15 mg in the morning and 5 mg in the afternoon or at night).

v. A search for the condition that precipitated the crisis, such as infection, should be undertaken. Treatment of the underlying cause should be instituted.

vi. Patients will not need mineralocorticoid replacement, because the renin-angiotensin-aldosterone axis is intact (Arlt 2009).

4.2. Anaphylaxis shock

Anaphylaxis is the quintessential disease of emergency medicine. The term anaphylaxis literally meaning "against protection" was introduced by Richet and Portier in 1902 (Brown 1995).

It is a potentially fatal illness with rapid onset that can affect young, healthy people. It must be diagnosed clinically, and is potentially curable if treated immediately (Golden 2007).

A systematic review of the literature has failed to demonstrate the effectiveness of any of these medications in the treatment of anaphylaxis (Ewan 2010).

Steroids are unlikely to be helpful in the treatment of acute anaphylaxis. They have a delayed onset of 4 to 6 hours. Steroids are thought to play a role in preventing rebound anaphylaxis; however, this has never been proven (Review Anaphylaxis in the emergency department 2008).

As with the antihistamines, despite their many theoretical benefits on mediator release and tissue responsiveness, there are no placebo-controlled trials to confirm the effectiveness of steroids in anaphylaxis.

Most clinicians however give prednisone 1 mg/kg up to 50 mg orally or hydrocortisone 1. 5-3 mg/kg IV particularly in patients with airway involvement and bronchospasm, based empirically on their important role in asthma (Soar 2008).

It is unclear if steroids prevent a biphasic reaction with recrudescence of symptoms following recovery, as supporting data are unconvincing (Lieberman 2005).

Steroids are of course fundamental to the management of recurrent idiopathic anaphylaxis (Ring 2002; Greenberger 2007).

5. Emergency drugs in general dental practice

5.1. Intracanal corticosteroid in root canal therapy

The application of antiinflammatory agents on exposed pulp tissue in an attempt to prevent or minimize inflammatory reaction and to favor healing has been investigated for a long time. Corticosteroid can be used as a dressing agent for deep cavities and exposed pulp tissue in order to control the inflammatory pulp response and reduce postoperative pain. The therapeutic effect of a corticosteroid agent seems to depend upon its potency, concentration and ability to diffuse into connective tissue (Holland 1991; Gordon Marshall 2002).

The results of studies that employ corticosteroids as a cavity liner support that these medications are effective in reducing or preventing postoperative thermal sensitivity. Researchers have shown that application of corticosteroid/ antibiotic association for short period of time was effective to control inflammation in the pulp tissue without determining changes in the healing process (Santini 1983).

Triamcinolone acetonide is a potent corticosteroid that could be used effectively to eliminate or at least reduce the severe inflammation that might occur secondary to endodontic treatment (Negm 2001).

5.2. Perioperative corticosteroid use in dentoalveolar surgery

Several authors have examined the effects of corticosteroids for prevention of pain and edema associated with oral surgery. Dental surgeons are often advised to use corticosteroids during and after third molar removal and other dentoalveolar surgery to reduce postsurgical edema. The most commonly used forms of corticosteroids in dentoalveolar surgery include dexamethasone (oral), dexamethasone sodium phosphate and dexamethasone acetate, and methylprednisolone acetate and methyl prednisolone sodium succinate. Dexamethasone has a longer duration of action than methlyprednisolone and is considered more potent (Alexander 2000).

Methylprednisolone has been used in a number of studies. Methylprednisolone is usually administered via the intramuscular or intravenous route though the possibility of topical (intraalveolar) application has been described, with a reduction in morbidity and possible side effects. This drug is five times more potent than cortisol, with scant associated saline retention and an intermediate duration of action (12-36 hours) (Micó-Llorens 2006; Leone 2007; Vegas-Bustamante 2008).

Based on the literature review, interim recommendations for the use of corticosteroids are proposed, including dosages and regimens that appear rational for oral, intramuscular, or intravenous corticosteroid administration before and after extractions and other dentoalveolar surgery. These largely empiric recommendations might require adjustment when evidence-based data become available in future studies

6. Adverse effects of steroids

Corticosteroids are chemical compounds of hormonal nature derived from cholesterol. Their biological power and actions depend on their chemical structure. Due to the remarkable anti-inflammatory and immunoregulatory effects of the corticosteroids, they have been employed as first step in the management of different diseases, and sometimes they are the only possible drug to use in daily medical practice. Despite their clinical efficacy, they can induce multiple severe adverse effects.

Adverse effects of corticosteroids may be due to local effects on the skin or mucosa at the site of or to systemic effects following absorption of the oral drugs. Systemic side effects are rarer than local side effects.

6.1. Systemic adverse effects

Systemic side effects occur because the steroids contained in the corticosteroid become absorbed into the blood stream and begin to affect other parts of the body, such as the adrenal gland (a gland that produces many of the body's natural steroids).

Systemic side effects can include (Lozada-Nur 1991; Bircher 1996):

- Hypothalamic-Pituitaryadrenal Axis and Secondary Adrenal
- Insufficiency
- Weight gain
- Osteoporosis
- Diabetes
- High Blood Pressure (hypertension)
- Psychological Effects
- Indigestion or Heartburn
- Cushing's Syndrome
- Moon Face
- Bone Damage
- Decreased Growth in Children
- Skin can become thin, easily bruised and slow to heal
- Avascular Necrosis (a painful bone condition)
- Glaucoma

6.2. Local adverse effects

While topical steroids have tremendous benefit in reducing inflammation, they also have significant side effects. Most of these side effects are seen with long-term use, but some may be noticed within days of starting therapy. The risk of side effects from topical corticosteroids is related to drug potency, duration of therapy, frequency of application and anatomical area. Local side effects can include (Key2003; Baid 2006):

- Tachyphylaxis
- Burning Mouth
- Hypogeusia

- Oral Hairy Leukoplakia
- Hypersensitive Reactions to the Drug
- Topical Steroid Allergy
- Skin Atrophy
- Striae - Stretch Marks
- Acne form/Rosacea like eruptions
- Candidosis
- Delayed Healing
- Fine Hair Growth

6.2.1. Special Considerations

Because corticosteroids cause the adrenal glands to slow or stop the production of cortisol, they cannot be discontinued abruptly. It takes some time for the adrenal glands to begin producing cortisol again. Gradually tapering the dose of corticosteroids allows the body to begin producing its own supply of cortisol again.

- Undertake weight bearing exercise (such as brisk walking)
- Stop smoking
- Avoid excess alcohol intake
- Contraindications for acute HSV Infection
- Creams are less effective in the mouth than ointments, and the ointment form is preferred.

7. Guidelines on the management of dental patients on corticosteroid therapy in community dental clinics

General dental procedures for patients receiving long-term steroid medication do not warrant supplementation with additional glucocorticoids.

The aims of these guidelines are to assist and support Dentists and Dental therapists when providing dental treatment to patients who are currently receiving, or who have received Corticosteroid therapy in the past twelve months.

7.1. For routine conservative dentistry or minor oral surgery (to include one simple extraction) under local anaesthesia

Although Opinions Conflict On Whether Any Significant Suppression Of Adrenal Function Occurs In Patients Taking Low Doses Of Steroids (Under 7. 5 Mg Prednisolone) Available Evidence Suggests That Supplementation Is Unnecessary For Local Anaesthetic Procedures.

7.2. For minor surgery under general anesthesia for patients undergoing general anesthesia for minor surgery

100 Mg Hydrocortisone Intramuscularly Should Be Administered And The Usual Glucocorticoid Medications Maintained.

7.3. For major surgery

100 Mg Hydrocortisone Delivered As A Bolus Pre-Operatively Followed By 50 Mg 8-Hourly For 48 Hours Is Adequate.

7.4. American Society of Anaesthesiologists (ASA) Physical Classification Status

1. A normal healthy patient
2. A patient with mild systemic disease
3. A patient with severe systemic disease
4. A moribund patient who is not expected to survive without surgery
5. A declared brain-dead patient whose organs are being removed for donor purposes.

Patients with ASA score 1 and 2 who are currently on or who have been on corticosteroids in the last year.

Patients with ASA score 3 and 4 who are currently on or who have been on corticosteroids in the last year.

Any patient that does not fit the above criteria or if the clinician is in any doubt then the patient should not be treated in the primary care setting and should be referred (Gibson 2004).

Author details

Masoumeh Mehdipour and Ali Taghavi Zenouz
Oral and Maxillofacial Medicine Department, Tabriz Faculty of Dentistry,
Tabriz University of Medical Sciences, Iran

8. References

Ad Hoc Working Group on Steroid-Sparing Criteria in Lupus. (2004). Criteria for Steroid-Sparing Ability of Interventions in Systemic Lupus Erythematosus: Report of a Consensus Meeting, Arthritis & Rheum, 50:3427

Adour KK, Wingerd J, Bell DN, Manhing JJ, Hurley JP. (1972). Prednisone treatment for idiopathic facial paralysis (Bell's palsy). N Engl J Med. 287: 1268–72.

Alexander RE, Throndson RR (2000). A review Of Perioperative Corticosteroid use In Dentoalveolar Surgery, Oral Surg Oral Med Oral Path . 90:406-15

Alstergren P, Appelgren A, Appelgren B, Kopp S, Lundeberg T, Theodorsson E. (1996). The effect on joint fluid concentration of neuropeptide Y by intra-articular injection of glucocorticoid in temporomandibular joint arthritis. Acta Odontol Scand. 54:1–7.

Arabshahi B, Dewitt EM, Cahill AM, Kaye RD, Baskin KM, Towbin RB, Cron RQ. (2005). Utility of corticosteroid injection for temporomandibular arthritis in children with juvenile idiopathic arthritis. Arthritis Rheum. 52:3563–3569.

Arlt W. (2009). The Approach to the Adult with Newly Diagnosed Adrenal Insufficiency J Clin Endocrinol Metab. 94 (4) :1059–1067

Bagan J, Lo Muzio L, Scully C. (2005). Mucosal disease series. Number III. Mucous membrane pemphigoid. Oral Dis. 11:197-218.

Baid SK, Nieman LK. (2006). Therapeutic doses of glucocorticoids: implications for oral medicine. Oral Dis. 12:436-42.

Bircher AJ, Pelloni F, Langauer Messmer S, Müller D. (1996). Delayed hypersensitivity reactions to corticosteroids applied to mucous membranes. Br J Dermatol. 35:310-3.

Borradori L, Bernard P. (2004). Vesiculobullous diseases: pemphoid group. eds. *Dermatology*. Philadelphia, PA: Mosby/Elsevier; 463-- 470

Brown AFT. (1995). Anaphylactic shock: Mechanisms and treatment. J Acc Emerg Med. 12:89-100.

Bruce A , Rogers RS III. (2007). New and old therapeutics for oral ulcerations. Arch Dermatol. 143: 519–23

Bystryn JC. Steinmann NM. (1996). The adjuvant therapy of pemphigus. Arch Dermatol. 132:203-12.

Cahill AM, Baskin KM, Kaye RD, Arabshahi B, Cron RQ, Dewitt EM et al. (2007). CT-guided percutaneous steroid injection for management of inflammatory arthropathy of the temporomandibular joint in children. AJR Am J Roentgenol. 188:182–186

Camisa C, Warner M. (1998). Treatment of pemphigus. Dermatol Nurs . 10 (2) :115-31.

Carbone M, Carrozzo M, Conrotto D, Garzino Demo P, Broccoletti R, Gandolfo S . (1997). Topical treatment of atrophic-erosive oral lichen planus with clobetasol in bioadhesive gel as well as chlorhexidine and miconazole in oral gel. Minerva stomatologica. 46 (7-8):423-8.

Carbone M, Conrotto D, Carrozzo M, Broccoletti R, Gandolfo S, Scully C. (1999). Topical corticosteroids in association with miconazole and chlorhexidine in the long-term managementof atrophic-erosive oral lichen planus: a placebo-controlledand comparative study between clobetasol and fluocinonide. Oral Dis . 5:44-9.

Cawson RA. (1968). Treatment of Oral Lichen Planus with Betamethasone. Br. Med. J. 2:86-89.

Chainani-Wu N, Silverman S Jr, Lozada-Nur F, Mayer P, Watson JJ. (2001). Oral lichen planus: patient profile, disease progression and treatment responses. J Am Dent Assoc. 132:901-9.

Chan CC, Paine M, O'Day J. (2001). "Steroid management in giant cell arteritis". Br J Ophthalmol 85 (9) :1061–4.

Chrousos GP. (2004). Adrenocorticosteroids and adrenocortical antagonists. In: Katzung BG, ed. Basic & Clinical Pharmacology. 9th ed. New York, NY: Lange Medical Books/McGraw-Hill. 641–660.

Cotell S, Robinson ND, Chan LS. (2000). Autoimmune blistering skin diseases . Am J Emerg Med . 18:288-99.

Dumas V, Roujeau JC, Wolkenstein P, Revuz J, Cosnes A. (1999). The treatment of mild pemphigus vulgaris and pemphigus foliaceus with a topical corticosteroid. Br J Dermatol. 140 (6) :1127-9.

Dworkin RH, Johnson RW, Breuer J, Gnann JW, Levin MJ, Backonja M, et al. (2007). Recommendations for the management of herpes zoster. Clin Infect Dis. 44 Suppl 1:S1-26.

Edwards CR, Baird JD, Frier B M, Shepherd J, Toft AD. (1995). Endocrine and metabolic diseases, including diabetes mellitus. In Edwards C R, Bouchier I A, Haslett C, Chilvers E R (eds) Davidson's principles and practice of medicine. 17th ed. pp 706-719. Edinburgh: ChurchillLivingstone

Edwards PC, Kelsch R. (2002). Oral Lichen Planus: Clinical Presentation and Management. J. C. D. 68:494-9.

Eisen D, Carrozzo M, Bagan Sebastian JV, Thongprasom K. (2005). Oral lichen planus: Clinical features and management. Oral Dis. 11:338-49.

Engström M, Berg T, Stjernquist-Desatnik A, Axelsson S, Pitkäranta A, Hultcrantz M et al. (2008). Prednisolone and valaciclovir in Bell's palsy: a randomised, double-blind, placebo-controlled, multicentre trial. Lancet Neurol. 7 (11) :993-1000.

Ewan PW, DuguéP, Mirakian R, Dixon TA, Harper JN, Nasser SM. (2010). BSACI guidelines for the investigation of suspected anaphylaxis during general anaesthesia. Clin Exp Allergy. 40 (1) :15.

Fassmann A, Dvo. akova N, Izakoviaova Holla L, Vanuk J, Wotke J. (2003). Manifestation of Pemphigus Vulgaris in the orofacial region. Case report. Scripta Medica (brno). 76:55–62.

Fellner MJ, Sapadin AN. (2001). Current therapy of pemphigus vulgaris. Mt Sinai J Med . 68 (4-5) :268–78.

Femiano F, Gombos F, Scully C. (2002). Pemphigus vulgaris with oral involvement: Evaluation of two different systemic corticosteroid therapeutic protocols. J EurAcadDermatolVenereol . 16 (4) :353-6.

Fernandes NC, Perez M. (2001). Treatment of pemphigus vulgaris and pemphigus foliaceus: experience with 71 patients over a 20 year period. Revista do Instituto de Medicina Tropical de Sao Paulo . 43 (1) , 33-36.

Field EA, Allan RB. (2003). Review article: oral ulceration – aetiopathogenesis, clinical diagnosisand management in the gastrointestinal clinic. Blackwell Publishing Ltd, Aliment

Fitzpatrick TB, Freedberg IM, Eisen AZ, Wolff K, Austen KF,Goldsmith LA, et al. (2008). Fitzpatrick's dermatology in general medicine (7th ed.). New York: McGraw-Hill.

Forman R, Koren G, Shear NH. (2002). Erythema mutliforme, Stevens-Johnson syndrome and toxic epidermal necrolysis in children: a review of 10 years' experience. Drug Saf. 25 (13) :965–972.

French L, Prins C. (2008). Erythema multiforme, Stevens-Johnson syndrome and toxic epidermal necrolysis. In: Bolognia JL, Jorizzo JL, Rapini RP, eds. Dermatology. 2nd ed. Philadelphia PA: Elsevier. 287–300.

Funauchi M, Ikoma S, Imada A, Kanamaru A. (1997). Combination of immune adsorption therapy and high dose methyl prednisolone in patients with lupus nephritis; possible indications in patients with early stage. J Clin Lab Immunol. 49: 47 – 57.

Gerwin N, Hops C, Lucke A. (2006). Intraarticular drug delivery in osteoarthritis. Advanced Drug Delivery Reviews. 58:226–242.

Gibson N, Ferguson JW. (2004). Steroid cover for dental patients on long-term steroid medication: proposed clinical guidelines based upon a critical review of the literature British Dental Journal . 197 (11) : 681–685

Gilden DH. (2004). Clinical Practice. Bell's palsy. The New England Journal of Medicine. 351 (13) :1323–31.

Golden DB. (2007). What is anaphylaxis? Curr Opin Allergy Clin Immunol. 7 (4) :331–6

Greenberger PA. (2007). Idiopathic anaphylaxis. Immunol Allergy Clin N Am 27:273-93.

Gonzalez-Moles MA, Morales P, Rodriguez-Archilla A, Isabel IR, Gonzalez-Moles S. (2002). Treatment of severe chronic oral erosive lesions with clobetasol propionate in aqueous solution. Oral Surg Oral Med Oral Pathol Oral Radiol Endod. 93:264-70.

Gordon Marshall J. (2002). Consideration of steroids for endodontic pain Endodontic Topics . 3, 41–51

Gray RJM, Davies SJ, Quayle AA. (1994). A clinical approach to temporomandibular disorders: Treatment planning, general guidelines and case histories. Br Dent J. 171: 171-178.

Greenspan JS, Yeoman CM, Harding SM. (1978). Oral Lichen Planus: A Double-Blind Comparison of Treatment with Betamethasone Valerate Aerosol and Pellets. Br. Dent. J. 144:83-84.

Grogan PM, Gronseth GS. (2001). Practice parameter: steroids, acyclovir, and surgery for Bell's palsy (an evidence-based review) : report of the Quality Standards Subcommittee of the American Academy of Neurology. Neurology. 56: 830-6.

Grover VK, Babu R, Bedi SPS. (2007). Steroid Therapy – Current Indications in Practice. Indian Journal of Anaesthesia. 51 (5) : 389-393

Harman KE, Albert S, Black MM. (2003). Guidelines for the managementof pemphigus vulgaris. Br J Dermatol. 149 (5) : 926-37.

Hashimoto T. (2008). Treatment strategies for pemphigus vulgaris in Japan. Expert OpinPharmacother. 9:1519-30.

Hato N, Yamada H, Kohno H, Matsumoto S, Honda N, Gyo K et al. (2007). Valacyclovir and prednisolone treatment for Bell s palsy: A multicenter, randomized, placebo-controlled study. Otology andNeurotology. 28:408–13.

Hayreh SS, Zimmerman B. (2003). Management of giant cell arteritis. Our 27-year clinical study: new light on old controversies. Ophthalmologica. 217:239–259

Hegarty AM, Hodgson TA, Lewsey JD, Porter SR. (2002). Fluticasone propionate spray and betamethasone sodium phosphate mouthrinse: a randomized crossover study for the treatment of symptomatic oral lichen planus. J AmAcad Dermatol. 47: 271 – 279.

Hench PS, Kendall EC, Slocumb CH, Polley HF. (1949). The effect of a hormone of the a drenal cortex (17-hydroxy-11-dehydrocorticosterone:compound E) and of pituitary adrenocorticotropic hormone on rheumatic arthritis. Proc Staff Meet Mayo Clin. 24:181

Hill G, Chauvenet AR, Lovato J, McLean TW. (2005). Recent steroid therapy increases severity of varicella infections in children with acute lymphoblastic leukemia. Pediatrics . 116 (4) :523–9.

Hiroshige K, Ikeda M, Hondo R. (2002). Detection of varicella zoster virus DNA in tear fluid and saliva of patients with Ramsay Hunt syndrome. Otol Neurotol. 23 (4) :602–7.

Hollander JL, Brown EM, Jessar RA, Brown CY. (1951). Hydrocortisone and Cortisone injected into arthritic joints: Comparative effect of and use of hydrocortisone as a local antiarthritic agent. JAMA. 147: 1629-1236.

Holland R, Okabe JA, Souza V, Saliba O. (1991). Diffusion of corticosteroid antibiotic solutions through human dentine. Rev Odontol UNESP. 20: 17-23.

Horten CP. (1953). The Treatment of Arthritic Temporomandibular Joints by Intra-articular Injection of Hydrocortisone. Oral Surg. 6: 826-829.

Horton B, Magath T, Brown G. (1932). An undescribed form of arteritis of the temporal vessels. Proc Staff Mtg MayoClin. 7:700-701.

Huff JC. (1992). Erythema multiforme and latent herpes simplex infection. Semin Dermatol. 11:207–10.

Hutchinson J. (1890). Diseases of the arteries. On a peculiar form of thrombotic arteritis of the aged which is sometimes productive of gangrene. ArchSurg. 1:323-9.

Hyvernat H, Roger PM, Pereira C, Saint-Paul MC, Vandenbos F, Bernardin G. (2005). Fatal varicella hepatitis in an asthmatic adult after short-term corticosteroid treatment. Eur J Intern Med. 16 (5) :361–2.

Ippolito A , Petri M. (2008). An Update on Mortality in Systemic Lupus Erythematosus, Clin Exp Rheumatol, 26 (5 Suppl 51) :S72-9.

Jacobson C, Cornell R, Savin R. (1986). A comparison of clobetasol propionate 0. 05% ointment and optimized betamethasone dipropionate 0. 05% ointment in the treatment of psoriasis. Cutis. 37:213-20.

Johnson RW. (2002). Consequences and management of pain in herpes zoster. J Infect Dis. 186 (suppl 1) :S83–S90

Joly P, Roujeau JC, Benichou J, Picard C, Dreno B, Delaporte E, et al. (2002). A comparison of oral and topical corticosteroids in patients with bullous pemphigoid. N Engl J Med. 346 (5) : 321-7.

Joly P, Benichou J, Lok C, Hellot MF, Saiag P, Tancrede-Bohin E et al. (2005). Prediction of survival for patients with bullous pemphigoid. Arch Dermatol. 141: 691-698.

Joly P, Roujeau JC, Benichou J, Delaporte E, D'Incan M, Dreno B et al. (2009). A comparison of two regimens of topical corticosteroids in the treatment of patients with bullous pemphigoid: A multicenter randomized study. J Invest Dermatol. 129 (7) : 1681-7.

Kakourou T, Klontza D, Soteropoulou F, Kattamis C. (1997). Corticosteroid treatment of erythema multiforme major (Stevens-Johnson syndrome) in children. Eur J Pediatr. 156:90–93.

Kardaun S, Jonkman M. (2007). Dexamethasone Pulse Therapy for Stevens-Johnson syndrome/toxic epidermal necrolysis. Acta Derm Venereol. 87:144–148.

Kasperkiewicz M, Enno Schmidt E. (2009). Current Treatment of Autoimmune Blistering Diseases. Current Drug Discovery Technologies, , 6, 270-280

Kelly DJ, Ahmad M, Brull SJ. (2001). Preemptive analgesia I: physiological pathways and pharmacological modalities. Can J Anaesth.:1000–10

Khare V. (2011). Discoid Lupus Erythematosus - A Case Report JIDA, Vol. 5, No. 1

Key SJ, Hodder SC, Davies R, Thomas DW, Thompson S. (2003). Perioperative corticosteroid supplementation and dento-alveolar surgery. Dent Update. 30:316-20.

Kinishi M, Amatsu M, Mohri M, Saito M, Hasegawa T, Hasegawa S. (2001). Acyclovir improves recovery rate of facial nerve palsy in Ramsay Hunt syndrome. Auris Nasus Larynx. 28 (3) :223–6. 9

Knudson RM, Kalaaji AN, Bruce AJ. . (2010). The management of mucous membrane pemphigoid and pemphigus. Dermatol Ther. 23:268-80.

Kopp S, Wenneberg B.(1981). Effects of occlusal treatment and intra-articular injections on temporomandibular pain and dysfunction. ActaOdontol Scand. 39:87–96.

Kotani N, Kushikata T, Hashimoto H, Kimura F, Muraoka M, Yodono M. et al. (2000).Intrathecal methyl prednisolone for intractable postherpetic neuralgia. N Engl J Med.; 343 (21):1514-9.

Lai DR, Chen HR. (1995). Clinical Evaluation of Different Treatment Methods for Oral Submucous Fibrosis. A 10-year experience with 150 cases, JOPM. 24, 402-614.

Lamoreux MR, Sternbach MR, Hsu WT. (2006). Erythema multiforme. Am Fam Physician. 74:1883–1888.

Larsson L. (1989). Anaphylactic shock after administration of triamcinolone acetonide in a 35 year old female. Scand J Rheamtol. 18: 441-444.

Lavelle W, Lavelle ED, Lavelle L. (2007). Intra-articular injections. Med Clin North Am. 91:241–250.

Leone M, Richard O, Antonini F, Rousseau S, Chabaane W, Guyot L, et al. (2007). Comparison of methylprednisolone and ketoprofen after multiple third molar extraction: a randomized controlled study. Oral Surg Oral Med Oral Pathol Oral Radiol Endod. 103:e7-9.

Lever WF, Schaumburg-Lever G. (1984). Treatment of pemphigus vulgaris. Results obtained in 84 patients between 1961 and 1982. Arch Dermato. 120 (1) :44–7.

Levin C, Maibach HI. (2002) :Topical corticosteroid-induced adrenocortical insufficiency: clinical implications. Am J Clin Dermatol. 3:141–7.

Lieberman P. (2005). Biphasic anaphylactic reactions. Ann Allergy Asthma Immunol . 95:217-26.

Lodi G, Scully C, Carrozzo M, Griffiths M, Sugerman PB, Thongprasom K. (2005). Current controversies in oral lichen planus: report of an international consensus meeting – Part 1. Viral infections and aetiopathogenesis. Oral Surg Oral Med Oral Pathol Oral Radiol Endod 100: 40-51.

Lo Muzio L, della Valle A, Mignogna MD, Pannone G, Bucci P, Bucci E, et al. (2001). The treatment of oral aphthous ulceration or erosive lichen planus with topical clobetasol propionate in three preparations: a clinical and pilot study on 54 patients. J OralPathol Med . 30:611-7.

Lozada –Nur F, Silverman S Jr. (1980). Topically applied fluocinonide in an adhesive base in the treatment of oral vesiculoerosive diseases. Arch Dermatol . 116:898-901.

Lozada-Nur F, Huang MZ, Zhou GA. (1991). Open preliminary clinical trial of clobetasol propionate ointment in adhesive paste for treatment of chronic oral vesiculoerosive diseases. Oral Surg Oral Med Oral Pathol . 71:283-7.

Lozada-Nur F, Miranda C, Maliksi R. (1994). Double-blind clinical trial of 0. 05% clobetasol propionate ointment in orobase and 0. 05% fluocinonide ointment in orobase in the treatment of patients with oral vesiculoerosive diseases. Oral Surg Oral Med Oral Pathol. 77: 598–604.

MacPhee IT, Sircus W, Farmer ED, Harkness RA, Cowley GC. (1968). Use of steroids in treatment of aphthous ulceration. Br Med J. 2:147-9.

Mamelak AJ, Eid MP, Cohen BA, Anhalt GJ. (2007). Rimximab therapy in severe juvenile pemphigus vulgaffs. Cutis. 80 (4) , 335–340.

Martinez AE, Atherton DJ. (2000). High-dose systemic corticosteroids can arrest recurrences of severe mucocutaneous erythema multiforme. Pediatr Dermatol. 17 (2) :87–90.

Mehdipour M, Taghavi Zenouz A, Bahramian A, Yazdani J, Poura- libaba F,Sadr K. (2010). Comparison of the Effect of Mouthwashes with and without Zinc and Fluocinolone on the Healing Process of Erosive Oral Lichen Planus. JODDD. 4 (1) :25-28

Mentink LF, Mackenzie MW, Tóth GG, Laseur M, Lambert FP, Veeger NJ, et al. (2006). Randomized controlled trial of adjuvant oral dexamethasone pulse therapy in pemphigus vulgaris: PEMPULS trial. Arch Dermatol. 142 (5) :570-6.

Merchant HW, Gangarosa LP, Glassman AB, Sobel RE. (1978). Betamethasone-17-benzoate in the treatment of recurrent aphthous ulcers. Oral Surg. 45:870-5.

Micó-Llorens JM, Satorres-Nieto M, Gargallo-Albiol J, Arnabat-Domínguez J, Berini-Aytés L, Gay-Escoda C. (2006). Efficacy of methylprednisolone in controlling complications after impacted lower third molar surgical extraction. Eur J Clin Pharmacol. 62:693-8.

Mondino BJ, Brown SI. (1981). Ocular cicatricial pemphigoid. Ophthalmology. 88:95-100.

Murakami S, Hato N, Horiuchi J, Honda N, Gyo K, Yanagihara N. (1997). Treatment of Ramsay Hunt syndrome with acyclovir-prednisone: significance of early diagnosis and treatment. Ann Neurol. 41:353-7.

Mutasim DF, Cincinatti. (2004). Management of Autoimmune Bullous Disease: Pharmacology and Therapeutics, J. Am. Acad. Dermatol. 51:859-77.

Natah SS, Konttinen YT. (2004). Recurrent Aphthous Ulcers Today: a review of the growing knowledge, IJOMS. 33:221-34.

Negm M M. (2001). Intracanal use of a Corticosteroid – antibiotic compound for the management of post treatment endodontic pain. Triplo. 92:435-9.

Oztas P, Onder M, Ilter N, Oztas MO. (2003). Childhood lichen planus with nail involvement: a case. Turkish J Pediatrics. 45:251-253.

Panjwani S. (2009). Early Diagnosis and Treatment of Discoid Lupus Erythematosus. J Am Board Fam Med. . 22 (2) :206-213.

Pavan-Langston D. (2008). Herpes zoster antivirals and pain management. Ophthalmology. 115:S13–S20

Pedersen A, Klausen B. (1984). Glucocorticosteroids and Oral Medicine, Oral Pathology & Medicine J. 13:1-15

Pimlott SJ, Walker DM. (1983). A controlled clinical trial of the efficacy of topically applied fluocinonide in the treatment of recurrent aphthous ulceration. Br Dent J. 154:174-7

Pipitone N, Boiardi L, Salvarini C. (2005). Are steroids alone sufficient for the treatment of giant cell arteritis? Best Pract Res Clin Rheumatol. 19:277–292

Prajapati V, Mydlarski PR. (2008). Advances in pemphigus therapy. Skin Therapy Lett. 13:4-7.

Rabiyi M, Sahebjamee M. (2003). Effect of aqueous triamcinolone actonide 0. 2% suspension in treatment oforal lichen planus. Journal Medical Faculty GuilanUniversity of Medical Sciences. 12: 6 – 14.

Rahman W, Rahman FZ. (2005). Major review – giant cell (temporal) arteritis: an overview and update. Surv Ophthalmol. 50:415–428

Ramsey MJ, Der Simonian R, Holtel MR, BurgessLPA. (2000). Corticosteroid treatment for idiopathic facialnerve paralysis: a meta-analysis. Laryngoscope. 110: 335–41.

Ratnam KV, Phay KL, Tan CK. (1990). Pemphigus therapy with oral prednisolone regimens: A 5-year study. Int J Dermatol. 29 (5) :363-7.

Rees TD, Binnie WH. (1996). Recurrent aphthous stomatitis. Dermatol Clin. 14:243-56.

Reich RF, Kerpel SM. (1998). Differential Diagnosis and Treatment of Ulcerative, Erosive and Vesiculobullous Lesions of Oral Mucosa, Oral and Maxillofacial Surgery Clinics of North America. 10: 95-129.

ReviewAnaphylaxis in the emergency department. (2008). a paediatric perspective. Curr Opin Allergy Clin Immunol. 8 (4) :321-9.

Ring J, Darsow U. (2002). Idiopathic anaphylaxis. Curr Allergy Asthma Reports . 2:40-5.

Robillard RB, Hilsinger RL Jr, Adour KK. (1986). Ramsay Hunt facial paralysis: clinical analyses of 185 patients. Otolaryngol Head Neck Surg. 1:292–7.

Ringold S, Torgerson TR, Egbert MA, Wallace CA. (2008). Intraarticular corticosteroid injections of the temporomandibular joint in juvenile idiopathic arthritis. J Rheumatol. 35:1157–1164.

Roed-Petersen B, Roed-Petersen J. (1992). Occlusive treatment of atrophic and erosive oral lichen planus with clobetasol propionate 0. 05% ointment (Dermovat) [Danish]. Tandlaegernes Tidsskr. 1:4- 7.

Ruocco E, Aurilia A, Ruocco V. (2001). Precautions and suggestions for pemphigus patients. Dermatology. 203 (3) :201–7.

Salvarani C, Cantini F, Bolardi L, Hunder GG. (2002). Polymyalgia rheumatica and giant-cell arteritis. N Engl J Med. 347:261–271

Santini A. (1983). Assessment of the pulpotomy technique in human first permanent mandibular molars. Br Dent J. 155: 151-4.

Setterfield JF, Black MM , Challacombe SJ. (2000). The management of oral lichen planus. Clin Exp Dermatol. 25: 176–82.

Schmader KE, Dworkin RH. (2008). Natural history and treatment of herpes zoster. J Pain. 9:S3–S9

Scully C, Bagan J. (2008). Oral mucosal diseases: erythema multiforme. Br J Oral Maxillofac Surg. 46:90–95.

Scully C, Lo Muzio L. (2008). Oral mucosal diseases: mucous membrane pemphigoid. Br J Oral Maxillofac Surg. 46:358-66.

Shin HT, Chang MW. (2001). Drug eruptions in children. Curr Probl Pediatr. 31:207–34.

Shafshak TS, Essa AY, Bakey FA. (1994). The possible contributing factors for the success of steroid therapy in Bell's palsy: a clinical and electrophysiological study. J Laryngol Otol. 108: 940-3.

Ship JA. (1996). Recurrent aphthous stomatitis. Oral Surg Oral Med Oral Pathol Oral Radiol Endod. 81:141-7.

Silbermann M, Moredohvich D, Toister Z, Azaria N. (1978). Mechanisms involved in mandibular condylopathy secondary to intra-articular injections of glucocorticoids. J Oral Surg. 36: 112-117.

Silverman S Jr, Gorsky M, Lozada-Nur F, Giannotti K. (1991). A prospective study of findings and management in 214 patients with oral lichen planus. Oral Surg Oral Med Oral Pathol Oral Radiol Endod. 72:665-70

Sirois D, Leigh JE, Sollecito TP. (2000). Oral pemphigus vulgaris preceding cutaneous lesions: recognition and diagnosis. J Am Dent Assoc. 131, 1156-1160.

Soar J, Pumphrey R, Cant A. (2008). Emergency treatment of anaphylactic reactions. Guidelines for health care providers. Resuscitation . 77:157-69

Sullivan FM, Swan IR, Donnan PT, Morrison JM, Smith BH, McKinstry B, et al. (2007). Early treatment with prednisolone or acyclovir in Bell's palsy. N Engl J Med. 357 (16) :1598-607.

Taverner D. (1954). Cortisone treatment of Bell's palsy. Lancet. ii:1052–4.

Thompson AC, Nolan A, Lamey J. (1989). Minor aphthous oral ulceration: a double-blind cross-over study of beclomethasone dipropionate aerosol spray. Scott Med J. 34:531

Thongprasom K, Luangjarmekorn L, Sererat T, Taweesap W. (1992). Relative efficacy of fluocinolone acetonide compared with triamcinolone acetonide in treatment of oral lichen planus.

Thongprasom K, Luengvisut P, Wongwatanakij A, Boonjatturus C. (2003). Clinical evaluation in treatment of oral lichen planus with topical fluocinolone acetonide: a 2-year follow-up. J Oral Pathol Med. 32: 315 – 322.

Thost A. (1911). Der chronische schleimhaut-pemphigus der oberen luftwege. Arch Laryng Rhinol. 25:459-78.

Toller PA. (1977). Use and misuse of intra-articular corticosteroids in treatment of temporomandibular joint pain. Proc Roy Soc Med. 70:461–463.

Toth GG, Jonkman MF. (2001). Therapy of pemphigus . Clin Dermatol. 19 (6) :761–7

Tht Yu J, Chong L, Kc Lee L. (2007). Pemphigoid, benign mucous membrane Hong Kong Med J. 13:157-60

Tyldesley WR, Harding SM. (1977). Betamethasone Valerate Aerosol in the Treatment of Oral Lichen Planus. Br. J. Dermatol. 96:659-662.

Uri N, Greenberg E, Kitzes-Cohen R, Doweck I. (2003). Acyclovir in the treatment of Ramsay Hunt syndrome. Otolaryngol Head Neck Surg. 129 (4) :379–81.

Valença MM, Valença LP, Lima MC. (2001). Idiopathic facial paralysis (Bell's palsy) : a study of 180 patients . Arquivos de Neuro-Psiquiatria. 59:733–9.

Van de Steene V, Kuhweide R, Vlaminck S, Casselman J. (2004). Varicella zoster virus: beyond facial paralysis. Acta Otorhinolaryngol Belg. 58 (1) :61–6

Van Wijck AJ, Opstelten W, Moons KG, van Essen GA, Stolker RJ, Kalkman CJ, et al. (2006). The PINE study of epidural steroids and local anaesthetics to prevent postherpetic neuralgia: a randomised controlled trial. Lancet; 367 (9506) :219-24.

Vegas-Bustamante E, Micó-Llorens J, Gargallo-Albiol J, Satorres-Nieto M, Berini-Aytés L, Gay-Escoda C. (2008). Efficacy of methylprednisolone injected into the masseter muscle following the surgical extraction of impacted lower third molars. Int J Oral Maxillofac Surg. 37:260-3.

Vincent SD, Lilly GE. (1992). Clinical, historic, and therapeutic features of aphthous stomatitis. Literature review and open clinical trial employing steroids. Oral Surg Oral Med Oral Pathol. 74:79-86.

Vincent SD, Fotos PG, Baker KA, Williams TP. (1990). Oral Lichen Planus: The Clinical, Historical, and Therapeutic Features of 100 Cases. Oral Surg. Oral Med. Oral Pathol. 70:165-171 .

Volcheck GW. (2004). Clinical evaluation and management of drug hypersensitivity. Immunol Allergy Clin North Am. 24:357–71.

Voute AB, Schulten EA, Langendijk PN, Kostense PJ, van der Waal I. (1993). Fluocinolone in an adhesive base for treatment of oral lichen planus. A double-blind, placebo controlled clinical study. Oral Surg Oral Med Oral Pathol. 75: 181 – 185.

Werth VP. (1996). Treatment of pemphigus vulgaris with brief , high-dose intravenous glucocorticoids. Arch Dermatol. 132:1435 – 1439

Westerhof W. (1989). Treatment of bullous pemphigoid with topical clobetasol propionate. J Am Acad Dermatol. 20: 458–61.

Weyand CM, Goronzy JJ. (2003). Medium- and large-vessel vasculitis. N Engl J Med. 349:160–169

Whitley RJ, Weiss H, Gnann JW Jr, Tyring S, Mertz GJ, Pappas PG et al. (1996). Acyclovir with and without prednisone for the treatment of herpes zoster. A randomized, placebo-controlled trial. The National Institute of Allergy and Infectious Diseases Collaborative Antiviral Study Group. Ann Intern Med. 125 (5) :376-83.

Williamson IG, Whelan TR. (1996). The clinical problem of Bell's palsy: is treatment with steroids effective? Br J Gen Pract. 46: 743-7.

Wise C. (2005). In: Kelley's Textbook of Rheumatology. Seventh. Harris ED Jr, Budd RC, Genovese MC, Firestein GS, Sargent JS, Sledge CB, editors. Elsevier Saunders; Philadelphia:pp. 695–696.

Wojnarowska F, Kirtschig G, Highet AS, Venning VA, Khumalo NP. (2002). Summary of Recommendations for Management of Bullous Pemphigoid. Br J Dermatol. 147: 214-221

Wolverton SE. (2007). Systemic corticosteroids. In: Wolverton SE, ed. Comprehensive Dermatologic Drug Therapy. 2nd ed. Philadelphia, PA: Saunders Elsevier. 127–161.

Woo SB, Sonis ST. (1996). Recurrent aphthous ulcers: a review of diagnosis and treatment. J Am Dent Assoc. 127:1202-13.

Wood MJ, Johnson RW, McKendrick MW, Taylor J, Mandal BK, Crooks J. (1994). A randomized trial of acyclovir for 7 days or 21 days with and without prednisolone for treatment of acute herpes zoster. N Engl J Med. 330 (13) :896-900.

Yazici H, Barnes CG. (1991). Practical treatment recommendations for pharmacotherapy of Behc¸et's syndrome. Drugs. 42:796–804.

Yeung AK, Goldman RD. (2005). Use of steroids for erythema multiforme in children. Can Fam Physician. 51 (11) :1481–1483.

Zegarelli EV, Kutscher AH, Mehrhof A. (1969). Long-lasting lozenges with triamcinolone acetonide. Treatment of erosive lichen planus of oral mucosa. N Y State J Med . 69:2463-4

Zegarelli DJ. (1980). Topical and intralesional steroid therapy of oral lichen planus. N Y State Dent J. 46:432, 434-432, 436.

Zegarelli DJ. (1983). Multimodality steroid therapy of erosive and ulcerative oral lichen planus. J Oral Med . 38:127-30.

Zimmermann R, Faure M, Claudy A. (1999). Prospective study of treatment of bullous pemphigoid by a class I topical corticosteroid. Ann Dermatol Venereol. 126: 13–16.

Chapter 6

Functional and Molecular Aspects of Glucocorticoids in the Endocrine Pancreas and Glucose Homeostasis

Alex Rafacho, Antonio C. Boschero and Henrik Ortsäter

Additional information is available at the end of the chapter

http://dx.doi.org/10.5772/50233

1. Introduction

As presented in the previous chapter, excessive exposure to endogenous or exogenous glucocorticoids (GCs) can disrupt glucose homeostasis in health individuals leading to glucose intolerance and/or insulin resistance (IR), and also aggravates the glucose metabolism in type 2 diabetic patients. In this context, we aim, in this chapter, to present and discuss the adaptive compensations in three levels: structural, functional and molecular - of the endocrine pancreas in response to the GC-induced IR and glucose intolerance that are required to maintain glycemia at physiological or near to physiological values. We will bring a comprehensive summary on experimental and clinical investigations performed in humans, rats and mice. Species differences will receive a special focus since the literature regarding humans, rats and mice responses to GC treatment indicates that there are species differences in both response to and sensitivity towards CGs.

2. Effect of glucocorticoids on the endocrine pancreas

GC hormones are secreted by the adrenal cortex under control of the HPA axis. This class of hormones plays an important role on energy homeostasis by modulating glucose, lipid and protein metabolism. The HPA axis may receive several inputs during some stressful conditions, such as fasting, physical activities as well as emotional episodes. In such conditions, the physiological GC actions guarantee adequate substrate supply for oxidative metabolism by increasing hepatic glucose production, lipolysis and proteolysis (Andrews & Walker, 1999).

Alterations in peripheral insulin sensitivity are reciprocally related to pancreatic islet function, in that insulin secretion is initially adaptively increased in response to conditions of IR (*e.g.*, obesity, pregnancy, pre-diabetes) (Kahn et al., 1993). As GCs induce IR, pancreatic β-cells initially also increase their insulin secretion capacity in response to GC treatment (Beard et al., 1984; Nicod et al., 2003; Ahrén, 2008; Rafacho et al., 2008; Rafacho et al., 2010). However, it is also known that GCs, by direct effects, can cause pancreatic β-cell dysfunction, which leads to attenuated GSIS (Lambillotte et al., 1997; Jeong et al., 2001; Ullrich et al., 2005; Zawalich et al., 2006; Roma et al., 2011). The crucial point is that, at least during short (2 to 15 days) periods of treatment, the direct negative effects of GCs are not reproduced on pancreatic β-cell during *in vivo* GC administration to normal subjects, and the derangement of β-cells during GC treatment seems to depend on predispositions such as genetic background (Ogawa et al., 1992), age (Novelli et al., 1999) as well as previous glucose intolerance and/or low insulin sensitivity (Wajngot et al., 1992; Ohneda et al., 1993; Henriksen et al., 1997; Larsson & Ahren, 1999; Besse et al., 2005). In the next topic, we will discuss in detail the endocrine pancreas and glucose homeostasis profile both in human and in rodent experimental models of GC treatment. In addition, results of *in vitro* studies in which primary β-cells or insulin-producing cells have been exposed to GCs will be discussed.

2.1. GC treatment and glucose tolerance, insulin sensitivity and β-cell function in humans

2.1.1. Acute GC effects in healthy individuals

The acute effects of GCs in healthy individuals, as judged by cortisol infusion (Shamoon et al., 1980) or by high doses of prednisolone (Kalhan & Adam, 1975; van Raalte et al., 2010), seem to be inhibitory for insulin secretion. This is based on the fact that circulating insulin levels during fasting state are not altered following GC treatment, despite the increase in blood glucose levels. The increase in glycemia is associated with decreased glucose uptake and clearance, whereas the rates of endogenous glucose production are unchanged (Shamoon et al., 1980). Glucose intolerance is observed during an oral glucose tolerance test (oGTT) in healthy individuals receiving a single oral dose of 1 mg dexamethasone (DEX) just prior to the oGTT. In the latter, glucose intolerance was also a result of decreased glucose clearance; while no differences in endogenous glucose production was observed too (Schneiter & Tappy, 1998). Although the literature concerning rapid GC effects on insulin secretion in healthy individuals is scarce, it seems that insulin secretion under glucose infusion is reduced (Shamoon et al., 1980) or unaltered (Schneiter & Tappy, 1998) in response to a glucose challenge, suggesting an acute inhibitory effect of the GCs on β-cells (Kalhan & Adam, 1975). It should also be mentioned that adaptive compensation to short GC exposures are transitory and usually reversible after discontinuation of steroid treatment (van Raalte et al., 2010).

2.1.2. GC effects during prolonged exposure in healthy individuals

Treatment of healthy subjects with high doses of DEX (2 to 4 days) or prednisolone (6 to 15 days) is associated with normoglycemia or modest increase in fasting blood glucose levels concomitant with significantly heightened circulating insulin concentrations during the post-absorptive state (Pagano et al., 1983; Beard et al., 1984; Grill et al., 1990; Schneiter & Tappy, 1998; Hollingdal et al., 2002; Willi et al., 2002; Nicod et al., 2003; Binnert et al., 2004; van Raalte et al., 2010), (see an overview in Table 1). The elevation of insulinemia indicates IR, a condition also confirmed after GC treatment (Pagano et al., 1983; Grill et al., 1990; Larsson & Ahren, 1999; Hollingdal et al., 2002; Willi et al., 2002; Nicod et al., 2003; Ahrén, 2008). The modest increase in fasting glycemia may be explained by direct effect of GCs on hepatic *de novo* glucose production or by a reduction of glucose uptake by peripheral tissues (*e.g.*, muscle, liver and adipose tissue). In this case, even high levels of insulin (Schneiter & Tappy, 1998) are insufficient to compensate for IR evoked by the steroid treatment. However, it must be stressed that most studies with GC administration for a short period in healthy volunteers do not show fasting hyperglycemia (Nicod et al., 2003; Binnert et al., 2004; Ahrén, 2008; van Raalte et al., 2010). Under glucose challenging by hyperglycemic-clamp (Beard et al., 1984; Nicod et al., 2003; Binnert et al., 2004) or an oGTT (Schneiter & Tappy, 1998; Hollingdal et al., 2002; Willi et al., 2002), insulin secretion is higher in GC-treated healthy subjects compared with control individuals. This increase in insulin secretion appears to be sufficient to maintain glucose homeostasis (Nicod et al., 2003; Binnert et al., 2004; Ahrén, 2008), suggesting that for the period of steroid exposure observed in the above studies the islets adjust their insulin release to overcome the IR imposed by GC treatment. However, we cannot exclude the possibility that at a more prolonged exposure (months or even years as in patients subjected to chronic GC therapies) β-cell dysfunction develops in face of sustained IR and/or by direct negative effects of GCs on β-cell function/viability resulting in dysregulation of glucose homeostasis.

The increased insulin secretion noted during GC treatment needs not necessarily result from a direct GC action on β-cells. This is suggested as several changes, such as in substrates, hormones, and/or neural influences that β-cells are exposed to, precluding a clear explanation of the factors causing increased islet function. Ahrén (Ahrén, 2008) performed an elegant experiment in which healthy women were subjected to oral DEX administration in a dose and period that resulted in IR, and insulin hypersecretion in response to arginine infusion. After 3 to 6 months, the same volunteers were treated with the same steroid regimen, but also received an intravenous infusion of a ganglionic antagonist (trimethaphan), which interrupts neural transmission. Arginine-stimulated insulin secretion was higher in DEX-treated individuals, as expected, but was markedly inhibited by the ganglionic antagonist. These data imply that a stimulus triggered by IR increases the parasympathetic tone to the islet β-cells to increase insulin secretion and this may contribute to the adaptive hypersecretion of insulin during IR (Ahrén, 2008). Whether this autonomic effect involves the classical neuropeptide acetylcholine, or any of the other parasympathetic neuropeptides, remains to be investigated (Ahrén, 2008).

In summary, the product of insulin secretion and peripheral insulin sensitivity, also called the disposition index, remains constant in healthy subjects exposed to GC treatment.

GC	Route	Dosing	Insulin sensitivity (IS) Glucose tolerance (GT)	Fasting glycemia	Fasting insulinemia	Insulin secretion	Reference
Pred	Oral	15 mg *b.i.d.* for 7 d	Decreased IS	Modest increase	Modest increase	-----	(Pagano et al., 1983)
Dex	Oral	3 mg *b.i.d.* for 2 1/2 d	-----	Modest increase	Increased	Increased	(Beard et al., 1984)
Dex	Oral	3 mg *b.i.d.* for 2 1/2 d	Decreased IS	Increased	Increased	Varied	(Grill et al., 1990)
Dex	Oral	4 mg for 5 d	Decreased IS	-----	-----	Increased	(Kautzky-Willer et al., 1996)
Dex	Oral	0.5 mg *q.d.* for 2 d and 1 mg at the 3rd d.	Decreased GT	Unaltered	Increased	Increased	(Schneiter & Tappy, 1998)
Pred	Oral	15 mg *b.i.d.* for 6 d	Decreased IS	Modest increase	Increased	Increased	(Hollingdal et al., 2002)
Dex	Oral	2 mg *b.i.d.* for 4 d	Decreased IS	Modest increase	Increase	Increased	(Willi et al., 2002)
Dex	Oral	0.5 mg *q.d.* for 2 d	Decreased IS	Unaltered	Increased	Increased	(Nicod et al., 2003)
Dex	Oral	0.5 mg *q.d.* for 2 d and 0.5 mg at the 3rd d	Decreased IS	Unaltered	Increased	Increased	(Binnert et al., 2004)
Dex	Oral	3 mg *b.i.d.* for 2 1/2 d	Decreased IS	Unaltered	Increased	Increased	(Ahrén, 2008)
Pred	Oral	30 mg for 15 d	Decreased IS Decreased GT	Increased	Tendency towards increase	Decreased	(van Raalte et al., 2010)

b.i.d.; twice a day (from Latin *bis in die*)**, d;** day, **q.d.;** four times each day (from Latin *quater die sumendus*), **Pred;** prednisolone, **Dex;** dexamethasone, **-----;** none

Table 1. Effects of prolonged GC treatment on glucose homeostasis in healthy volunteers.

2.1.3. GC effects in susceptible subjects

Administration of GCs to individuals with any degree of susceptibility towards glucose intolerance, but still normoglycemic, before treatment with GCs, such as those with low insulin sensitivity (Larsson & Ahren, 1999) or with low insulin response to glucose (Wajngot et al., 1992), obese women (Besse et al., 2005) and first-degree relatives of patients with type 2 diabetes *mellitus* (T2DM) (Henriksen et al., 1997), fails to induce the adaptive islet compensation observed in healthy subjects. Thus, in such individuals GC treatment may disrupt glucose homeostasis and cause hyperglycemia. The derangements that contribute to glucose intolerance include reduction in glucose-dependent or arginine-induced insulin release (Larsson & Ahren, 1999), increased glucose production and decreased glucose clearance (Wajngot et al., 1992), and reduction in whole body glucose disposal (Besse et al., 2005). Therefore, the enhancement in β-cell response, required to accommodate the GC-induced IR state, is impaired in these subjects.

2.1.4. Obstacles for the investigation of β-cell function in humans

The prolonged period of GC therapy utilized in clinical practice may surpass the short period used for experimental approaches in human studies that often is restricted to 2-15 days of GC treatment (van Raalte et al., 2009). Thus, the data from human experimental models, although of great relevance, fail to mimic the conditions of clinical practice. Elaboration of chronic GC protocols to investigate β-cell function in human volunteers is not feasible in consideration of the risk to develop irreversible adverse effects, ethical issues, as well as the nature of *ex vivo* and *in vitro* tools available for the mechanistic comprehension of β-cell function and growth (van Raalte et al., 2009). Yet, patients exhibiting excess of endogenous or exogenous GCs generally develop other side effects or altered circulating factors that could mask the GC effects on β-cell function (Dessein & Joffe, 2006).

Taken together, acute GC administration seems to exert an inhibitory effect on insulin secretion, while prolonged exposure induces alterations in β-cell function as an adaptive compensation to surpass GC-induced IR. However, susceptible subjects are prone to develop β-cell dysfunction with subsequent impairment of glucose homeostasis. Considering that mechanistic investigations require *ex vivo* and *in vitro* approaches, and that rodent models exhibit similar responses as humans in terms of insulin secretion and glucose homeostasis profile, use of experimental rodent models has been important for understanding β-cell function during GC treatments.

2.2. GC treatment and glucose tolerance, insulin sensitivity and β-cell function in rodents

The effects of GCs on insulin secretion have been assessed *in vivo* and *ex vivo* in rats and mice and show that the compensatory islet responses in rats are similar to those observed in human volunteers. The importance of endogenous GCs was demonstrated in rats (Borelli et al., 1982) with bilateral adrenalectomy. These rats exhibit impaired insulin secretion *in vivo* in response to glucose, which is corrected by GC replacement. The endocrine pancreas adaptations to GC administration are not similar between rats and mice and for this reason we will first discuss the literature obtained with rat models and then proceed to mouse models.

2.2.1. Acute GC effects in normal rats

When administered acutely (4 to 6 hours), DEX causes a modest decrease in insulin sensitivity (Qi et al., 2004) or increased rate of glucose disappearance (Stojanovska et al.,

1990). This remains controversial, but at any rate it is accompanied by normoglycemia (Stojanovska et al., 1990; Qi et al., 2004) together with normal (Qi et al., 2004) or increased plasma insulin values (Stojanovska et al., 1990). These data reveal no deleterious effect of DEX on the insulinogenic index (the ratio between insulinemia and glycemia) when the steroid is acutely administered in rats.

2.2.2. Glucose tolerance and insulin sensitivity in GC-treated rats

The majority of the studies using rat models are performed with prolonged exposure to GCs and DEX is the compound preferentially employed. The protocols vary in dose (0.01 to 5 mg/kg, *b.w.*), duration (1 day to 8 weeks) and administration route (subcutaneous, intramuscular, intraperitoneal, oral), gender, age, and strain (Lee et al., 1989; O'Brien et al., 1991; Koranyi et al., 1992; Ohneda et al., 1993; Wang et al., 1994; Novelli et al., 1999; Holness & Sugden, 2001; Karlsson et al., 2001; Choi et al., 2006; Wierup et al., 2006; Rafacho et al., 2008; Rafacho et al., 2011) (Table 2). Similar to humans, normal rats treated with DEX had decreased peripheral insulin sensitivity. This GC-induced IR is time-, dose- and age-dependent (Novelli et al., 1999; Rafacho et al., 2008; Rafacho et al., 2011) and is a common effect in GC-treated rats. This is supported by the fact that most studies showed fasting hyperinsulinemia, an indicator of IR (Lee et al., 1989; Stojanovska et al., 1990; Koranyi et al., 1992; Novelli et al., 1999; Zakrzewska et al., 1999; Barbera et al., 2001; Holness & Sugden, 2001; Karlsson et al., 2001; Severino et al., 2002; Choi et al., 2006; Giozzet et al., 2008; Rafacho et al., 2008; Rafacho et al., 2010). This rise in circulating insulin concentrations fully compensates for peripheral IR in normal rats and prevents any increase in blood glucose concentrations (Lee et al., 1989; Koranyi et al., 1992; Ogawa et al., 1992; Novelli et al., 1999; Zakrzewska et al., 1999; Barbera et al., 2001; Holness & Sugden, 2001; Severino et al., 2002; Choi et al., 2006; Giozzet et al., 2008; Rafacho et al., 2008; Rafacho et al., 2010), except in normal elderly rats (Novelli et al., 1999) or when the highest experimental doses (1 mg/kg. *b.w.*) and/or duration (four days or more) of DEX administration are used. However, these latter experimental conditions provoke only a slight elevation in blood glucose levels that do not exceed an average value of 7.5 mM (Stojanovska et al., 1990; Holness & Sugden, 2001; Holness et al., 2005; Rafacho et al., 2008; Rafacho et al., 2010). The glucose tolerance in GC-treated rats also varies depending on the dose, duration or predisposing factors (*e.g.*, pregnancy, obesity and aging) (Novelli et al., 1999; Holness & Sugden, 2001). Normal male adult rats receiving 0.1, 0.5 or 1 mg/kg *b.w.* of DEX for 1 to 3 days do not exhibit glucose intolerance during a glucose load; however, when these rats are submitted to 5 days of DEX treatment at 1 mg/kg *b.w.* they become glucose intolerant (Rafacho et al., 2008). Thus, for low doses and/or short periods of GC administration, the elevation in insulin secretion is sufficient to prevent any derangement in glucose homeostasis. However, for higher doses and/or prolonged periods of GC treatment, these normal rats are unable to fully compensate for the metabolic demand and glucose intolerance appears, despite the marked increase in insulin response to glucose. Whether increased levels of lipids, like non-esterified fatty acids (NEFA), contribute to this metabolic perturbation deserves investigation, but there is already evidence that increased lipolysis may affect insulinogenic index under GC-induced IR in normal rats (Novelli et al., 2008). It is also important to mention that GC-treated elderly rats (Novelli et al., 1999), high-fat diet rats (Holness et al., 2005) or pregnant rats (Holness & Sugden, 2001) become intolerant to glucose after a sugar challenge that is associated with a decreased insulinogenic index. Notably, all above alterations by GC treatment are transitory and normalized after discontinuation of steroid administration in healthy rats (Rafacho et al., 2010).

GC R	Dosing	Insulin sensitivity (IS) Glucose tolerance (GT)	Fasting glycemia	Fasting insulinemia	Insulin secretion	Reference
Dex----	5 μg *b.i.d.* for 3 or 4 d in male SD	Decreased IS	Modest increase	Increased	Increased	(Stojanovska et al., 1990)
Dex*i.p*	2 mg/kg *b.w.* for 7 d in female SD	-----	-----	-----	Increased 1st phase, but not 2nd in isolated islets	(O'Brien et al., 1991)
Dex*i.p.*	5 mg/kg for 24 d (male and female?)	Decreased IS in normal animals	Unaltered	-----	Increased	(Ogawa et al., 1992)
Dex----	0.125 mg/kg *b.w. b.i.d.* for 4 d in male SD	-----	Unaltered	Increased	-----	(Koranyi et al., 1992)
Dex*s.c.*	4 mg/kg *b.w.* for 10 d -----	-----	-----	-----	Increased	(Wang et al., 1994)
Dex*s.c.*	0,125 mg/kg *b.w.* for 13 d in 3-, 18- and 26-month old in male SD	-----	Unaltered for 3-month old and marked increase for 18- and 26-month old	Increased in age-dependent manner	Increased mainly in young animals and in less extent in olders	(Novelli et al., 1999)
Dex*i.p.*	2 mg/kg *b.w.* for 12 d in female SD	-----	Fed moderate hyperglycemia	Fed increase	Increased	(Karlsson et al., 2001)
Dex*s.c.*	100 μg /kg *b.w* for 6 d in non-pregnant Wistar	Modest decrease in GT	Unaltered	Increased	Increased	(Holness & Sugden, 2001)
Dex*s.c.*	1 μg b.i.d. for 4 wk	Decreased IS	Unaltered	Increased	Increased	(Severino et al., 2002)
Dexoral	10 or 100 μg /kg *b.w.* for 8 wk in male SD	Decreased IS	Unaltered	Increased for both	-----	(Choi et al., 2006)
Dex*i.p.*	0.1, 0.5 or 1 mg/kg *b.w.* for 5 d on Wistar	Decreased IS in all Decreased GT (0.5 and 1 mg)	Modest increase with high dose	Dose-dependent increase	Increased dose dependently	(Rafacho et al., 2008)

GC R	Dosing	Insulin sensitivity (IS) Glucose tolerance (GT)	Fasting glycemia	Fasting insulinemia	Insulin secretion	Reference
Dex*i.p*	0.125 mg/kg *b.w.* for 20 d in SD	Decreased IS	Unaltered	Increased	Increased	(Novelli et al., 2008)
Dex*i.p.*	0.2 mg/kg *b.w.* for 2 d in male Wistar	-----	Modest increase	Increased	Increased	(Sood & Ismail-Beigi, 2010)
Dex*i.p.*	1 mg/kg *b.w.* for 1, 3 or 5 d in male Wistrar	Decreased IS - 3 and 5 d Decreased GT – 5 d	Tendency towards on 5 d	Time-dependent increase	Increased in all	(Rafacho et al., 2011)

R; route, **b.i.d.;** twice a day (from Latin *bis in die*), **d;** day, **Dex;** dexamethasone, **SD;** Sprague-Dawley, -----; none

Table 2. Effects of prolonged GC treatment in normal rats on endocrine pancreas parameters.

2.2.3. Ex vivo insulin secretion by isolated islets from GC-treated rats

Islet insulin secretion in response to several stimuli, especially glucose, has been found to be reduced (Ogawa et al., 1992; Ohneda et al., 1993), unchanged (Chuthaputti & Fletcher, 1987; O'Brien et al., 1991) or increased (Wang et al., 1994; Novelli et al., 1999; Barbera et al., 2001; Karlsson et al., 2001; Giozzet et al., 2008; Rafacho et al., 2008; Rafacho et al., 2009; Rafacho et al., 2010; Sood & Ismail-Beigi, 2010; Rafacho et al., 2011) in GC-treated rats. The abrogation of insulin secretion by glucose is observed in Wistar rats vulnerable to GC treatment (that develop a diabetic profile after steroid treatment) (Ogawa et al., 1992) or in a Zucker fatty strain (*fa*/*fa*) (Ogawa et al., 1992; Ohneda et al., 1993). In islets from these rats, a chronological association between reductions in glucose transporter (GLUT)-2 immunolocalization in β-cells and glucose uptake in islets with the development of hyperglycemia is found (Ohneda et al., 1993). The reduction of GLUT2 could however not fully explain the total loss of GSIS in these rats if one considers that the remaining β-cells with intact GLUT2 distribution maintain a normal insulin response to glucose. These findings, if reproduced in humans, speak against the use of GCs in conditions where the insulin demand is already increased prior to GC treatment.

The most prominent functional islet adaptation, when rats are challenged with steroids, is the increased insulin response to glucose. This adaptation most likely occurs to compensate for GC-induced IR. This enhancement of β-cell function, also observed in humans, is anticipated in healthy individuals and guarantees a regular disposition index (the product of insulin secretion and peripheral insulin sensitivity). Figure 1 shows an overview of some already known mechanisms involved in this enhanced islet function and the proposed modes of interference by GC treatment. The β-cell possesses a unique signal transduction system dependent on metabolism of fuel stimuli to initiate insulin secretion (Matschinsky, 1996). Glycolytic and oxidative metabolism accelerates the generation of adenosine triphosphate (ATP). A rise in the cytosolic ATP/adenosine diphosphate (ADP) ratio is believed to close metabolically sensitive K^+ channels (K_{ATP} channels), leading to depolarization of the β-cell membrane. This activates voltage-gated Ca^{2+} channels and elevates intracellular Ca^{2+} concentration ($[Ca^{2+}]_i$), and culminates in the exocytosis of insulin-containing granules. In addition, elevation of $[Ca^{2+}]_i$ activates a number of potentiating signaling pathways, including protein kinase A (PKA) and protein kinase C (PKC), which amplify insulin release (Nesher et al., 2002).

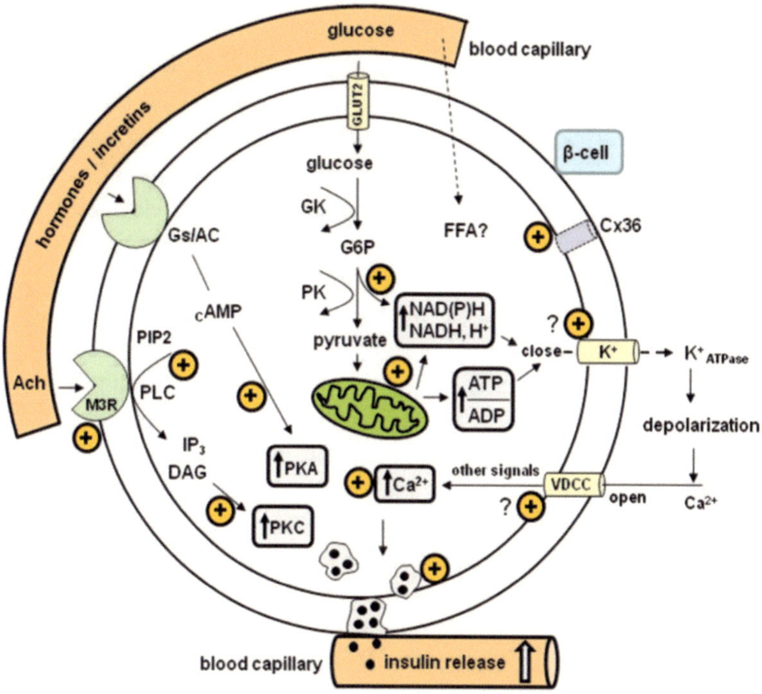

Figure 1. Insulin secretory process in β-cells from GC-treated rats. The known components involved in the adaptive increase in β-cell function after GC treatment are highlighted with a positive signal (orange circle), which indicates increased content or activity of the component after GC treatment. Most notably, increased glucose metabolism and cholinergic pathway activity cause increased calcium influx and insulin secretion. Abbreviations: AC, adenylyl cyclase; Ach, acetylcholine; ADP, adenosine diphosphate; ATP, adenosine triphosphate; cAMP, cyclic adenosine monophosphate; Cx36, connexin 36; DAG, diacylglycerol; FFA, free fatty acids; G6P, glucose-6-phosphatase; Gs. G-coupled stimulatory protein; GK, glucokinase; GLUT2, glucose transporter 2; IP3, inositol trisphosphate; M3R, muscarinic receptor type 3; NADH, nicotinamide dinucleotide; NAD(P)H, nicotinamide adenonine dinucleotide phosphate; PIP2, phosphatidylinositol bisphosphate; PK, pyruvate kinase; PKA, protein kinase A; PKC, protein kinase C; PLC, phospholipase C; VDCC, voltage-dependent calcium channel. Modified from Nussey & Whitehead, 2001; Endocrinology: An integrated approach, box 2.19 (Nussey & Whitehead, 2001).

The establishment of any direct GC effects on β-cells under *in vivo* conditions is difficult, since systemic metabolic consequences of GC treatment (*e.g.*, circulating factors changing such glucose, NEFA, and other metabolites and hormones) probably interfere with GC-mediated changes in β-cell function (van Raalte et al., 2009). Islets isolated from GC-treated rats have enhanced glucose responsiveness (Novelli et al., 1999; Barbera et al., 2001; Karlsson et al., 2001; Rafacho et al., 2008; Sood & Ismail-Beigi, 2010), higher glucose sensitivity (lower EC_{50} values to glucose) (Giozzet et al., 2008; Rafacho et al., 2008), and exhibit pronounced first and second phase insulin secretion in response to glucose (Rafacho et al., 2008; Rafacho et al., 2011). The glycolytic components seem not to be involved in such augmented insulin response, since mRNA and protein contents of GLUT2, glucokinase (GK) and pyruvate kinase (PK) are unaltered in islets from DEX-treated rats (Rafacho et al., 2010; Sood & Ismail-Beigi, 2010). However, these data do not exclude that GK and/or PK activities may be elevated since enzymatic activities have not been measured directly. Indirect determination of reduced nicotinamide adenine dinucleotide phosphate [NAD(P)H] generation and mitochondrial function, by NAD(P)H autofluorescence and rhodamine 123 fluorescence, respectively, indicate increased glucose metabolism in islets from GC-treated rats (Rafacho et al., 2010). These authors did not determine the islet ATP content but found augmented $[Ca^{2+}]_i$ in response to glucose that was not a result of elevated basal $[Ca^{2+}]_i$. The glucose-induced elevation in $[Ca^{2+}]_i$ appeared not to involve significant changes in K_{ATP} channels or voltage-gated Ca^{2+} channels response, since islets from DEX-treated rats perfused with high K^+ or tolbutamide did not show higher $[Ca^{2+}]_i$ compared to control islets. These data give a clear indication of enhanced glucose sensitivity in islets from GC-treated rats. The amplifying pathway of GSIS, which involves activation of Ca^{2+}-dependent kinases, is altered in GC-treated rat islets. DEX-treated rats have high islet content of phosphorylated PKCα protein that is associated with increased number of docked insulin-containing granules (Rafacho et al., 2010) as well as higher insulin secretion in response to the PKC activator phorbol 12-myristate 13-acetate (PMA) (Rafacho et al., 2010). In addition, the cholinergic pathway, mediated by phospholipase C (PLC)/inositol triphosphate (IP3) / PKC signals, contributes to such an increase in β-cell function in GC-treated rats. The insulin secretion and $[Ca^{2+}]_i$ are increased in response to cholinergic stimulation in islets from GC-treated rats (Rafacho et al., 2008; Rafacho et al., 2010). It is known that DEX-treated rats exhibit higher islet content of muscarinic receptor type 3 (M3R) and PLC β1. These islets are less responsive to cholinergic blockade during dynamic insulin secretion experiments in the presence of stimulatory concentrations of glucose and cholinergic agonists (Angelini et al., 2010). Corroborating this hypothesis, vagus dennervation partially abrogated the hyperinsulinemic profile in DEX-treated rats (Angelini et al., 2010). Notwithstanding the important role of glucose metabolism and cholinergic signals for the increased β-cell function in GC-treated rat models, the involvement of non-glucidic insulin secretagogues (amino acids and NEFA) (Novelli et al., 1999; Rafacho et al., 2010), non-metabolic signals (Rafacho et al., 2010), cyclic adenosine monophosphate (cAMP)-dependent protein kinases (Rafacho et al., 2010), and gap junctional intercellular communications (formed by connexin 36 protein in β-cells) (Rafacho et al., 2007) are also observed in these rats. All this information indicates that several factors are involved in augmentation of the insulin secretion response in islets isolated from GC-treated rats. It was recently demonstrated that insulin hypersecretion precedes any discernible indication of IR in DEX-treated rats (Rafacho et al., 2011). After 24 hours of DEX administration, rats become hyperinsulinemic and exhibit increased GSIS concomitant with normal blood glucose values, normal lipidemia, and without any evidence of IR. As the treatment continues, IR unfolds and islets become more responsive to glucose. A possible explanation for the early increase of insulin release may reside in central nervous system (CNS) signals. Direct administration of DEX to the CNS appears to increase parasympathetic system activity, resulting in augmented plasma insulin levels (Zakrzewska et al., 1999). This observation is in agreement with the results obtained with ganglionic antagonist infusion in DEX-induced IR and insulin hypersecretion in human volunteers as described before (Ahrén, 2008). Of note, all these altered *ex vivo* islet responses are transitory and reversible after discontinuation of GC treatment (Karlsson et al., 2001; Wierup et al., 2006; Rafacho et al., 2010); however, great caution is required in translating these observation to human applications.

2.2.4. Structural changes in pancreatic islets in response to GC treatment in rats

Compensatory islet hypertrophy in response to GC treatment *in vivo* was first described in the eighties (Jonas et al., 1983; Tomita et al., 1984; Zwicker & Eyster, 1993). The mechanisms involved in islet hypertrophy were elucidated several years later (Rafacho et al., 2007; Rafacho et al., 2008; Rafacho et al., 2009). Activation of cell cycle progression machinery in normal rats in response to GC treatment is probably associated with the degree of IR that in turn is correlated to dose and/or duration of GC administration (Rafacho et al., 2009; Rafacho et al., 2011) and does not involve direct effects of GCs on β-cells, since it is known that steroids inhibit β-cell proliferation and promote β-cell death *in vitro* (Weinhaus et al., 2000; Liu et al., 2006; Ranta et al., 2006; Nicoletti-Carvalho et al., 2010). Instead, increased levels of circulating hormones and/or substrates, such as glucose, insulin, insulin-growth factor (IGF)-1, glucagon-like peptide (GLP)-1 and other circulating growth factors, may be responsible for promotion of β-cell growth in GC-treated rats [for review see references (Heit et al., 2006) and (Vasavada et al., 2006)]. β-cell proliferation is significantly increased after 5 days of DEX treatment in a positive reciprocity with steroid dose (1.0 mg/kg > 0.5 mg/kg *b.w.*), but absent when IR is modest as in 5-days 0.1 mg/kg *b.w.* DEX treatment (Rafacho et al., 2009). The same correlation between IR degree and β-cell proliferation is observed when analyzed during time-course studies. After 1 day GC treatment, no changes in β-cell proliferation are observed and IR is not discernible. However, as GC treatment continues (3 to 5 days), IR develops and and the increase in β-cell proliferation is correlated with the degree of IR (Rafacho et al., 2011). With some combinations of GC treatment, β-cell hypertrophy is also observed (Choi et al., 2006; Rafacho et al., 2009). Thus, β-cell hypertrophy and/or proliferation accounts for increased β-cell mass upon GC treatment (Choi et al., 2006; Rafacho et al., 2010, Rafacho, 2009). This augmentation in β-cell mass is associated with increased islet protein content of insulin receptor substrate (IRS)-2, phosphorylated serine-threonine kinase (PKB), cyclin D (Cd)-2, cyclin-dependent kinase (Cdk)-4, phosphorylated retinoblastoma protein (pRb), but not with activation of extracellular-regulated kinase (Erk)-1/2 (Rafacho et al., 2008; Rafacho et al., 2009). Considering that plasma insulin concentrations increase in a GC dose- and/or time-dependent manner, it is conceivable that circulating insulin is one candidate mediator of β-cell growth. In addition, these GC-induced IR models do not exhibit changes in β-cell death (Rafacho et al., 2009; Rafacho et al., 2010) and almost all morphological changes are transitory and reversible after 10 days discontinuation of steroid treatment, suggesting an unacknowledged plasticity in the regulation of β-cell growth.

Taken altogether, like in humans, rats subjected to prolonged steroid treatment develop increased β-cell function as an adaptive compensation to surpass GC-induced IR. Susceptible strains; however, are prone to develop β-cell dysfunction that results in impaired glucose homeostasis. The β-cell growth accompanies the requirement for insulin in a direct relation with IR and demonstrates a great plasticity of endocrine pancreas to face fluctuations in metabolic demand.

2.3. Functional and structural changes in pancreatic islets in GC-treated mice

Less is known about *in vivo* GC effects in normal mice than in rats. Acute administration of hydrocortisone (300 mg/kg *b.w.*) to male Swiss mice inhibits insulin secretion (Longano & Fletcher, 1983) with reduced insulinogenic index already after 1 h of steroid administration. The insulin secretion in response to *i.v.* glucose load is also suppressed in this hydrocortisone model and may involve increased sympathetic drive. In response to prolonged DEX treatment (2½ days, with a dose equivalent to 1 mg/kg *b.w.*) islets isolated from normal adult mice show a modest decrease in insulin response to either 5.5 mM or 16.7 mM glucose. However, when the increment in insulin release between 5.5 mM and 16.7 mM glucose is calculated, a higher insulin response in DEX-treated animals as compared to vehicle treated mice is noted. As blood glucose and insulinemia were not determined in this experiment (Ling et al., 1998), which could indicate any deleterious GC effects on glucose homeostasis, caution should be exerted as to making conclusions about GC effects in normal mice.

Most of the data obtained with mouse models come from studies in genetically obese, leptin deficient mice (*ob/ob*) that display IR (Table 3). Obese mice treated with 25 μg DEX for 1 to 2½ days (at a dose equivalent to 0.5 mg/kg *b.w.*) exhibit increased islet glucose cycling (dephosphorylation of glucose-6-phosphate [G6P] to glucose by glucose-6-phosphatase [G6Pase]) both at 5.5 mM and at 16.7 mM glucose, but at the same time unaltered islet glucose oxidation and utilization. These results are associated with diminished or inhibited GSIS (Figure 2) (Khan et al., 1992; Khan et al., 1995). In an attempt to extrapolate these observations and determine whether they are caused by direct islet effects of GC *in vivo*, a transgenic mouse that overexpresses the GR specifically in β-cells was generated (Delaunay et al., 1997). These mice also displayed increased glucose cycling, mild glucose intolerance, decreased insulinogenic index and GSIS, but remained normoglycaemic (Delaunay et al., 1997; Ling et al., 1998). DEX treatment increased glucose cycling and the impairment of GSIS in this transgenic model. Again, islet glucose utilization and oxidation in the transgenic mice were comparable to those in control animals, demonstrating that the enhanced glucose flux trough G6Pase does not alter glucose utilization. Moreover, glucose cycling is neglible in normal rodents (≈ 3%) and appears not to be a plausible explanation of the inhibitory effect of insulin release by DEX (Khan et al., 1992). The impact of direct GC effects in β-cells is better demonstrated in 11- to 12-month-old transgenic mice (GR-overexpressing at β-cells). At this age, mice developed hyperglycemia and hypoinsulinemia, glucose intolerance, borderline IR (not significant), and decreased GSIS both *in vivo* and *ex vivo*. The reduction of GSIS was abolished after incubation of islets with an antagonist of α2-adrenergic receptor (α2-AdrR) that is associated with increased islet mRNA and α2-AdrR density. No alterations in GLUT2 distribution or in β-cell apoptosis were detected (Davani et al., 2004). Thus, the adrenergic signals (Figure 2) may participate in this impaired β-cell response caused by acutely or for more prolonged periods GC treatment. The transgenic approach revealed valuable information regarding the specific GC effects upon β-cells, but it does not take into account the overall metabolic GC effects. Studies conducted in adult mice treated with GCs, where peripheral effects of GCs are preserved, have shown increased circulating insulin levels when IR is apparent, but investigation of β-cell function and structure was not done (Thomas et al., 1998; Karatsoreos et al., 2010). In summary, acute GC treatment induces reduction of β-cell function in mice and this effect is accelerated in susceptible mice (old, obese or GR-overexpressing), which is in agreement with the deleterious effects of GCs on β-cell function known from studies with predisposed human individuals and in certain rat models. Nevertheless, GC effects on β-cell function and growth in normal mice are not known and merit further investigation.

GC	R	Dosing	Insulin sensitivity (IS) Glucose tolerance (GT)	Fasting glycemia	Fasting insulinemia	Insulin secretion	Reference
Dex	*i.p.*	1 or 2 d of 25 μg for ob/ob mice weighing around 50 g	-----	Unaltered in both	Unaltered in 48 h, but not determined in 24 h	Decreased (24 h) or inhibited (48 h)	(Khan et al., 1992)
Dex	*i.p.*	2 ½ d of 25 μg for ob/ob mice weighing more than 50 g	-----	-----	-----	-----	(Khan et al., 1995)
-----	-----	Transgenic adult mice	Mild decrease in GT	Unaltered	Modest decrease only in 1 from 2 groups analyzed	Decreased	(Delaunay et al., 1997)
Dex	*i.p.*	25 μg for 2 ½ d in normal or transgenic adult weighing around 25 g	-----	Unaltered between transgenic and controls	-----	Decreased in normal and transgenic	(Ling et al., 1998)
-----	-----	12-15 month-old transgenic mice	Tendency towards decrease in IS Decreased GT	Increased	Decreased	Decreased	(Davani et al., 2004)

d; day, **Dex;** dexamethasone, **R;** route, **Transgenic;** glucocoticoid receptor overexpression under rat insulin promoter 1, **-----;** none

Table 3. Effects of prolonged GC treatment in *ob/ob* or transgenic mice on endocrine pancreas parameters.

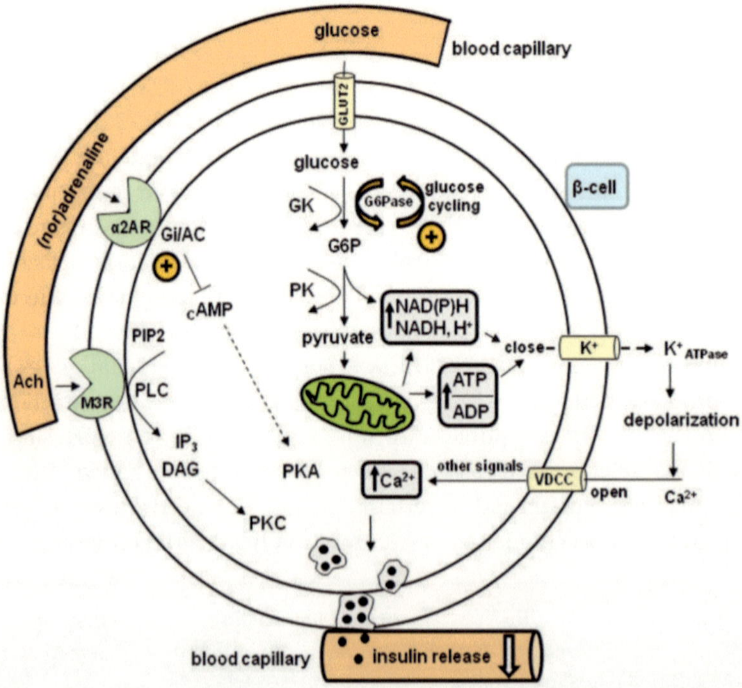

Figure 2. Insulin secretory process in β-cells from GC-treated mice. The known components involved in the reduced β-cell function are highlighted with a positive signal (orange circle), which indicates increased content or activity of the component after GC treatment. Most notably is the increased adrenergic activity that seems to inhibit insulin secretion. Abbreviations: AC, adenylyl cyclase; Ach, acetylcholine; ADP, adenosine diphosphate; ATP, adenosine trisphosphate; cAMP, cyclic adenosine monophosphate; DAG, diacylglycerol; G6P, glucose-6-phosphatase; Gi, G-coupled inhibitory protein; GK, glucokinase; GLUT2, glucose transporter 2; IP3, inositol trisphosphate; M3R, muscarinic receptor type 3; NADH, nicotinamide dinucleotide; NAD(P)H, nicotinamide adenonine dinucleotide phosphate; PIP2, phosphatidylinositol bisphosphate; PK, pyruvate kinase; PKA, protein kinase A; PKC, protein kinase C; PLC, phospholipase C; VDCC, voltage-dependent calcium channel. Modified from Nussey & Whitehead, 2001; Endocrinology: An integrated approach, box 2.19 (Nussey & Whitehead, 2001).

2.4. Direct glucocorticoid effects on insulin secretion and β-cell growth in islets and β-cell lines

In vitro, as *in vivo*, it is difficult to determine with accuracy the specific factors involved in the GC effects on β-cell function. This is because *in vitro* culture does not mimic perfectly the metabolic *milieu* of an intact system *in vivo*. For example, the timing, duration and level of exposure to GC compounds, the concentration range of serum and/or glucose in the culture medium, the concentration and variety of insulin secretagogues chosen, and the β cell (isolated islets, dispersed islet β-cells, β-cell lines) and species (human, hamster, rat or mouse islets) vary (Santerre et al., 1981; Lambillotte et al., 1997; Myrsén-Axcrona et al., 1997; Fabregat et al., 1999; Jeong et al., 2001; Shao et al., 2004; Arumugam et al., 2008; Swali et al., 2008; Roma et al., 2011). Despite the repercussions of these variables, *in vitro* insights have been of great importance to elucidate the direct effects of GCs on insulin secretion.

2.4.1. Acute GC effects

Rodent-derived islets or dispersed β-cells have diminished or inhibited insulin response to non-metabolizable and metabolizable secretagogues, especially to glucose, both after acute (minutes) (Billaudel & Sutter, 1979; Barseghian & Levine, 1980) or prolonged (hours to days) GC exposure (Lambillotte et al., 1997; Weinhaus et al., 2000; Jeong et al., 2001; Zawalich et al., 2006). In the presence of three different concentrations (physiological and supraphysiological), corticosterone does not affect rat islet insulin secretion under basal glucose conditions, whereas, in response to 16.7 mM glucose, insulin release is inhibited. This study emphasizes that physiological corticosterone concentrations (0.02 and 0.2 mg/L) have strong negative impact on insulin secretion (Billaudel & Sutter, 1979). In the same trend, it was shown that cathecolaminergic signals may play a role in this process, since phentolamine, an α-AdrR blocking agent, ameliorated the strong inhibitory effect of corticosterone on insulin release (Barseghian & Levine, 1980). This immediate negative effect of corticosterone on insulin release is not reproduced by the synthetic GC DEX in isolated mouse (Lambillotte et al., 1997) or rat islets (Zawalich et al., 2006). Thus, acute GC effects on insulin release appear to be more evident with natural corticosterone used at physiological concentrations.

2.4.2. Hours to days GC effects

The inhibition of insulin secretion by GCs begins after 3 to 6 hours (Lambillotte et al., 1997; Weinhaus et al., 2000; Zawalich et al., 2006). The mechanisms by which this occurs are not completely understood, but several components are already identified as shown in a schematic overview and the proposed loci of interference by GCs in Figure 3. Details regarding GC compounds used, concentrations, duration of treatment, and main effects on β-cell function are described in Table 4. The GC-induced reduction in GSIS could not be attributed to decreases in insulin content since it was unchanged or augmented (Pierluissi et al., 1986; Gremlich et al., 1997; Lambillotte et al., 1997; Zawalich et al., 2006), although reduction was also observed under certain conditions (Jeong et al., 2001). It has been shown that presence of DEX in islet or β-cell culture medium induces reduction (Gremlich et al., 1997) or no change (Shao et al., 2004) in GLUT 2 protein content, decrease in β-cell GK (Shao et al., 2004) and pyruvate dehydrogenase (PDH) (Arumugam et al., 2010) activities, and increased pyruvate dehydrogenase kinase (PDK)-2 mRNA content (Arumugam et al., 2010). Despite alterations of these proximal metabolic components, the failure of β-cells' response to glucose does not appear to involve a defect in the recognition of glucose, because no changes in the rate of glucose oxidation (Lambillotte et al., 1997; Zawalich et al., 2006), oxygen consumption (Ortsäter et al., 2005), NAD(P)H production (Lambillotte et al., 1997), or $[Ca^{2+}]_i$ (Lambillotte et al., 1997) have been observed. There are controversies related to Ca^{2+} influx in response to glucose or non-glucidic stimuli (Myrsén-Axcrona et al., 1997; Koizumi & Yada, 2008), but in spite of elevation or reduction in Ca^{2+} influx, there is consensus that Ca^{2+} oscillations are impaired, which may harm the distal events of secretion dependent of finely tuned Ca^{2+} handling.

GC	Dose and period, and β-cell source	Main results	Reference
Cort	0.02, 0.2 or 20 mg/l along first min in isolated rat islets	With 4.2 mM glucose, Cort did not affect IS, but with 16.7 mM glucose IS was inhibited by the three Cort concentrations tested during static incubation, and by the two physiological during islets perifusion	(Billaudel & Sutter, 1979)
Cort	Physiological Cort concentrations along first in rat pancreas	Acutely inhibit the IS induced by both glucose and arginine. Phentolamine, an α-adrenergic blocking agent, diminished the strong inhibitory effect of Cort on IS	(Barseghian & Levine, 1980)
Dex	0.1-1.0 μM for 6, 48 or 96 h in hamster β-cell line (HIT)	Inhibited the IS to the culture medium after 48 or 96 h, but not to 6 h	(Santerre et al., 1981)
Dex Pred Hydr	0.063, 0.63 or 6.3 μM for 1, 2 or 3h in rat islets	No alteration at 2 mM glucose, but reduced GSIS (20 mM) when cultured with 6.3 μM Dex for 1, 2 or 3h or 2 h with 0.063 μM or 630 μM for islet culture. The reduced GSIS under 6.3 μM for 2 h culture was also seen with 7.5, 10, 12.5, 15, 20 and 30 mM glucose. These responses were re-established after 4 h. Pred and Hydr also induced decreased GSIS and none of these drugs elicit a decrease in islet insulin content	(Pierluissi et al., 1986)
Dex Pred Hydr	24 h in HIT-T15 or RIN-5AH cells	Dex, Pred and Hydr induced an increase of α2-AdrR in HIT cells that was prevented by the GR antagonist RU38486. 1μM Dex also induced increased expression of receptor in RIN-5 cells	(Hamamdzic et al., 1995)
Dex	1 μM for 18 h in mouse islets	Dex had inhibitory effect from the 3rd h incubation. Cultured islets in presence of Dex 1 μM had higher insulin content than control and the reversibility of GSIS in islets treated with 0.25 μM dex was observed after 3 h of DEX discontinuation. 20 mM glucose in the medium or the presence of KIC did not change the inhibitory effect of Dex; however, PMA, cAMP or inhibition of α2-AdrR was able to attenuate or reversed the negative action of 18 h 1 μM Dex. The presence of pertussis toxin abolished the negative effect of Dex. IS continues inhibited even after stimulation with tolbutamide, high glucose and diazoxide. Glucose oxidation and NAD(P)H were similar between both islet groups in presence of 3 or 15 mM glucose. Dex islets had reduced response under high glucose during the dynamic protocol and the pattern of calcium oscillations were changed in Dex islets. IS and calcium influx were also lower in response to Cch in Dex islets	(Lambillotte et al., 1997)
Dex	1 μM for 48 h in rat islets	Dex induced a decrease in GLUT2 protein expression in a glucose-dependent manner that is blunted by RU486. Addition of palmitic acid had no additive effect on the reduction of GLUT2 protein	(Gremlich et al., 1997)

GC	Dose and period, and β-cell source	Main results	Reference
		expression compared to Dex alone. Dex induced an inhibition of GSIS that was also evidenced by palmitic acid alone or in combination with Dex. The total islet insulin content were decreased in response to the palmitic acid whereas were increased by Dex. The effect of Dex was inhibited by RU486	
Dex	100 nM for 1 to 5 d in RINm5 cells	Dex induced an increase in NPY mRNA expression in a time-dependent manner. It also induced an increase in NPY immunoreactivity. Dex treated cells had less IS to the medium, whereas increased NPY release. IS in several conditions was reduced in cells treated with Dex. The D-glyceraldehyde-induced raise in $[Ca^{2+}]_i$ was impaired after Dex treatment. Also, the increase in cytosolic calcium when stimulated with KCl was lowered by Dex.	(Myrsén-Axcrona et al., 1997)
Dex	1 nM – 1 μM during 6 d culture in 5 d neonate rat islets	After 6 d culture, 10 nM to 1 μM Dex markedly reduced the content of IS to the medium in control and in PRL-treated islets. Dex (100 nM) exerted its effects since the 1st day culture and abolished the positive effects of PRL when incubated together with PRL. Six d of 100 nM Dex inhibited the IS from 2.8 to 7.2 or 13.5mM glucose alone or in combination with PRL, but did not induce a decrease in total islet insulin content	(Weinhaus et al., 2000)
11-DHC	50 or 500 nM 11-DHC for 20 h in ob/ob mouse islets	Incubation of β cells in the presence of 11-DHC led to a dose-dependent inhibition of IS. Inhibition of 11β-HSD1 activity by carbenoxolone reversed inhibition of IS	(Davani et al., 2004)
Dex	1, 10 or 100 nM for 1 to 6 h in rat islets	IS decreased in a time- and dose-dependent manner being significant already after the 1st h incubation within 10 or 100 nM Dex, but not for 1 nM until the 6th h culture. The 1st, but not 2nd phase GSIS were reduced in response to 10 or 100 nM Dex (Dex were exposed only during perifusion). The islet insulin content was higher in islets from 1, 10 and 100nM culture after 1 h treatment and reduced for only 100 nM after 6 h. After 6, but not 1 h, 10 and 100 nM Dex reduced the pre-proinsulin mRNA content.	(Jeong et al., 2001)
Dex	50 ng/ml -1ug/ml for 24 h in MIN6 cells	Dex from 50 ng to 1mg/ml inhibited IS to the culture medium after 24 h. Dex (100 nM) inhibited GSIS in a time-dependent fashion from the 6 h to 48 h treatment. Dex (100nM) did not change GK protein content, but inhibited GK activity from the 6 h ahead and did not affect the GLUT2 protein content during long term treatments. Even in response to KIC Dex-treated cells had inhibited IS. Dex induces a	(Shao et al., 2004)

GC	Dose and period, and β-cell source	Main results	Reference
		reduction in cAMP content that was prevented by the presence of the inhibitor of the PDE. The increase in PDE activity was confirmed after Dex treatment	
Dex	100 nM for 4h in mouse islets or INS1 cells. For IHC, mice received 1 injection of 10 mg/kg *b.w.* Dex and killed 24 h after	After 4 h 100 nM Dex it was observed increased mRNA expression of Kv-1.5 (repolarizing K channel). This was associated with increased SGK1 mRNA and protein expression in a time-dependent manner (INS1 cells) and immunoreactivity in mice islet pancreas. All analysis in cells was abrogated by the presence of RU486. The activity of Kv-1.5 channel was increased after Dex treatment and mediated by SGK1, that was associated to reduced $[Ca^{2+}]_i$ peaks in response to glucose. The inhibited GSIS in DEX-treated INS1 cells and mouse islets were reverted by the presence of K channel inhibitors TEA and MSD. Presence of diazoxide and high KCL also reversed the insulin secretion in DEX-treated INS1 cells. SGK1 knockout mice did not present the same reduction in GSIS.	(Ullrich et al., 2005)
11-DHC	5, 50 or 500 nM 11-DHC for 48 h in *ob/ob* mouse islets	Islets from the ob/ob mouse contained almost twofold more 11β-HSD1 protein than islets from the C57BL/6J mouse. When islets from ob/ob mice were cultured with 50 nM 11-DHC, the 11β-HSD1 levels doubled compared with islets cultured in the absence of DHC. Selective inhibition of 11β-HSD1 attenuated DHC-induced increase in 11β-HSD1 levels, as did an antagonist of the GR. In individually perfused *ob/ob* mouse islets, early and late phases of GSIS were dose-dependently inhibited by 11-DHC. Whereas inclusion of 11β-HSD1 inhibitors restored, addition of the GR antagonist attenuated the DHC-mediated inhibition of GSIS.	(Ortsäter et al., 2005)
Dex	100 nM for 3 d in BRIN-BD 11 cells	DEX-treated cells lacked responsiveness to glucose and membrane depolarisation, and both PKA and PKC secretory pathways were desensitised.	(Liu et al., 2006)
Dex	1 μM concomitant or for 3 h previous culture in rat islets	Dex (included in the perifusion solution) has no effect on GSIS. Previous incubation with Dex markedly decrease the 1st and the 2nd phases IS under 15 mM glucose. This result was not associated to reduction in insulin content or glucose oxidation. IS was also reduced in response to TPA or KCl in Dex islets. Dex also reduces the agonist-induced inositol phosphate accumulation in islets, but did not change the protein content of 5 different PLC protein isoforms. Significant reductions in glucose-induced IP accumulation accompanied the reduction	(Zawalich et al., 2006)

GC	Dose and period, and β-cell source	Main results	Reference
		in GSIS. Islet exposed to Dex for 3 h contained protein amounts of PLC isoforms and PKCα comparable to control islets. No impairment in label incorporation, used to monitor PLC activation under these conditions, was observed	
Dex Cort	10 - 500 ng/ml Cort or 1μg/ml Dex for 3 d in dispersed rat β-cells	Cort (10 to 500 ng/ml) decreased the Ca^{2+} response to glucose in β-cells, which were GR dependent (Ru486). Dex (1ug/ml, but not 10 ng/ml) reduced Ca^{2+} response to glucose in β-cells. Co-incubation of Cort with aldosterone revealed a protective role for aldosterone.	(Koizumi & Yada, 2008)
Dex	100 nM for 1 d in INS1 cells	Dex upregulated the expression of SGK1 in INS1 cells and increased plasma membrane Na+/K+ ATPase activity.	(Ullrich et al., 2007)
Dex Hydr	100 nM Dex for 20 h in INS1 cells	Dex upregulated FoxO1, PGC1α, PPARγ, CPT-1, and UCP-2 mRNAs inhibited GSIS in INS1 cells. Hydr had similar effects.	(Arumugam et al., 2008)
Dex Cort 11-DHC	For 2 h in mouse islets	11β-HSD1 co-localized with glucagon in the periphery of murine and human islets, but not with insulin or somatostatin. Incubation (2 h) of islets from normal mice to Dex resulted in a dramatic reduction of IS in a dose-dependent manner that was GR-dependent (RU486). Cort (50 nM) and 11-DHC (11β-HSD1-mediated) induced inhibition of GSIS. Dex, Cort and 11-DHC also decreased glucagon release, and the effect of 11-DHC was partially prevented by enzyme inhibitor	(Swali et al., 2008)
Dex	100 nM Dex for 48 h in rat islets or 3 h in 100 nM Dex in RINm5F cells	Dex time- and dose-dependently increased total FoxO1 mRNA and protein content together with decreased phosphorylation levels in RINm5F cells as well as islets. Presence of IGF-1 reverses these changes. Dex induced a nuclear localization of FoxO1. The mRNA content of FoxO1 were reduced in RINm5F cells after knockdown, which resulted in increased mRNA and protein levels of the PDX1 in cells cultivated in presence of Dex. Islets infected with Adenovirus-Foxo1-SiRNA had decreased FoxO1 protein content and had ameliorated GSIS.	(Zhang et al., 2009)
Dex	100 nM Dex for 24h in rat islets or INS1 cells	Dex did not alter PC protein or activity levels. Dex reduced PDH activity and had increased PDK2 mRNA in islets and INS-1 cells.	(Arumugam et al., 2010)
Dex	1 μM for 3 d in rat islets	Dex increased the ROS, decreased viability and GSIS, but did not change calcium handling. Dex treatment also resulted in reduction of catalase and synaptotagmine VII mRNA content.	(Roma et al., 2011)
Pred	Most effects achieved by 700	PRED inhibited GSIS and decreased both PDX1 and	(Linssen et

GC	Dose and period, and β-cell source	Main results	Reference
	nM after 20 h in INS1 cells	insulin expression, leading to a marked reduction in cellular insulin content. These PRED-induced detrimental effects were GR-mediated (RU486). PRED induced a GR-mediated activation of both ATF6 and IRE1/XBP1 pathways but was found to reduce the phosphorylation of PERK and its downstream substrate eIF2α. These modulations of ER stress pathways were accompanied by upregulation of calpain 10, increased cleaved caspase 3 and β-cell apoptosis.	al., 2011)

Dex; dexamethasone, **Pred;** prednisolone, **Cort;** corticosterone, **GSIS;** glucose-stimulated insulin secretion, **Hydr;** hydrocorticosterone, **IS;** insulin secretion, **11-DHC;** 11-hydroxysteroid dehydrogenase

Table 4. Effects of GCs *in vitro* on insulin secretion from islets, dispersed islet β-cells or β-cell lines.

The insulin secretory dysfunction induced by GCs is not solely restricted to glucose. Additional effects may contribute to β-cell dysfunction; impairment of insulin secretion in response to α-ketoisocaproate (KIC), tolbutamide, or high K^+ concentration after DEX treatment is also observed (Lambillotte et al., 1997; Shao et al., 2004; Liu et al., 2006), suggesting that factors distal to oxidative phosphorylation (KIC) or metabolism-independent signals (tolbutamide, high K^+) may also be involved in the adverse GC effects on the insulin secretory process. DEX may also modulate the inward repolarizing K^+ currents by upregulating $K_v1.5$ ion channels as well as Na^+/K^+ ATPase activity, which appear to be mediated through activation of the serum- and GC-inducible kinase (SGK1)-1 (Ullrich et al., 2005; Ullrich et al., 2007). These repolarizing currents may limit Ca^{2+} influx and insulin secretion. Downstream steps in the insulin secretory machinery also seem involved in the direct GC derangements in β-cells. Zawalich and colleagues (Zawalich et al., 2006) demonstrated that DEX pretreatment of rat islets impairs insulin secretion by decreasing activation of the PLC/PKC signaling pathway. Moreover, GCs increase the mRNA content and α-2AdrR protein density in β-cell lines (Hamamdzic et al., 1995), which may explain the lower cyclic adenosine monophosphate (cAMP) levels and attenuated GSIS (Shao et al., 2004). This latter event is prevented by phosphodiesterase (PDE) inhibitors, which aligns well with the upregulated PDE activity by DEX treatment (Shao et al., 2004), although controversy remains (Lambillotte et al., 1997). Overall, it appears that GCs act at distal sites by diminishing the efficacy of $[Ca^{2+}]_i$ on the secretory response by interfering with the amplifying pathway, although we cannot exclude their possible negative effects also in the mechanisms involved in the rapid first phase insulin secretion (Jeong et al., 2001). The interference of GCs in distal sites of the insulin secretory machinery may explain the wide spectrum of non-glucose insulin secretagogues being inhibited by GCs (Lambillotte et al., 1997; Myrsén-Axcrona et al., 1997; Shao et al., 2004; Liu et al., 2006).

2.4.3. Recent insights into GC effects on insulin secretion in vitro.

The mRNA content of Forkhead box O (FoxO)-1, peroxisome proliferator activator receptor (PPAR)-γ coactivator (PGC)-1α and uncoupling protein (UCP)-2 were upregulated in primary islets after 20 hours of DEX treatment (Arumugam et al., 2008). From these observations, it is expected that GC-induced derangements of GSIS can include limited production of cellular ATP due to UCP-2 mediated uncoupling of oxidative phosphorylation. In addition, increased PGC1-α action, which is associated with elevated fat acid oxidation, could induce impairments in insulin secretory process mediated by lack of critical lipid mediators involved in the amplifying pathway (Herrero et al., 2005). The GC-induced increment in total FoxO1 mRNA and protein content, as well as decreased levels of FoxO-1 phosphorylation in a rat insulinoma cell line (RINm5F), are time-and dose-dependent effects and appear to be mediated by the IGF-1 pathway (Zhang et al., 2009). Using molecular tools, it was demonstrated that lack of FoxO-1 ameliorates the DEX-induced impairment of GSIS in β-cell lines, an effect associated with increased levels of pancreatic duodenal homeobox (PDX)-1. It was recently demonstrated that presence of 1 μM DEX for 3 consecutive days in primary islet culture results in increased generation of reactive oxygen species (ROS) (Roma et al., 2011). This study also revealed impaired generation of NAD(P)H and reduced GSIS, decreased gene expression of catalase (an antioxidant enzyme) and synaptotagmin VII, without alteration in Ca^{2+} handling. These DEX effects were attenuated by N-acetylcysteine (NAC) (Roma et al., 2011), further supporting a role for ROS in mediating the cytotoxic effects of GCs. The role of endoplasmic reticulum (ER) homeostasis has also been investigated in the context of prednisolone-induced β-cell dysfunction. It has been observed that PDX-1 expression and cellular insulin content are reduced by steroid treatment (700 nM for 20 hours) in INS-1E cells, which resulted in inhibition of GSIS (Linssen et al., 2011). Prednisolone exerts its effects by activation of activating transcription factor (ATF)-6 and inositol requiring enzyme (IRE)-1/X-box binding protein (XBP)-1 pathways and by decreasing the phosphorylation of protein kinase RNA-activated (PKR)-like eukaryotic initiation factor 2α kinase (PERK) and its downstream substrate eukaryotic initiation (eIF2)-α. Thus, β-cell dysfunction induced by GCs may be, at least partially, attributed to ER dyshomeostasis. These mechanisms are depicted in Figure 3.

2.4.4. 11β-hydroxysteroid dehydrogenase type 1 and pancreatic islets

The enzyme 11β-hydroxysteroid dehydrogenase type 1 (11β-HSD1) catalyzes the conversion of inactive 11-dehydrocorsticosterone (11-DHC) to active corticosterone in rodents and it was found in pancreatic islets isolated from *ob/ob* mice and humans (Davani et al., 2000). Incubation of β-cells in the presence of 11-DHC leads to a dose-dependent attenuation of GSIS, indicating that cellular activation of 11-DHC may play a role in GC-induced β-cell dysfunction and that 11β-HSD1 may potentiate the detrimental effect of GCs on β-cell function. The protein content of 11β-HSD1 is higher in islets from *ob/ob* mice, compared to C57BL/6J mice, and is further increased when *ob/ob* islets are cultured in presence of 11-DHC (Ortsäter et al., 2005). GSIS in islets from *ob/ob* mice (but not from normal mice) was dose-dependently inhibited in presence of 11-DHC, an effect prevented by addition of selective 11β-HSD1 inhibitors or GR antagonist RU486 (Ortsäter et al., 2005). Recently, it was demonstrated that 11β-HSD1 is mainly localized to pancreatic α-cells both in mouse and human islets (Swali et al., 2008). In that study, mouse islets had lower glucagon or insulin secretion when cultured in presence of DEX, corticosterone or 11-DHC; the effect of 11-DHC was partially prevented by an 11β-HSD1 inhibitor. These data suggest that the ability of α-cells to generate active GC within the islet impacts on insulin and glucagon secretion by three distinct mechanisms: (1) directly at the level of the α-cells, modulating glucagon secretion; (2) by decreasing glucagon secretion, which may decrease insulin secretion via glucagon receptors expressed on the β-cells and (3) by GC production by α-cells acting in a paracrine manner, regulating insulin secretion from neighbouring β-cells (Swali et al., 2008). Although the overall conclusion of these findings is that 11β-HSD1 plays a negative role in pancreatic β-cell function, it should be noted that the complete lack of 11β-HSD1 expression in β-cells is associated with mild β-cell impairment (Turban et al., 2012). In addition, moderate β-cell specific overexpression of 11β-HSD1 can protect against the diabetogenic effects of a high-fat diet. These data lend support to the notion that GCs under certain conditions can promote β-cell function (Hult et al., 2009; Rafacho et al., 2010).

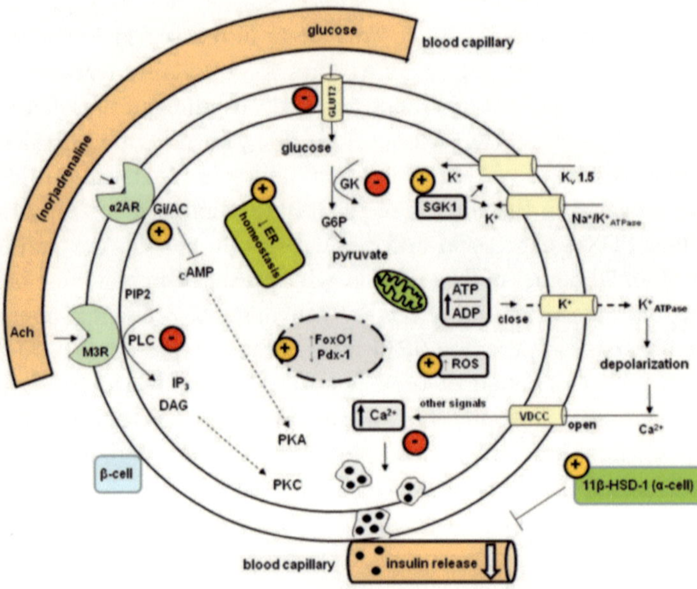

Figure 3. Direct GC effects on the insulin secretory process in β-cells. The known components involved in the direct effects of GCs on the β-cell insulin secretory process are highlighted with a positive signal (orange circle – indicates GCs stimulate that action) or negative signal (red circle – indicates GCs inhibit that action). Most notably, GCs impair β-cell glucose metabolism, favor repolarizing K^+ currents, decrease PKA and PKC activation, induce ER dyshomeostasis and increased FoxO1 protein content that altogether impair calcium handling and inhibits insulin secretion. Abbreviations: AC, adenylyl cyclase; Ach, acetylcholine; ADP, adenosine diphosphate; ATP, adenosine trisphosphate; cAMP, cyclic adenosine monophosphate; Cx36, connexin 36; DAG, diacylglycerol; ER, endoplasmic reticulum; FFA, free fatty acids; FoxO1, Forkhead box O; G6P, glucose-6-phosphatase; Gs, G-coupled stimulatory protein; GK, glucokinase; GLUT2, glucose transporter 2; IP3, inositol trisphosphate; $K_{v1.5}$, voltage-dependent K^+ channel; M3R, muscarinic receptor type 3; PDX-1, pancreatic duodenal homeobox; PIP2, phosphatidylinositol bisphosphate; PKA, protein kinase A; PKC, protein kinase C; PLC, phospholipase C; SGK-1, serum- and glucocorticoid inducible kinase-1; VDCC, voltage-dependent calcium channel, 11-βHSD-1, 11-β hydroxysteroid dehydrogenase type 1. Modified from Nussey & Whitehead, 2001; Endocrinology: An integrated approach, box 2.19 (Nussey & Whitehead, 2001) and from van Raalte et al., 2009; Eur J Clin Invest 2009, 39(2):page 87, Figure 3 (van Raalte et al., 2009).

2.4.5. *Effects of GCs on β-cell growth in vitro*

It was demonstrated in the seventies that 10 μg/ml DEX exerts inhibitory effects on β-cell proliferation in rat pancreatic monolayer cells (Chick, 1973). Several years later, it was found that 100 nM DEX negatively interferes with the positive effects of prolactin on β-cell growth both in mouse islet cells and INS-1 cells (Weinhaus et al., 2000). The direct effects of DEX on β-cell proliferation and β-cell death are GR-mediated and involve the activation of caspase-3, mitochondrial depolarization, reduction of Bcl-2 protein content, increase of Hsp90 protein, increased calcineurin activity with attendant elevation in dephosphorylated BAD protein levels, and inhibition of IRS-2, PKB and ERK phosphorylations (Ranta et al., 2006; Avram et al., 2008; Ranta et al., 2008). Exendin-4, an agonist of GLP-1 receptor, and IGF-1 protect β-cells against DEX-induced β-cell death. In a recent study, specific knockdown of mitogen-activated protein kinase (MAPK) phosphatase (MKP)-1 in RINm5F and MIN6 insulinoma cells, counteracted the down-regulation of ERK1/2 protein phosphorylation and the reduction of β-cell proliferation induced by DEX (Nicoletti-Carvalho et al., 2010). Prednisolone also induces β-cell apoptosis in INS-1E cells through up-regulation of calpain 10 and increased cleavage of caspase-3 (Linssen et al., 2011). In their entirety, these data, summarized in Table 5, clearly demonstrate the negative effects of GCs on β-cell growth that contrasts to those observed when GCs are administered *in vivo*.

GC	Dose and period, and β-cell source	Main results	Reference
Dex	10 μg/ml for 4 d in rat pancreatic monolayer cells	Reduced β-cell proliferation	(Chick, 1973)
Dex	100 nM for 24 h to 3 d in rat islet	Dex alone did not induce significant decrease in β-cell proliferation, but markedly decreased the positive effect of PRL on β-cell proliferation. Dex for 24 h to 3 d induced an increase in islet cell death even in the presence of PRL.	(Weinhaus et al., 2000)
Dex	100 nM for 1 or 4 d in mouse β-cells or INS1 cells	Dex induced mouse islet cells or INS1 cells death that was GR-dependent (RU486). Dex induced caspase 3 activity in INS1 cells. Dex reduced mRNA and protein content of Bcl-2 and decrease of mitochondrial polarization. Dex-induced cell death was associated to increased calcineurin activity and increased BAD dephosphorylation (all reverted by RU486 or calcineurin inhibitors). Exendin-4 protects islet cells and INS1 cells from Dex-induced cell death via activation of PKA.	(Ranta et al., 2006)
Dex	100 nM for 1 d in INS-1 cells	Dex inhibited cell growth, BrdU incorporation and induced apoptosis. Dex induced cell death was partially antagonizedal by IGF-1. Despite increased IRS-2 protein, IRS-2 tyrosine phosphorylation stimulated by IGF-1 was inhibited by Dex. Dex treatment reduced basal PKB phosphorylation. However, IGF-1-mediated ERK phosphorylation was affected.	(Avram et al., 2008)
Dex	100 nM for 1 to 4 d in INS-1 cells	In INS-1 cells cultured up to 4 d with Dex, the percentage of apoptosis increased from 1% to 10.9%. FK506 inhibited dex-	(Ranta et al., 2008)

GC	Dose and period, and β-cell source	Main results	Reference
		mediated cell death. Apoptosis was significantly higher at glucose concentrations that induce $[Ca^{2+}]_i$ oscillations than at low, non-stimulatory glucose. Calcineurin activity was unaltered after Dex treatment. However, Dex treatment significantly increased enzyme activity at submaximal, physiological Ca^{2+} concentrations. Dex did not stimulate the Ca^{2+}-dependent protease calpain, known to activate calcineurin by cleavage. In Dex-treated cells Hsp90 protein, a component of the GR known to stimulate calcineurin,was increased while calcineurin protein levels were unchanged. In immunoprecipitates with calcineurin antibodies, Hsp90 was only detected in Dex-treated cell homogenates.	
Dex	100nM Dex for 3 d culture both for MIN6 or Rin5 cells	Dex reduced phospho-ERK1/2 and increased MKP-1 expression in RINm5F and MIN-6 cells. Inhibition of transduction with cycloheximide and inhibition of phosphatases with orthovanadate efficiently blocked DEX-induced downregulation of phospho-ERK1/2. In addition, specific knockdown of MKP-1 with siRNA suppressed the downregulation of phospho-ERK1/2 and the reduction of proliferation induced by DEX.	(Nicoletti-Carvalho et al., 2010)

Dex; dexamethasone

Table 5. Effects of GC *in vitro* on cell growth in islets, dispersed islet β-cells or β-cell lines.

3. Conclusions

Collectively, direct effects of GCs on β-cell function *in vitro* are opposite to those observed when the GCs are administered *in vivo* to healthy individuals (especially humans and rats), which does not exclude that *in vivo* GCs might exert their known negative effects on β-cells, *e.g.* by increasing 11β-HSD1 activity, induce apoptosis and eventually obscure glucose sensing. However, based on data summarized herein, it seems clear that these direct effects of steroids on the β-cells are overwhelmed by the compensatory adaptations provoked by the GC-induced IR *in vivo*. Whether continuation of GC treatment for long periods (weeks to years) in healthy individuals results in impaired β-cell function is still a matter of debate; nevertheless, it is reasonable to say that since short treatments in susceptible subjects (obese, low-insulin responders, first-degree relatives of patients with T2DM, pregnant, etc) clearly demonstrate β-cell dysfunction, great caution should be exerted as to use GC therapies in high doses and/or with prolonged duration. The direct effects of GCs are achieved through classical ligand-GR mechanisms, since selective inhibition of GR prevents most GC-induced impairments of β-cells *in vitro* (Hamamdzic et al., 1995; Gremlich et al., 1997; Lambillotte et al., 1997; Ullrich et al., 2005; Ranta et al., 2006; Koizumi & Yada, 2008; Swali et al., 2008; Linssen et al., 2011) and *in vivo* (Ohneda et al., 1993). The extent of non-genomic actions of GCs on insulin secretion is not yet clear. However, rapid effects observed by physiological GC concentrations seem to involve sympathetic autonomic signals (Longano & Fletcher,

1983), whereas synthetic compounds with GC activity do not elicit acute modifications in β-cell responses to insulin secretagogues (Lambillotte et al., 1997; Zawalich et al., 2006). The real involvement of 11β-HSD1 on pancreatic islets *milieu* as well as the effects of GCs on pancreatic α-cells and its paracrine consequences on pancreatic β-cell function remain to be investigated.

Author details

Alex Rafacho

Department of Physiological Sciences, Centre of Biological Sciences, Universidade Federal de Santa Catarina, Brazil

Antonio C. Boschero

Department of Structural and Functional Biology, Universidade Estadual de Campinas, Brazil

Henrik Ortsäter

Department of Clinical Science and Education, Södersjukhuset, Karolinska Insititutet, Sweden

Acknowledgement

H. Ortsäter is funded by the Swedish Society for Medical Research. A. C. Boschero is funded by FAPESP and CNPq. A. Rafacho is funded by CNPq and FAPESC. The authors have no conflict of interest to disclose.

4. References

Ahrén, B. (2008). Evidence that autonomic mechanisms contribute to the adaptive increase in insulin secretion during dexamethasone-induced insulin resistance in humans. *Diabetologia* Vol. 51, No. 6, pp. 1018-1024

Andrews, R.C., & Walker, B.R. (1999). Glucocorticoids and insulin resistance: old hormones, new targets. *Clin Sci (Lond)* Vol. 96, No. 5, pp. 513-523

Angelini, N., Rafacho, A., Boschero, A.C., & Bosqueiro, J.R. (2010). Involvement of the cholinergic pathway in glucocorticoid-induced hyperinsulinemia in rats. *Diabetes Res Clin Pract* Vol. 87, No. 2, pp. 184-191

Arumugam, R., Horowitz, E., Lu, D., Collier, J.J., Ronnebaum, S., Fleenor, D., & Freemark, M. (2008). The interplay of prolactin and the glucocorticoids in the regulation of beta-cell gene expression, fatty acid oxidation, and glucose-stimulated insulin secretion: implications for carbohydrate metabolism in pregnancy. *Endocrinology* Vol. 149, No. 11, pp. 5401-5414

Arumugam, R., Horowitz, E., Noland, R.C., Lu, D., Fleenor, D., & Freemark, M. (2010). Regulation of islet beta-cell pyruvate metabolism: interactions of prolactin, glucose, and dexamethasone. *Endocrinology* Vol. 151, No. 7, pp. 3074-3083

Avram, D., Ranta, F., Hennige, A.M., Berchtold, S., Hopp, S., Haring, H.U., Lang, F., & Ullrich, S. (2008). IGF-1 protects against dexamethasone-induced cell death in insulin secreting INS-1 cells independent of AKT/PKB phosphorylation. *Cell Physiol Biochem* Vol. 21, No. 5-6, pp. 455-462

Barbera, M., Fierabracci, V., Novelli, M., Bombara, M., Masiello, P., Bergamini, E., & De Tata, V. (2001). Dexamethasone-induced insulin resistance and pancreatic adaptive response in aging rats are not modified by oral vanadyl sulfate treatment. *Eur J Endocrinol* Vol. 145, No. 6, pp. 799-806

Barseghian, G., & Levine, R. (1980). Effect of corticosterone on insulin and glucagon secretion by the isolated perfused rat pancreas. *Endocrinology* Vol. 106, No. 2, pp. 547-552

Beard, J.C., Halter, J.B., Best, J.D., Pfeifer, M.A., & Porte, D., Jr. (1984). Dexamethasone-induced insulin resistance enhances B cell responsiveness to glucose level in normal men. *Am J Physiol* Vol. 247, No. 5 Pt 1, pp. E592-596

Besse, C., Nicod, N., & Tappy, L. (2005). Changes in insulin secretion and glucose metabolism induced by dexamethasone in lean and obese females. *Obes Res* Vol. 13, No. 2, pp. 306-311

Billaudel, B., & Sutter, B.C. (1979). Direct effect of corticosterone upon insulin secretion studied by three different techniques. *Horm Metab Res* Vol. 11, No. 10, pp. 555-560

Binnert, C., Ruchat, S., Nicod, N., & Tappy, L. (2004). Dexamethasone-induced insulin resistance shows no gender difference in healthy humans. *Diabetes Metab* Vol. 30, No. 4, pp. 321-326

Borelli, M.I., Garcia, M.E., Gomez Dumm, C.L., & Gagliardino, J.J. (1982). Glucocorticoid-induced changes in insulin secretion related to the metabolism and ultrastructure of pancreatic islets. *Horm Metab Res* Vol. 14, No. 6, pp. 287-292

Chick, W.L. (1973). Beta cell replication in rat pancreatic monolayer cultures. Effects of glucose, tolbutamide, glucocorticoid, growth hormone and glucagon. *Diabetes* Vol. 22, No. 9, pp. 687-693

Choi, S.B., Jang, J.S., Hong, S.M., Jun, D.W., & Park, S. (2006). Exercise and dexamethasone oppositely modulate beta-cell function and survival via independent pathways in 90% pancreatectomized rats. *J Endocrinol* Vol. 190, No. 2, pp. 471-482

Chuthaputti, A., & Fletcher, H.P. (1987). Effect of hydrocortisone on terbutaline stimulated insulin release from isolated pancreatic islets. *Res Commun Chem Pathol Pharmacol* Vol. 57, No. 3, pp. 329-341

Davani, B., Khan, A., Hult, M., Martensson, E., Okret, S., Efendic, S., Jornvall, H., & Oppermann, U.C. (2000). Type 1 11β-hydroxysteroid dehydrogenase mediates glucocorticoid activation and insulin release in pancreatic islets. *J Biol Chem* Vol. 275, No. 45, pp. 34841-34844.

Davani, B., Portwood, N., Bryzgalova, G., Reimer, M.K., Heiden, T., Ostenson, C.G., Okret, S., Ahren, B., Efendic, S., & Khan, A. (2004). Aged transgenic mice with increased glucocorticoid sensitivity in pancreatic beta-cells develop diabetes. *Diabetes* Vol. 53 Suppl 1, No., pp. S51-59

Delaunay, F., Khan, A., Cintra, A., Davani, B., Ling, Z.C., Andersson, A., Ostenson, C.G., Gustafsson, J., Efendic, S., & Okret, S. (1997). Pancreatic β cells are important targets for the diabetogenic effects of glucocorticoids. *J Clin Invest* Vol. 100, No. 8, pp. 2094-2098

Dessein, P.H., & Joffe, B.I. (2006). Insulin resistance and impaired beta cell function in rheumatoid arthritis. *Arthritis Rheum* Vol. 54, No. 9, pp. 2765-2775

Fabregat, M.E., Fernandez-Alvarez, J., Franco, C., Malaisse, W.J., & Gomis, R. (1999). Dexamethasone-induced changes in FAD-glycerophosphate dehydrogenase mRNA, content and activity, and insulin release in human pancreatic islets. *Diabetes Nutr Metab* Vol. 12, No. 6, pp. 388-393

Giozzet, V.A., Rafacho, A., Boschero, A.C., Carneiro, E.M., & Bosqueiro, J.R. (2008). Dexamethasone treatment in vivo counteracts the functional pancreatic islet alterations caused by malnourishment in rats. *Metabolism* Vol. 57, No. 5, pp. 617-624

Gremlich, S., Roduit, R., & Thorens, B. (1997). Dexamethasone induces posttranslational degradation of GLUT2 and inhibition of insulin secretion in isolated pancreatic β cells. Comparison with the effects of fatty acids. *J Biol Chem* Vol. 272, No. 6, pp. 3216-3222.

Grill, V., Pigon, J., Hartling, S.G., Binder, C., & Efendic, S. (1990). Effects of dexamethasone on glucose-induced insulin and proinsulin release in low and high insulin responders. *Metabolism* Vol. 39, No. 3, pp. 251-258

Hamamdzic, D., Duzic, E., Sherlock, J.D., & Lanier, S.M. (1995). Regulation of alpha 2-adrenergic receptor expression and signaling in pancreatic beta-cells. *Am J Physiol* Vol. 269, No. 1 Pt 1, pp. E162-171

Heit, J.J., Karnik, S.K., & Kim, S.K. (2006). Intrinsic regulators of pancreatic β-cell proliferation. *Annu Rev Cell Dev Biol* Vol. 22, No., pp. 311-338

Henriksen, J.E., Alford, F., Ward, G.M., & Beck-Nielsen, H. (1997). Risk and mechanism of dexamethasone-induced deterioration of glucose tolerance in non-diabetic first-degree relatives of NIDDM patients. *Diabetologia* Vol. 40, No. 12, pp. 1439-1448

Herrero, L., Rubi, B., Sebastian, D., Serra, D., Asins, G., Maechler, P., Prentki, M., & Hegardt, F.G. (2005). Alteration of the Malonyl-CoA/Carnitine Palmitoyltransferase I Interaction in the β-Cell Impairs Glucose-Induced Insulin Secretion. *Diabetes* Vol. 54, No. 2, pp. 462-471

Hollingdal, M., Juhl, C.B., Dall, R., Sturis, J., Veldhuis, J.D., Schmitz, O., & Porksen, N. (2002). Glucocorticoid induced insulin resistance impairs basal but not glucose entrained high-frequency insulin pulsatility in humans. *Diabetologia* Vol. 45, No. 1, pp. 49-55

Holness, M.J., Smith, N.D., Greenwood, G.K., & Sugden, M.C. (2005). Interactive influences of peroxisome proliferator-activated receptor alpha activation and glucocorticoids on pancreatic beta cell compensation in insulin resistance induced by dietary saturated fat in the rat. *Diabetologia* Vol. 48, No. 10, pp. 2062-2068

Holness, M.J., & Sugden, M.C. (2001). Dexamethasone during late gestation exacerbates peripheral insulin resistance and selectively targets glucose-sensitive functions in beta cell and liver. *Endocrinology* Vol. 142, No. 9, pp. 3742-3748

Hult, M., Ortsäter, H., Schuster, G., Graedler, F., Beckers, J., Adamski, J., Ploner, A., Jornvall, H., Bergsten, P., & Oppermann, U. (2009). Short-term glucocorticoid treatment increases insulin secretion in islets derived from lean mice through multiple pathways and mechanisms. *Mol Cell Endocrinol* Vol. 301, No. 1-2, pp. 109-116

Jeong, I.K., Oh, S.H., Kim, B.J., Chung, J.H., Min, Y.K., Lee, M.S., Lee, M.K., & Kim, K.W. (2001). The effects of dexamethasone on insulin release and biosynthesis are dependent on the dose and duration of treatment. *Diabetes Res Clin Pract* Vol. 51, No. 3, pp. 163-171.

Jonas, L., Putzke, H.P., & Hahn von Dorsche, H. (1983). The islands of Langerhans in rats (Rattus norvegicus, Forma alba) following administration of prednisolone - semi-quantitative light and electron microscopy study. *Anat Anz* Vol. 154, No. 4, pp. 273-282

Kahn, S.E., Prigeon, R.L., McCulloch, D.K., Boyko, E.J., Bergman, R.N., Schwartz, M.W., Neifing, J.L., Ward, W.K., Beard, J.C., Palmer, J.P., & et al. (1993). Quantification of the relationship between insulin sensitivity and beta-cell function in human subjects. Evidence for a hyperbolic function. *Diabetes* Vol. 42, No. 11, pp. 1663-1672

Kalhan, S.C., & Adam, P.A. (1975). Inhibitory effect of prednisone on insulin secretion in man: model for duplication of blood glucose concentration. *J Clin Endocrinol Metab* Vol. 41, No. 3, pp. 600-610

Karatsoreos, I.N., Bhagat, S.M., Bowles, N.P., Weil, Z.M., Pfaff, D.W., & McEwen, B.S. (2010). Endocrine and physiological changes in response to chronic corticosterone: a potential model of the metabolic syndrome in mouse. *Endocrinology* Vol. 151, No. 5, pp. 2117-2127

Karlsson, S., Ostlund, B., Myrsen-Axcrona, U., Sundler, F., & Ahren, B. (2001). Beta cell adaptation to dexamethasone-induced insulin resistance in rats involves increased glucose responsiveness but not glucose effectiveness. *Pancreas* Vol. 22, No. 2, pp. 148-156

Kautzky-Willer, A., Thomaseth, K., Clodi, M., Ludvik, B., Waldhausl, W., Prager, R., & Pacini, G. (1996). Beta-cell activity and hepatic insulin extraction following dexamethasone administration in healthy subjects. *Metabolism* Vol. 45, No. 4, pp. 486-491

Khan, A., Hong-Lie, C., & Landau, B.R. (1995). Glucose-6-phosphatase activity in islets from ob/ob and lean mice and the effect of dexamethasone. *Endocrinology* Vol. 136, No. 5, pp. 1934-1938

Khan, A., Ostenson, C.G., Berggren, P.O., & Efendic, S. (1992). Glucocorticoid increases glucose cycling and inhibits insulin release in pancreatic islets of ob/ob mice. *Am J Physiol* Vol. 263, No. 4 Pt 1, pp. E663-666

Koizumi, M., & Yada, T. (2008). Sub-chronic stimulation of glucocorticoid receptor impairs and mineralocorticoid receptor protects cytosolic Ca2+ responses to glucose in pancreatic beta-cells. *J Endocrinol* Vol. 197, No. 2, pp. 221-229

Koranyi, L., Bourey, R., Turk, J., Mueckler, M., & Permutt, M.A. (1992). Differential expression of rat pancreatic islet beta-cell glucose transporter (GLUT 2), proinsulin and islet amyloid polypeptide genes after prolonged fasting, insulin-induced hypoglycaemia and dexamethasone treatment. *Diabetologia* Vol. 35, No. 12, pp. 1125-1132

Lambillotte, C., Gilon, P., & Henquin, J.C. (1997). Direct glucocorticoid inhibition of insulin secretion. An in vitro study of dexamethasone effects in mouse islets. *J Clin Invest* Vol. 99, No. 3, pp. 414-423.

Larsson, H., & Ahren, B. (1999). Insulin resistant subjects lack islet adaptation to short-term dexamethasone-induced reduction in insulin sensitivity. *Diabetologia* Vol. 42, No. 8, pp. 936-943

Lee, H.C., Bonner-Weir, S., Weir, G.C., & Leahy, J.L. (1989). Compensatory adaption to partial pancreatectomy in the rat. *Endocrinology* Vol. 124, No. 3, pp. 1571-1575

Ling, Z.C., Khan, A., Delauny, F., Davani, B., Ostenson, C.G., Gustafsson, J.A., Okret, S., Landau, B.R., & Efendic, S. (1998). Increased glucocorticoid sensitivity in islet beta-cells: effects on glucose 6-phosphatase, glucose cycling and insulin release. *Diabetologia* Vol. 41, No. 6, pp. 634-639.

Linssen, M.M., van Raalte, D.H., Toonen, E.J., Alkema, W., van der Zon, G.C., Dokter, W.H., Diamant, M., Guigas, B., & Ouwens, D.M. (2011). Prednisolone-induced beta cell dysfunction is associated with impaired endoplasmic reticulum homeostasis in INS-1E cells. *Cell Signal* Vol. 23, No. 11, pp. 1708-1715

Liu, H.K., Green, B.D., McClenaghan, N.H., McCluskey, J.T., & Flatt, P.R. (2006). Deleterious effects of supplementation with dehydroepiandrosterone sulphate or dexamethasone on rat insulin-secreting cells under in vitro culture condition. *Biosci Rep* Vol. 26, No. 1, pp. 31-38

Longano, C.A., & Fletcher, H.P. (1983). Insulin release after acute hydrocortisone treatment in mice. *Metabolism* Vol. 32, No. 6, pp. 603-608

Matschinsky, F. (1996). A lesson in metabolic regulation inspired by the glucokinase glucose sensor paradigm. *Diabetes* Vol. 45, No., pp. 223-241

Myrsén-Axcrona, U., Karlsson, S., Sundler, F., & Ahren, B. (1997). Dexamethasone induces neuropeptide Y (NPY) expression and impairs insulin release in the insulin-producing cell line RINm5F. Release of NPY and insulin through different pathways. *J Biol Chem* Vol. 272, No. 16, pp. 10790-10796

Nesher, R., Anteby, E., Yedovizky, M., Warwar, N., Kaiser, N., & Cerasi, E. (2002). Beta-cell protein kinases and the dynamics of the insulin response to glucose. *Diabetes* Vol. 51 Suppl 1, No., pp. S68-73

Nicod, N., Giusti, V., Besse, C., & Tappy, L. (2003). Metabolic adaptations to dexamethasone-induced insulin resistance in healthy volunteers. *Obes Res* Vol. 11, No. 5, pp. 625-631

Nicoletti-Carvalho, J.E., Lellis-Santos, C., Yamanaka, T.S., Nogueira, T.C., Caperuto, L.C., Leite, A.R., Anhe, G.F., & Bordin, S. (2010). MKP-1 mediates glucocorticoid-induced ERK1/2 dephosphorylation and reduction in pancreatic ss-cell proliferation in islets from early lactating mothers. *Am J Physiol Endocrinol Metab* Vol. 299, No. 6, pp. E1006-1015

Novelli, M., De Tata, V., Bombara, M., Lorenzini, A., Masini, M., Pollera, M., Bergamini, E., & Masiello, P. (1999). Insufficient adaptive capability of pancreatic endocrine function in dexamethasone-treated ageing rats. *J Endocrinol* Vol. 162, No. 3, pp. 425-432

Novelli, M., Pocai, A., Chiellini, C., Maffei, M., & Masiello, P. (2008). Free fatty acids as mediators of adaptive compensatory responses to insulin resistance in dexamethasone-treated rats. *Diabetes Metab Res Rev* Vol. 24, No. 2, pp. 155-164

Nussey, S., & Whitehead, S. (2001). Endocrinology: An Integrated Approach. Oxford, BIOS Scientific Publishers Limited.

O'Brien, T.D., Westermark, P., & Johnson, K.H. (1991). Islet amyloid polypeptide and insulin secretion from isolated perfused pancreas of fed, fasted, glucose-treated, and dexamethasone-treated rats. *Diabetes* Vol. 40, No. 12, pp. 1701-1706

Ogawa, A., Johnson, J.H., Ohneda, M., McAllister, C.T., Inman, L., Alam, T., & Unger, R.H. (1992). Roles of insulin resistance and β-cell dysfunction in dexamethasone-induced diabetes. *J Clin Invest* Vol. 90, No. 2, pp. 497-504

Ohneda, M., Johnson, J.H., Inman, L.R., & Unger, R.H. (1993). GLUT-2 function in glucose-unresponsive β-cells of dexamethasone-induced diabetes in rats. *J Clin Invest* Vol. 92, No. 4, pp. 1950-1956

Ortsäter, H., Alberts, P., Warpman, U., Engblom, L.O., Abrahmsén, L., & Bergsten, P. (2005). Regulation of 11 β-hydroxysteroid dehydrogenase type 1 and glucose-stimulated insulin secretion in pancreatic islets of Langerhans. *Diabetes Metab Res Rev* Vol. 21, No. 4, pp. 359-366

Pagano, G., Cavallo-Perin, P., Cassader, M., Bruno, A., Ozzello, A., Masciola, P., Dall'omo, A.M., & Imbimbo, B. (1983). An in vivo and in vitro study of the mechanism of prednisone-induced insulin resistance in healthy subjects. *J Clin Invest* Vol. 72, No. 5, pp. 1814-1820

Pierluissi, J., Navas, F.O., & Ashcroft, S.J. (1986). Effect of adrenal steroids on insulin release from cultured rat islets of Langerhans. *Diabetologia* Vol. 29, No. 2, pp. 119-121

Qi, D., Pulinilkunnil, T., An, D., Ghosh, S., Abrahani, A., Pospisilik, J.A., Brownsey, R., Wambolt, R., Allard, M., & Rodrigues, B. (2004). Single-dose dexamethasone induces whole-body insulin resistance and alters both cardiac fatty acid and carbohydrate metabolism. *Diabetes* Vol. 53, No. 7, pp. 1790-1797

Rafacho, A., Abrantes, J.L., Ribeiro, D.L., Paula, F.M., Pinto, M.E., Boschero, A.C., & Bosqueiro, J.R. (2011). Morphofunctional alterations in endocrine pancreas of short- and long-term dexamethasone-treated rats. *Horm Metab Res* Vol. 43, No. 4, pp. 275-281

Rafacho, A., Cestari, T.M., Taboga, S.R., Boschero, A.C., & Bosqueiro, J.R. (2009). High doses of dexamethasone induce increased β-cell proliferation in pancreatic rat islets. *Am J Physiol Endocrinol Metab* Vol. 296, No. 4, pp. E681-689

Rafacho, A., Giozzet, V.A., Boschero, A.C., & Bosqueiro, J.R. (2008). Functional alterations in endocrine pancreas of rats with different degrees of dexamethasone-induced insulin resistance. *Pancreas* Vol. 36, No. 3, pp. 284-293

Rafacho, A., Marroqui, L., Taboga, S.R., Abrantes, J.L., Silveira, L.R., Boschero, A.C., Carneiro, E.M., Bosqueiro, J.R., Nadal, A., & Quesada, I. (2010). Glucocorticoids in vivo induce both insulin hypersecretion and enhanced glucose sensitivity of stimulus-secretion coupling in isolated rat islets. *Endocrinology* Vol. 151, No. 1, pp. 85-95

Rafacho, A., Quallio, S., Ribeiro, D.L., Taboga, S.R., Paula, F.M., Boschero, A.C., & Bosqueiro, J.R. (2010). The adaptive compensations in endocrine pancreas from glucocorticoid-treated rats are reversible after the interruption of treatment. *Acta Physiol (Oxf)* Vol. 200, No. 3, pp. 223-235

Rafacho, A., Ribeiro, D.L., Boschero, A.C., Taboga, S.R., & Bosqueiro, J.R. (2008). Increased pancreatic islet mass is accompanied by activation of the insulin receptor substrate-2/serine-threonine kinase pathway and augmented cyclin D2 protein levels in insulin-resistant rats. *Int J Exp Pathol* Vol. 89, No. 4, pp. 264-275

Rafacho, A., Roma, L.P., Taboga, S.R., Boschero, A.C., & Bosqueiro, J.R. (2007). Dexamethasone-induced insulin resistance is associated with increased connexin 36 mRNA and protein expression in pancreatic rat islets. *Can J Physiol Pharmacol* Vol. 85, No. 5, pp. 536-545

Ranta, F., Avram, D., Berchtold, S., Dufer, M., Drews, G., Lang, F., & Ullrich, S. (2006). Dexamethasone induces cell death in insulin-secreting cells, an effect reversed by exendin-4. *Diabetes* Vol. 55, No. 5, pp. 1380-1390

Ranta, F., Dufer, M., Stork, B., Wesselborg, S., Drews, G., Haring, H.U., Lang, F., & Ullrich, S. (2008). Regulation of calcineurin activity in insulin-secreting cells: stimulation by Hsp90 during glucocorticoid-induced apoptosis. *Cell Signal* Vol. 20, No. 10, pp. 1780-1786

Roma, L.P., Oliveira, C.A., Carneiro, E.M., Albuquerque, G.G., Boschero, A.C., & Souza, K.L. (2011). N-acetylcysteine protects pancreatic islet against glucocorticoid toxicity. *Redox Rep* Vol. 16, No. 4, pp. 173-180

Santerre, R.F., Cook, R.A., Crisel, R.M., Sharp, J.D., Schmidt, R.J., Williams, D.C., & Wilson, C.P. (1981). Insulin synthesis in a clonal cell line of simian virus 40-transformed hamster pancreatic beta cells. *Proc Natl Acad Sci U S A* Vol. 78, No. 7, pp. 4339-4343

Schneiter, P., & Tappy, L. (1998). Kinetics of dexamethasone-induced alterations of glucose metabolism in healthy humans. *Am J Physiol* Vol. 275, No. 5 Pt 1, pp. E806-813

Severino, C., Brizzi, P., Solinas, A., Secchi, G., Maioli, M., & Tonolo, G. (2002). Low-dose dexamethasone in the rat: a model to study insulin resistance. *Am J Physiol Endocrinol Metab* Vol. 283, No. 2, pp. E367-373

Shamoon, H., Soman, V., & Sherwin, R.S. (1980). The influence of acute physiological increments of cortisol on fuel metabolism and insulin binding to monocytes in normal humans. *J Clin Endocrinol Metab* Vol. 50, No. 3, pp. 495-501

Shao, J., Qiao, L., & Friedman, J.E. (2004). Prolactin, progesterone, and dexamethasone coordinately and adversely regulate glucokinase and cAMP/PDE cascades in MIN6 beta-cells. *Am J Physiol Endocrinol Metab* Vol. 286, No. 2, pp. E304-310

Sood, A., & Ismail-Beigi, F. (2010). Effect of dexamethasone on insulin secretion: examination of underlying mechanisms. *Endocr Pract* Vol. 16, No. 5, pp. 763-769

Stojanovska, L., Rosella, G., & Proietto, J. (1990). Evolution of dexamethasone-induced insulin resistance in rats. *Am J Physiol* Vol. 258, No. 5 Pt 1, pp. E748-756

Swali, A., Walker, E.A., Lavery, G.G., Tomlinson, J.W., & Stewart, P.M. (2008). 11β-Hydroxysteroid dehydrogenase type 1 regulates insulin and glucagon secretion in pancreatic islets. *Diabetologia* Vol. 51, No. 11, pp. 2003-2011

Thomas, C.R., Turner, S.L., Jefferson, W.H., & Bailey, C.J. (1998). Prevention of dexamethasone-induced insulin resistance by metformin. *Biochem Pharmacol* Vol. 56, No. 9, pp. 1145-1150

Tomita, T., Visser, P., Friesen, S., & Doull, V. (1984). Cortisone-induced islet cell hyperplasia in hamsters. *Virchows Arch B Cell Pathol Incl Mol Pathol* Vol. 45, No. 1, pp. 85-95

Turban, S., Liu, X., Ramage, L., Webster, S.P., Walker, B.R., Dunbar, D.R., Mullins, J.J., Seckl, J.R., & Morton, N.M. (2012). Optimal elevation of beta-cell 11beta-hydroxysteroid dehydrogenase type 1 is a compensatory mechanism that prevents high-fat diet-induced beta-cell failure. *Diabetes* Vol. 61, No. 3, pp. 642-652

Ullrich, S., Berchtold, S., Ranta, F., Seebohm, G., Henke, G., Lupescu, A., Mack, A.F., Chao, C.M., Su, J., Nitschke, R., Alexander, D., Friedrich, B., Wulff, P., Kuhl, D., & Lang, F.

(2005). Serum- and glucocorticoid-inducible kinase 1 (SGK1) mediates glucocorticoid-induced inhibition of insulin secretion. *Diabetes* Vol. 54, No. 4, pp. 1090-1099

Ullrich, S., Zhang, Y., Avram, D., Ranta, F., Kuhl, D., Haring, H.U., & Lang, F. (2007). Dexamethasone increases Na+/K+ ATPase activity in insulin secreting cells through SGK1. *Biochem Biophys Res Commun* Vol. 352, No. 3, pp. 662-667

Wajngot, A., Giacca, A., Grill, V., Vranic, M., & Efendic, S. (1992). The diabetogenic effects of glucocorticoids are more pronounced in low- than in high-insulin responders. *Proc Natl Acad Sci U S A* Vol. 89, No. 13, pp. 6035-6039

van Raalte, D.H., Nofrate, V., Bunck, M.C., van Iersel, T., Elassaiss Schaap, J., Nassander, U.K., Heine, R.J., Mari, A., Dokter, W.H., & Diamant, M. (2010). Acute and 2-week exposure to prednisolone impair different aspects of beta-cell function in healthy men. *Eur J Endocrinol* Vol. 162, No. 4, pp. 729-735

van Raalte, D.H., Ouwens, D.M., & Diamant, M. (2009). Novel insights into glucocorticoid-mediated diabetogenic effects: towards expansion of therapeutic options? *Eur J Clin Invest* Vol. 39, No. 2, pp. 81-93

Wang, Z.L., Bennet, W.M., Wang, R.M., Ghatei, M.A., & Bloom, S.R. (1994). Evidence of a paracrine role of neuropeptide-Y in the regulation of insulin release from pancreatic islets of normal and dexamethasone-treated rats. *Endocrinology* Vol. 135, No. 1, pp. 200-206

Vasavada, R.C., Gonzalez-Pertusa, J.A., Fujinaka, Y., Fiaschi-Taesch, N., Cozar-Castellano, I., & Garcia-Ocana, A. (2006). Growth factors and beta cell replication. *Int J Biochem Cell Biol* Vol. 38, No. 5-6, pp. 931-950

Weinhaus, A.J., Bhagroo, N.V., Brelje, T.C., & Sorenson, R.L. (2000). Dexamethasone counteracts the effect of prolactin on islet function: implications for islet regulation in late pregnancy. *Endocrinology* Vol. 141, No. 4, pp. 1384-1393

Wierup, N., Bjorkqvist, M., Kuhar, M.J., Mulder, H., & Sundler, F. (2006). CART regulates islet hormone secretion and is expressed in the beta-cells of type 2 diabetic rats. *Diabetes* Vol. 55, No. 2, pp. 305-311

Willi, S.M., Kennedy, A., Wallace, P., Ganaway, E., Rogers, N.L., & Garvey, W.T. (2002). Troglitazone antagonizes metabolic effects of glucocorticoids in humans: effects on glucose tolerance, insulin sensitivity, suppression of free fatty acids, and leptin. *Diabetes* Vol. 51, No. 10, pp. 2895-2902

Zakrzewska, K.E., Cusin, I., Stricker-Krongrad, A., Boss, O., Ricquier, D., Jeanrenaud, B., & Rohner-Jeanrenaud, F. (1999). Induction of obesity and hyperleptinemia by central glucocorticoid infusion in the rat. *Diabetes* Vol. 48, No. 2, pp. 365-370

Zawalich, W.S., Tesz, G.J., Yamazaki, H., Zawalich, K.C., & Philbrick, W. (2006). Dexamethasone suppresses phospholipase C activation and insulin secretion from isolated rat islets. *Metabolism* Vol. 55, No. 1, pp. 35-42

Zhang, X., Yong, W., Lv, J., Zhu, Y., Zhang, J., Chen, F., Zhang, R., Yang, T., Sun, Y., & Han, X. (2009). Inhibition of forkhead box O1 protects pancreatic β-cells against dexamethasone-induced dysfunction. *Endocrinology* Vol. 150, No. 9, pp. 4065-4073

Zwicker, G.M., & Eyster, R.C. (1993). Chronic effects of corticosteroid oral treatment in rats on blood glucose and serum insulin levels, pancreatic islet morphology, and immunostaining characteristics. *Toxicol Pathol* Vol. 21, No. 5, pp. 502-508

Chapter 7

Adherence to Guidelines and Its Effect on Glycemic Control During the Management of Type 2 Diabetes in Turkey: The ADMIRE Study

Ilhan Satman, Sazi Imamoglu, Candeger Yilmaz and ADMIRE Study Group*

Additional information is available at the end of the chapter

http://dx.doi.org/10.5772/51294

1. Introduction

Type 2 diabetes is a progressive chronic disease that causes serious complications and decreases the life expectancy. According to 1997-98 population-based survey (TURDEP-I), the prevalence of diabetes was 7.2% in adult population of Turkey [1]. The second survey which was recently completed (TURDEP-II), indicated that the prevalence of diabetes increased by 90% within last 12 years and reached to 13.7% (undiagnosed 7.5%), which means that almost 6.5 million adults have diabetes in Turkey [2].

Intensive control of glycemia and cardiovascular risk factors can significantly reduce the rate of acute and chronic complications, and increase the life expectancy and quality of life in patients with diabetes [3–6]. Early diagnosis, correct and intensive antidiabetes treatment, and effective follow-up were recommended to decrease the risk of complications [7]. Despite extensive evidence of benefits of tight glycemic control, large proportions of people with diabetes do not achieve target glycemic control.

The use of clinical guidelines is the best strategy for the effective control of diabetes. There are multiple diabetes practice guidelines based on published data or derived from expert consensus and provide specific recommendations to diagnose diabetes and to achieve and maintain glycemic control. Previous studies reported non-adherence to evidence-based guidelines, which was based on physician factors, patient factors, and organizational factors [8–11].

The national guidelines have particular importance to address local requirements. Therefore, Diabetes Study Group of The Society of Endocrinology and Metabolism of Turkey (SEMT) developed 'Clinical Practice Guidelines for Diagnosis, Treatment, and Follow-up of Diabetes and Its Complications' in 2006, which are reviewed and updated biannually [12–14]. In comparison with 'American Diabetes Association (ADA) Clinical Practice Recommendations', the SEMT guidelines include more detailed information on diagnosis and follow-up of diabetes and its complications in addition to general information on diabetes. Furthermore, diabetes management on special and co-morbid conditions such as pregnancy, surgery, travel, vaccination, hypertension, hyperlipidemia, coronary artery disease was explained in detail in the SEMT guidelines. While target glycated hemoglobin A1c (A1C) is ≤6.5% in the SEMT guidelines, it is <7% in ADA guidelines [15]. The treatment algorithm in the SEMT guidelines has also some differences than that of ADA/European Association for the Study of Diabetes (EASD) guidelines [16]: initially lifestyle modification + MET treatment; if A1C target is not reached in 2-3 months, other oral antidiabetics for A1C <8.5% or insulin treatment for A1C >8.5%; if initial A1C >10%, insulin or combination regimens are suggested from the beginning. If target A1C is not still obtained, basal-bolus insulin is started and MET treatment is retained if possible.

The perception and use of SEMT guidelines by physicians in Turkey, however, are unknown.

Therefore, we aimed to determine the physicians' adherence to the SEMT diabetes guidelines in a study entitled "Adherence of physicians to guidelines for the management of type 2 diabetes: The ADMIRE study". The main objectives of the ADMIRE study were to evaluate physicians' adherence to SEMT diabetes guidelines, to determine the factors affecting physicians' adherence, to evaluate the impact of physicians' adherence to guidelines on glycemic control in diabetes mellitus, and to prospectively evaluate the impact of education of physicians on the adherence to guidelines.

2. Patients and methods

2.1. Study design

2.1.1. Retrospective phase

This was a patient-based, multi-centre, and non-interventional study. The study was composed of two phases: a retrospective phase and a prospective phase.

For the retrospective phase, 200 Internal Medicine or Family Medicine physicians who involved in medical care of patients with type 2 diabetes were randomly selected to represent all geographical regions and hospital types. Of these physicians, 180 agreed to participate in the ADMIRE Study Group. The medical records of 1,790 patients with type 2 diabetes (mean age, 58.7±10.9 years; female, 61.7%; duration of diabetes, 7.7±7.5 years, mean body mass index [BMI], 30.1±5.6 kg/m^2; chronic complications, 58.6%) followed by 180 physicians during last 12 months were reviewed to determine whether the patients were followed and treated according to SEMT guidelines. The number of visits was at least 4 for 1,149 (64.2%) patients.

The effects of following patient- and physician-related factors on adherence to guidelines were analyzed using data from retrospective phase: patients' age, gender, diabetes duration,

BMI, presence and number of chronic complications, physicians' specialty, and type of institution were considered as variables affecting guideline adherence.

2.1.2. Prospective phase

In this phase, physicians were educated on the basis of data obtained from retrospective phase. Before the education, 883 type 2 diabetes patients (female, 61.7%; mean age, 55.3±10.4 years, duration of diabetes, 7.1±6.9 years, BMI, 30.4±5.4 kg/m^2) who were under control by study physicians were included in the study during two months of recruitment period. These patients were followed up for four months including initial and control visits. Afterwards, recruitment of patients was stopped and physicians received education. The educations included one-day comprehensive training course with case presentations and distribution of a DVD and booklets on several complications of diabetes mellitus. Along with a hard copy of SEMT diabetes guidelines, and online access to education materials for three months. After the education of physicians, 1,613 type 2 diabetes patients (female 58.7%, mean age, 56.7±10.8 years, duration of diabetes, 7.3±6.3 years, BMI, 30.3±5.3 kg/m^2) who were under control by study physicians were included in the study during two months and then were followed up for four months with a control visit. Total duration of prospective phase was 15 months.

The change in adherence of physicians to SEMT guidelines and glycemic control with education of physicians was evaluated. Furthermore, the effect of education on the rate of patients with regard to physicians' adherence to guidelines for treatment of diabetes was determined.

2.2. Parameters for adherence to guidelines

Adherence to SEMT guidelines was assessed in three domains of medical history, physical examination, and laboratory evaluations; each domain was scored on a 10-point scale (0 for non-adherence, 10 for full adherence). The score for adherence to guidelines for overall diagnosis and follow-up procedures was calculated by multiplying the arithmetic mean of the adherence scores for medical history, physical examination, and laboratory evaluation by 10, and changed between 0 and 100.

2.3. Glycemic control parameters

The relation between the degree of adherence to SEMT guidelines and glycemic control of patients was evaluated. The glycemic control parameters were A1C ≤6.5% (≤48 mmol/mol), fasting blood glucose (FBG) levels 70–120 mg/dL, and 2-hour postprandial blood glucose (PPBG) levels <140 mg/dL.

2.4. Statistical analyses

Study data was summarized with descriptive statistics (number, percentages, mean, standard deviation). Spearman's simple correlation coefficient (*r*) was calculated for the correlation of between degree of adherence to guidelines and the levels of A1C, FBG, and PPBG. Student t test and analysis of variance (ANOVA) followed by post-hoc Tukey test were used to compare continuous data of two and three groups, respectively. Chi-square test or Mantel-Haenszel chi-square test was used for comparison of discrete data between groups. Statistical level of significance was defined as $p<0.05$.

3. Results

3.1. Physicians' adherence to guidelines on retrospective phase

Evaluation of physicians' adherence to SEMT guidelines regarding medical history, physical examination, and laboratory evaluation showed that diagnosis and follow-up procedures were >75% compliant with SEMT guidelines for 869 patients (48.5%) (Table 1). Full physicians' adherence to medical history, physical examination, and laboratory aspects of SEMT guidelines were met in 68.6%, 8.3%, and 19.2% of the patients, respectively. The mean adherence scores for medical history, physical examination, and laboratory aspects of SEMT guidelines were 8.83±2.21, 5.86±2.98, and 6.29±2.68, respectively.

Physicians were adherent to guidelines in 565 patients (54.2%) for antidiabetic treatment. They applied insufficient treatment for 468 patients (44.9%) and unnecessarily aggressive treatment for 10 patients (1.0%). Management was adherent to guidelines in 859 patients (79.2%) for antihypertensive treatment, and in 578 patients (76.0%) for antilipid treatment approaches (Figure 1).

3.2. Factors affecting physicians' adherence on retrospective phase

Patients' age, gender, diabetes duration, BMI, presence and number of chronic complications were patient-related factors; type of institution and specialty were physician-related factors whose effects on scores for adherence to guidelines were studied. For older patients and males, physicians' adherence to guidelines was higher for laboratory evaluations. All aspects of guideline adherence were poor in patients with short duration (<5 years) of diabetes and in the absence of chronic complications. Furthermore, physicians in state institutions and family practitioners had lower adherence scores for physical examination and laboratory evaluation (Table 2).

3.3. Impact of adherence to guidelines on glycemic control on retrospective phase

Degree of overall adherence for diagnosis and follow-up procedures to guidelines did not correlate with glycemic control parameters except a negative correlation with FBG levels in visit 2. However, there was a weak inverse correlation between physical examination adherence score and A1C ($r=-0.058$, $p=0.045$), FBG ($r=-0.049$, $p=0.050$), and PPBG ($r=-0.073$, $p=0.030$) levels in visit 1. There was also negative correlation between adherence to guidelines for laboratory evaluation and FBG in visit 1 ($r=-0.051$, $p=0.039$) and visit 2 ($r=-0.093$, $p=0.001$) and between adherence to guidelines for medical history and FBG in visit 2 ($r=-0.073$, $p=0.008$) and A1C in visit 3 ($r=-0.097$, $p=0.007$) (Table 3).

	n		%
Medical history[a]			
0	39		2.2
2	30		1.7
4	65		3.6
6	111		6.2
8	317		17.7
10	1,228		68.6
Mean score		8.83±2.21	
Physical examinations[b]			
0	134		7.5
1	80		4.5
2	89		5.0
3	112		6.3
4	135		7.5
5	177		9.9
6	189		10.6
7	220		12.3
8	232		13.0
9	273		15.3
10	149		8.3
Mean score		5.86±2.98	
Laboratory evaluation[c]			
0	146		8.2
3.3	254		14.2
6.7	1,046		58.4
10	344		19.2
Mean score		6.29±2.68	
Overall diagnosis and follow-up procedures[d]			
<50	283		15.8
50-75	638		35.6
>75	869		48.5
Mean score		69.94±20.27	

[a] Adherence to guidelines was evaluated on a 10-point scale with 2-point for each of five items (diabetes symptoms, acute complications, chronic complications, cardiovascular risk factors, family history) that should be questioned for medical history.

[b] Adherence to guidelines was evaluated on a 10-point scale with 1 or 0 point respectively for performing or not performing each of the following 10 physical examination items: height, weight, waist circumference, blood pressure and heart rate measurements; thyroid, abdominal, neurological, foot and fundus examination.

[c] Adherence to guidelines was evaluated on a 10-point scale with 3.33 points for each of three laboratory tests (lipid profile, creatinine, and urinalysis).

[d] Adherence to guidelines for overall diagnosis and follow-up procedures was evaluated on a 100-point scale, it was obtained by multiplying the mean of adherence scores for medical history, physical examination, and laboratory evaluation by 10.

Table 1. Physicians' adherence to SEMT guidelines regarding medical history, physical examination, and laboratory evaluation. Data are given as number of patients and % or mean±standard deviation of score.

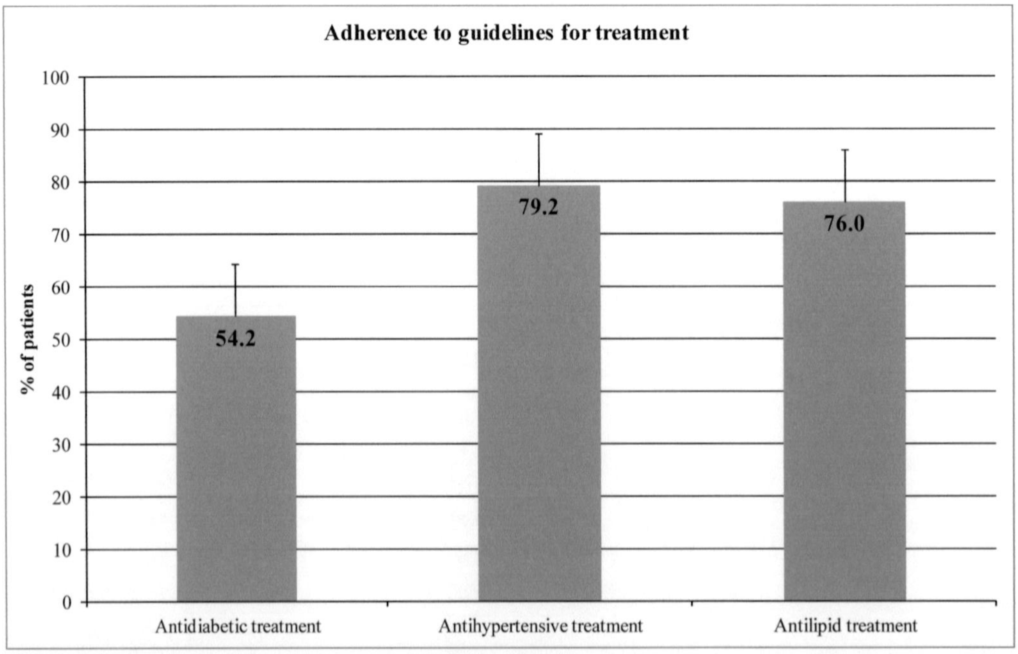

Figure 1. Physicians were adherent to guidelines for treatment.

			Scores for adherence to SEMT guidelines			
			Medical history	Physical examinations	Laboratory evaluation	Overall diagnosis and follow-up procedures
Patient-related factors						
Age (years)	<40		9.4±1.5	5.7±3.0	6.4±2.9	71.4±20.0
	40-49		8.8±2.2	5.6±3.0	6.2±2.8[a]	68.9±21.1
	50-59		8.8±2.2	5.8±3.1	6.6±2.8	70.8±21.6
	60-69		8.9±2.1	6.0±3.0	6.8±2.7	72.2±21.0
	≥70		8.7±2.4	6.0±2.8	6.9±2.6	72.1±20.3
		p	0.322	0.515	***0.020***	0.272
Gender	Male		8.9±2.2	5.9±3.0	6.8±2.7	72.1±20.8
	Female		8.8±2.2	5.8±3.0	6.5±2.8	70.6±21.0
		p	0.469	0.666	***0.021***	0.139
Diabetes duration (years)	0-5		8.7±2.3[b]	5.4±3.0[c]	6.3±2.9[c]	68.1±22.0[c]
	6-10		9.0±1.9	6.2±2.9	6.9± 2.6	74.0±19.3
	11-15		8.9±2.1	6.5±2.8	7.4±2.6	75.9±19.6

			Scores for adherence to SEMT guidelines			
			Medical history	Physical examinations	Laboratory evaluation	Overall diagnosis and follow-up procedures
Patient-related factors						
	16-20		9.4±1.2	6.7±2.9	7.3±2.7	78.2±19.1
	>20		8.9±2.1	6.5±2.8	7.3±2.5	75.6±18.9
		p	***0.003***	***<0.001***	***<0.001***	***<0.001***
Body mass index (kg/m^2)	<25		9.3±1.7	7.8±1.9	7.3±2.1	81.3±13.8
	25-26		9.5±1.5	8.0±1.8	7.5±2.2	83.6±13.4
	27-29		9.3±1.6	7.9±1.9	7.4±2.5	82.1±15.3
	30-39		9.5±1.3	8.0±1.7	7.3±2.4	82.7±13.6
	≥40		9.6±0.9	8.2±1.7	7.4±2.2	84.2±11.2
		p	0.278	0.635	0.922	0.619
Chronic complications (number of systems involved)	None		9.4±1.4[d]	5.9±2.9[e]	6.6±2.7[e]	72.9±18.2[e]
	1 system		9.1±1.8	6.2±2.9	6.8±2.8	73.8±19.1[e]
	2 systems		9.4±1.2	6.4±2.8	6.9±2.7	75.8±17.2
	>2 systems		9.4±1.2	6.6±2.8	7.4±2.5	77.6±17.4
		p	***0.020***	***0.007***	***0.001***	***0.003***
History of chronic complications	Yes		9.3±1.5	6.3±2.8	7.0±2.7	75.4±18.2
	No		9.4±1.4	5.9±2.9	6.6±2.7	72.9±18.2
		p	0.096	***0.002***	***0.002***	***0.008***
Physician-related factors						
Type of institution	State		8.7±1.9	5.5±2.6[g]	6.4±2.3[g]	68.7±18.7
	Private		9.1±1.5	6.4±2.4	6.7±2.3	73.9±17.7
	University		8.8±1.6	7.5±2.4	8.2±2.0	81.8±18.8
		p	0.550	***0.008***	***0.041***	***0.035***
Specialty	Family practice		9.0±1.4	5.1±2.5[h]	5.7±2.1[h]	65.9±16.1[h]
	Internal medicine		8.7±1.9	5.7±2.5	6.7±2.4	70.2±19.6[h]
	Endocrinology		9.6±1.8	7.9±1.7	7.9±1.4	84.5±8.7
		p	0.096	***<0.001***	***0.003***	***0.002***

[a] p<0.05 versus 60-69 years and ≥70 years of age; [b] p<0.05 versus 16-20 years diabetes duration; [c] p<0.05 versus all other diabetes duration groups; [d] p<0.05 versus 1 system involvement; [e] p<0.05 versus >2 systems involvement; [g] p<0.05 versus university; [h] p<0.05 versus endocrinology.

Table 2. Effect of patient- and physician-related factors on scores for adherence to guidelines. Data are given as mean±standard deviation of score.

Adherence to guidelines		Visit 1			Visit 2			Visit 3			Visit 4		
		A1C level	FBG level	PPBG level	A1C level	FBG level	PPBG level	A1C level	FBG level	PPBG level	A1C level	FBG level	PPBG level
Medical history	r	-0.023	0.024	-0.003	-0.043	-0.073	-0.046	-0.097	-0.026	-0.054	-0.059	0.016	-0.040
	p	0.428	0.326	0.918	0.209	***0.008***	0.197	***0.007***	0.385	0.159	0.137	0.635	0.342
Physical examination	r	-0.058	-0.049	-0.073	-0.019	-0.044	-0.064	-0.062	-0.042	-0.042	-0.036	0.012	0.042
	p	***0.045***	***0.050***	***0.030***	0.585	0.111	0.073	0.086	0.163	0.281	0.360	0.731	0.318
Laboratory evaluation	r	-0.017	-0.051	-0.033	0.024	-0.093	-0.027	0.028	-0.024	-0.006	0.077	0.040	0.111
	p	0.571	***0.039***	0.323	0.477	***0.001***	0.442	0.441	0.425	0.878	0.051	0.239	***0.008***
Overall diagnosis and follow-up	r	-0.046	-0.039	-0.053	-0.013	-0.091	-0.062	-0.053	-0.043	-0.036	-0.001	0.030	0.063
	p	0.116	0.118	0.111	0.702	***0.001***	0.080	0.144	0.152	0.350	0.983	0.372	0.131

A1C: Glycated hemoglobin A1c; FBG: Fasting blood glucose, PPBG: 2-hour postprandial blood glucose.

Table 3. Correlation coefficients (Spearman's r) between degree of adherence to SEMT guidelines and the levels of A1C, FBG, and PPBG

The minimum levels of A1C, FBG, and PPBG were significantly associated with the degree of general adherence to guidelines ($p<0.05$, Table 4). The minimum levels of A1C, FBG, and PPBG were significantly lower in >75% adherence to SEMT guidelines.

	Adherence to SEMT guidelines			p
	<50	50–75	>75	
A1C (%)				
Minimum	7.8±1.9	7.6±1.8	7.4±1.8	***0.021***
Maximum	8.7±2.1	8.7±2.0	8.8±2.1	0.315
FBG (mg/dL)				
Minimum	154.0±61.7	149.71±62.2	139.8±51.2	***<0.001***
Maximum	202.2±82.4	212.8±86.0	207.6±83.7	0.232
PPBG (mg/dL)				
Minimum	201.3±89.1	195.9±69.6	180.9±69.9	***0.001***
Maximum	248.9±93.8	246.7±87.9	250.6±90.6	0.809

A1C: Glycated hemoglobin A_{1c}; FBG: Fasting blood glucose, PPBG: 2-hour postprandial blood glucose.

Data are given as mean±standard deviation.

Table 4. The relation between the degree of adherence to SEMT guidelines for overall diagnosis and follow-up procedures and minimum and maximum levels of A1C, FBG, and PPBG during previous year

3.4. Impact of education of physicians prospectively on the adherence to guidelines

After the education of physicians, adherence scores to SEMT guidelines significantly increased for medical history, physical examination, and overall diagnosis and follow-up procedures ($p<0.001$), however, adherence score decreased significantly for laboratory evaluation ($p<0.001$) (Table 5). This might be caused due to the time limit between visits. Patients may not have yet their laboratory control or could not provide test results to their physicians.

The percentage of patients whose physicians comply with guidelines for antidiabetic ($p<0.001$), antihypertensive ($p<0.001$) and antilipid ($p=0.002$) treatment were increased significantly with the education (Table 6).

However, rate of patients under glycemic control was similar before and after the education of physicians. Furthermore the level of adherence to SEMT guidelines for overall diagnosis and follow-up procedures had no effect on glycemic control before or after the education, except that significantly more patients whose physician adhere to guidelines >75% had FBG <120 mg/dL in control visit before education ($p<0.013$) (Table 7).

	Before education		After education		p
	n	%	*n*	%	
Medical history[a]					***<0.001***
0	35	4.0	141	8.7	
2	109	12.3	51	3.2	
4	160	18.1	0	0.0	
6	106	12.0	0	0.0	
8	116	13.1	54	3.3	
10	359	40.6	1,370	84.8	
Mean score	6.79±3.24		8.81±3.08		***<0.001***
Physical examinations[b]					***<0.001***
0	14	1.6	122	7.5	
1	21	2.4	1	0.1	
2	20	2.3	7	0.4	
3	112	12.7	12	0.7	
4	417	47.1	50	3.1	
5	147	16.6	351	21.7	
6	36	4.1	194	12.0	
7	6	0.7	22	7.5	
8	23	2.6	41	2.5	
9	14	1.6	167	10.3	
10	75	8.5	549	34.0	
Mean score	4.65±2.12		7.02±2.95		***<0.001***
Laboratory evaluation[c]					***<0.001***
0	58	6.6	235	14.5	
3.3	93	10.5	171	10.6	
6.7	473	53.4	859	53.2	
10	261	29.5	351	21.7	
Mean score	6.86±2.71		6.07±3.11		***<0.001***
Overall diagnosis and follow-up procedures[d]					***<0.001***
<50	225	25.4	203	12.6	
50-75	481	54.4	416	25.7	
>75	179	20.2	997	61.7	
Mean score	61.03±17.36		72.99±25.30		***<0.001***

[a] Adherence to guidelines was evaluated on a 10-point scale with 2-point for each of five items (diabetes symptoms, acute complications, chronic complications, cardiovascular risk factors, family history) that should be questioned for medical history.

[b] Adherence to guidelines was evaluated on a 10-point scale with 1 or 0 point respectively for performing or not performing each of the following 10 physical examination items: height, weight, waist circumference, blood presssure and heart rate measurements; tyroid, abdominal, neurological, foot and fundus examination.

[c] Adherence to guidelines was evaluated on a 10-point scale with 3.33 points for each of three laboratory tests (lipid profile, creatinine, and urinalysis).

[d] Adherence to guidelines for overall diagnosis and follow-up procedures was evaluated on a 100-point scale, it was obtained by multiplying the mean of adherence scores for medical history, physical examination, and laboratory evaluation by 10.

Table 5. Physicians' adherence to SEMT guidelines during prospective phase of the study before and after education of physicians on guidelines. Data are given as number of patients and % or mean±standard deviation of score.

Adherence to guidelines	Before education		After education		p
	n	%	*n*	%	
Antidiabetic treatment					
Incompliant	283	40.0	440	32.5	***<0.001***
Insufficient treatment	253	35.7	301	22.2	
Unnecessary treatment	30	4.2	139	10.3	
Compliant	425	60.0	914	67.5	
Antihypertensive treatment					
Incompliant	181	21.4	183	12.7	***<0.001***
Compliant	664	78.6	1,253	87.3	
Antilipid treatment					
Incompliant	100	13.6	118	9.2	***0.002***
Compliant	634	86.4	1,170	90.8	

Table 6. Number and percentage of patients in terms of physicians' adherence to SEMT guidelines for treatment of diabetes patients during prospective phase of the study before and after education of physicians on guidelines

Beside this, A1C of the patients followed up after the education significantly decreased at control visit compared to baseline. Similarly the percentage of the patients at target A1C significantly increased at control visit compared to baseline, after the education.

4. Discussion and conclusion

The use of diabetes guidelines meeting national requirements is the most effective way to improve quality in practice; however, they must be effectively disseminated and implemented to obtain this goal. On the other hand, national studies mostly reported suboptimal level of physicians' adherence to the guidelines [10, 11, 17, 18]. Similarly, we found that only for half of the diabetes patients, diagnosis and follow-up procedures were >75% compliant with current SEMT guidelines; and for 54.2% patients, antidiabetic treatment were adherent to guidelines.

Lack of knowledge, reluctance to change practice, clinical inertia, time constraints, difficulties with referral systems, patient nonadherence for various reasons and deficiencies in healthcare system are some of the barriers affecting physicians' adherence to guidelines [19–21]. Among these factors, clinical inertia is defined as "recognizing the problem but failure to act" by health care professionals in primary care [22–29]. The key issues in the

	Before education						After education					
	A1C (≤%6.5)		FBG (<120 mg/dL)		PPBG (<140 mg/dL)		A1C (≤%6.5)		FBG (<120 mg/dL)		PPBG (<140 mg/dL)	
	First visit	Control visit	First visit	Control visit	First visit	Control visit	First visit	Control visit	First visit	Control visit	First visit	Control visit
Adherence to SEMT guidelines for overall diagnosis and follow-up procedures												
<50	30 (15.3)	28 (19.6)	30 (16.4)	25 (21.7)	11 (9.1)	15 (22.4)	57 (28.4)	17 (30.4)	12 (23.1)	9 (45.0)	8 (21.1)	7 (36.8)
50-75	80 (17.8)	90 (23.6)	83 (17.7)	117 (32.2)	46 (13.7)	52 (18.6)	81 (20.0)	64 (28.1)	67 (18.7)	50 (27.2)	19 (8.0)	20 (15.9)
>75	30 (16.9)	39 (23.9)	32 (18.0)	57 (36.3)	20 (12.7)	29 (21.2)	191 (19.5)	182 (28.2)	206 (21.4)	203 (31.9)	105 (13.9)	100 (20.0)
Total	140 (17.0)	157 (22.9)	145 (17.5)	199 (31.3)	77 (12.6)	96 (19.9)	329 (20.8)	263 (28.3)	285 (20.7)	262 (31.2)	132 (12.8)	127 (19.7)
p	0.674	0.381	0.691	***0.013***	0.416	0.988	***0.016***	0.821	0.546	0.778	0.364	0.742

A1C: Glycated hemoglobin A_{1c}; FBG: Fasting blood glucose, PPBG: 2-hour postprandial blood glucose.

Table 7. The rate of patients under glycemic control before and after the education of physicians on guidelines on glycemic control with respect to adherence to SEMT guidelines. Data are given as number of patients (%).

	Before		After	
	Baseline	Control	Baseline	Control
A1C (%)	8.68	7.98	8.39	7.69
FPG (mg/dL)	190.9	158.2	178.4	150.1
PPG (mg/dL)	247.9	200.9	240.2	199.5
Patients on target A1C (≤6.5%) (%)	17.0	22.9	20.8	28.3
Patients on target FBG (<120 mg/dL) (%)	17.5	31.3	20.7	31.2

Table 8. Glycemic control before and after the education.

management of people with type 2 diabetes include early detection of problems, realistic goal setting, improved patient adherence, better knowledge and understanding of pharmaco-therapeutic treatment options and prompt intervention. Clinical inertia is due to at least three problems: overestimation of care provided; use of "soft" reasons to avoid intensification of therapy; and lack of education, training, and practice organization aimed at achieving therapeutic goals. Health care professionals must need to overcome clinical inertia and need to intensify therapy in an appropriate and timely manner. Using guidelines in the management of diabetes patients and continuous education of diabetes care providers are effective ways to overcome clinical inertia [24, 29]. In a 3-year trial on 345 internal medicine residents, feedback on performance given to medical resident primary care providers improved provider behaviour and lowered A1C levels [27]. We think that lower adherence of guidelines by the physicians who provide care for younger (<50 year old) patients, males, and patients with short duration (<5 years) of diabetes and patients without complications in the ADMIRE study might be linked to clinical inertia in this group of patients.

Furthermore characteristics of patients and physicians can also influence clinical decision making and guideline adherence. McKinlay et al. showed that adherence to guidelines varied according to patients' age and gender and physicians' years of experience [30]. We also found that guideline adherence was influenced by patient-related factors such as gender, diabetes duration, and comorbid conditions. Unfortunately, new onset diabetes patients were less likely to receive best practice. Physician specialty and institution type were also contributing factors for guideline adherence; family practitioners and physicians in state institutions had lower adherence scores.

Although overall adherence for diagnosis and follow-up procedures to guidelines did not affect the glycemic control, weak inverse correlations were noted between physical examination, laboratory evaluation and medical history adherence scores and the levels of

A1C, FBG, and PPBG in some visits. Even if the correlation coefficients were too low to speak about, glycemic control is better maintained with increasing adherence to guidelines. Yet, the minimum levels of A1C, FBG, and PPBG were significantly lower with the increasing degree of general adherence to guidelines. On the other hand, poorer adherence scores for laboratory evaluation in our study may be because of the short duration following the educational session. Due to non-interventional design of the study, we think that some of the patients could not be able to come to a control visit or might have missed their appointment.

In a controlled study, Gerstein et al. [31] evaluated the effect of a national continuing medical education (CME) program designed to improve family physicians' implementation of diabetes-specific clinical practice guidelines. They found that compared to controls, participants who attended CME programs had improved their attitude, and knowledge. Moreover self-reported practice pattern of physicians regarding diabetes after one month but not after one year was also improved. Thus the education of physicians is effective to disseminate practice guidelines, but needs to be repeated periodically. We also hypothesized that specific training of physicians on SEMT guidelines would increase the adherence and improve patient outcomes. We provide to participating physicians one-day educational session along with a DVD and a hard copy of the guidelines. Adherence to SEMT guidelines significantly increased for overall diagnosis and follow-up procedures with the education. Compliance to guidelines for treatment of diabetes patients was also increased after education of physicians. However, glycemic control of patients was similar before and after the education, which may be due to relatively short duration (four months) of follow-up of patients.

The major limitation of this study is that the effect of other factors on the adherence to guidelines such as patient nonadherence to appointments, failure to comply with requested laboratory evaluations or system-related factors could not be eliminated. However, this study has particular importance in terms of type 2 diabetes knowledge: it showed that local guidelines are crucial to improve the clinical care of patients and to increase life-expectancy and quality of life of patients. However, continuous education of physicians on these guidelines should be recognized as a necessity rather than an individual optional behaviour. For example setting regulations to physicians to receive CME periodically on a compulsory manner may be beneficial.

4.1. Conclusions and recommendations

The following conclusions and recommendations were inferred from the ADMIRE study:

1. The physician adherence to diabetes guidelines is suboptimal in Turkey.
2. Patients with old age, established disease and multiple chronic complications received better care which is in compliance with guidelines.
3. Patients with short duration of diabetes, younger age, no complication, and males received less attention, this may be attributed to clinical inertia of care providers.

4. Specialists and physicians practicing in university settings followed guidelines better than family practitioners and physicians practicing in state institutions.
5. Glycemic control is better maintained with increasing physicians' adherence to guidelines.
6. Education of physicians on SEMT guidelines significantly increased their adherence to guidelines.
7. A better glycemic control is provided, unnecessary treatment is decreased and more rational treatment preferences are observed, after education.

As a conclusion, the educational programs targeted towards family practitioners and state institutions, may improve guideline adherence and patients' outcome. These programs should emphasize the preventive aspect of diabetes management rather than symptom-based treatment approach, Better adherence to diabetes guidelines provide better glycemic control and, thus lower the number of chronic complications and slow the natural course (progression) of the disease.

Appendix

ADMIRE study group*:

Taner Akdere, Cihansah Akdogan, Hatice Sule Akin, S. Ahmet Akin, Baris Akinci, Sertug Akkorlu, Ersin Akpinar, Derya Gunes Aksoy, Kamuran Aksoy, Osman Tevfik Aksoy, Ahmet Hamdi Aktan, Kursat Alam, Pervin Algan, Nuri Nazif Altiner, Derya Altintig, Abdullah Aricioglu, Cengiz Arslan, Erhan Atav, Serdar Ay, Teslime Ayaz, Akin Aydemir, Mehmet Aydemir, Neslihan Aydin, Mehmet Deniz Ayli, Serkan Bakirdogen, Mehmet Bastemir, Halil Basturkmen, Hur Baybuga, Zeynep Baykal, Taner Bayraktaroglu, Serdar Baysoy, Recep Bentli, Ali Ayberk Besen, Mehmet Besen, Dogan Nasir Binici, Serife Nur Boysan, Nafiz Bozdemir, Cemal Akin Bozoglu, Mustafa Budak, Selahattin Cakiroglu, Tolga Cakmak, Ayse Kargili Carlioglu, Taner Cavusoglu, Aslan Celebi, Murat Celik, Mustafa Cesur, Onur Cubukcu, Kursat Dal, Aysegul Gok Dalbeler, Askin Demirci, Hakan Demirci, Oguz Demirtas, Ibrahim Dinc, M.Aydin Dincer, Halil Dogan, Cemil Dolay, Erdal Duman, Halil Duran, Metin Durandurdu, Ercan Dursunoglu, Berna Dalmis Ekiz, Evren Eraytac, M. Emin Erdem, Fuat Erdemir, Seref Eren, Munire Erengul, Tayyibe Erkenez, Necip Ersan, Oznur Ertas, Cengiz Erten, Sebahattin Erten, Osman Eseler, Hurrem Ezergul, Mehmet Gemici, Hakan Gocturk, Erdem Gokdeniz, Sait Gonen, Ahmet Gozeten, Mehmet Gumus, Mehmet Gunay, Osman Sadi Gunaydin, Eren Gurkan, Idil Hallac, Aysin Harmanda, Taner Hasan, Ayhan Haspulat, Aysen Helvaci, Metin Ilhan, Nevzat Iliman, Ibrahim Ince, Ismet Onder Isik, Can Iyiiz, Aytac Kosova Iyikavak, Ibrahim Kahraman, Seyfi Kamberoglu, Gulgun Kandogan, Ayse Gul Karacam, Mahmut Celal Karakoc, Murat Karakurt, Nesibe Karakus, Abdullah Katki, Fatih Oner Kaya, Sebnem Gider Kaya, Sezgi Sevinc Kayikcioglu, Kamuran Kaynar, Yasemin Turkmen Kemal, Sakir Ozgur Keskek, Osman Keskin, Murat Kilic, Surur Kip, Guven Koc, Ozgur Kocabas, Serdal Korkmaz, Ahmet Kovac, Selim Kum, Hatice Kurdak, Ali Kutlucan, Baha Moral, Ilhan Murat, Ayhan

Mutlu, Selim Nalbant, Ayse Aysin Oge, Bulent Oguz, Ozer Oktayer, Iris Kavalali Oktem, Hasan Onat, Halil Ugur Oney, Mehmet Renan Ozakgun, M. Kemal Ozbek, Sevgi Ozcan, Ibrahim Ozdes, Adem Ozkara, Meryem Tek Ozokcu, Kemal Ozsahin, Mine Ozturk, Mustafa Ozturk, Pervin Pehlivan, Erol Pektas, Bekir Pocan, Hayri Polat, Halil Rakici, Esra Saatci, Huseyin Saglam, Ozlem Sahan, Hakan Sari, Ramazan Sari, Hakan Ziya Satir, Ilhan Satman, Mehmet Seker, Hakki Selcuk, H. Atilla Sengul, Ayhan Sonmez, Halil Sozmen, Yaser Suleymanoglu, Mustafa Gurkan Taskale, Alisan Taspinar, Nihat Tekden, Melek Tezcan, Mustafa Togan, Osman Nuri Topal, Fusun Topcugil, Tufan Tukek, Nezih Tuncay, Mehmet Turk, Idil Atac Turkmen, Sibel Ergun Turkmen, Pelin Tutuncuoglu, Asli Dogruk Unal, Tugrul Unat, Mehtap Erkmen Uyar, Ceyhun Varim, Mumin Varol, Feryal Atmaca Yalcin, Hamiyet Yilmaz Yasar, Hamza Yazici, Mehmet Yildiz, Zeki Yildiz, Zerrin Yildizbas, Mahmut Yilmaz, Mehmet Kaan Yilmaz, Hikmet Yuce, Yasar Yucel, Arif Yuksel, Iskender Yuksel, Adem Yurumez, Sefik Zeytunlu

Author details

Ilhan Satman
Division of Endocrinology & Metabolism, Department of Internal Medicine, Istanbul Faculty of Medicine, Istanbul University,Istanbul, Turkey

Sazi Imamoglu
Division of Endocrinology & Metabolism, Department of Internal Medicine, Uludag University Faculty of Medicine, Bursa, Turkey

Candeger Yilmaz
Division of Endocrinology & Metabolism, Department of Internal Medicine, Ege University Faculty of Medicine, Izmir, Turkey

ADMIRE Study Group
ADMIRE Study Group members are listed in the Appendix

Acknowledgement

We thank to the members of the ADMIRE Study Group for their valuable contributions (see Appendix). Special thanks to Dr. Oktay Ozdemir and Murat Kirtis for their assistance with the preparation of the manuscript. We also thank to sanofi-Turkey for providing unrestricted and unconditioned grant for the study.

This study was partly published/presented in the following journals/meetings:

Original article:

1. Satman İ, İmamoğlu Ş, Yılmaz C, ADMIRE Study Group. Adherence of physicians to SEMT guidelines for the management of type 2 diabetes in Turkey: ADMIRE study. Turk J Endocrin Metab (Turk JEM) 2010; 14: 66-72.

Presentations:

2. Satman I, Imamoglu S, Yilmaz C, Ozkaya RD, Ozdemir O. Adherence of internists and family physicians to SEMT guidelines for type 2 diabetes mellitus in Turkey. 11th ECE 2009, 25-29 April 2009, Istanbul, Turkey, Poster No. 295.
3. Satman I, Yilmaz C, Imamoglu S. Interrelationship among chronic complications, adherence of guidelines and degree of metabolic control in type 2 DM patients in Turkey. 91th Annual Meeting ENDO 09, 10-13 June 2009, Washington DC, USA, Poster No. 515.
4. Satman I, Imamoglu S, Yilmaz C. Relationship between adherence of physicians and the degree of glycaemic control in type 2 DNM patients in Turkey. 69th Scientific Session of ADA, 5-9 June 2009, New Orleans, USA, Poster No. 900.
5. Satman I, Imamoglu S, Yilmaz C and ADMIRE Study Group. Factors related with the adherence of physicians to diabetes guidelines in type 2 DM patients in Turkey. ECE 2011, 30 April-04 May 2011, Rotterdam, The Netherlands, Poster No. 672.
6. Satman I, Imamoglu S, Yilmaz C. Impact of adherence to guidelines on glycemic control and chronic complications in Turkey. 71st Scientific Session of ADA, 24-28 June 2011, New Orleans, USA, Poster No. 1189-P.
7. Satman I, Imamoglu S, Yilmaz C. Relationship between adherence of physicians to SEMT diabetes guidelines and degree of glycemic control in type 2 DM patients in Turkey. 93rd Annual Meeting ENDO 09, 4-7 June 2011, Boston, USA, Poster No. P2-758.
8. Satman I, Imamoglu S, Yilmaz C and ADMIRE Study Group. Türkiye'de Hekimlerin Tip 2 Diyabette TEMD Kılavuzuna Uyum Derecesi ile Glisemik Kontrol Arasındaki İlişkinin Değerlendirilmesi: ADMIRE Çalışması Birinci Aşama Sonuçları. 32nd Congress of Endocrinology and Metabolism Diseases of Turkey (TEMD) 2010, 13-17 October 2010, Antalya, Turkey.
9. Satman I, Imamoglu S, Yilmaz C and ADMIRE Study Group. Comparison of the Methods for Evaluation of Adherence to Type 2 DM Guidelines: Retrospective Chart Review vs. Prospective Patient Follow-up. World Diabetes Congress (WDC), IDF 2011, 4-8 December 2011, Dubai.

ADMIRE Study was performed by Diabetes Study Group of The Society of Endocrinology and Metabolism of Turkey (SEMT), with an unrestricted educational grant from sanofi.

5. References

[1] Satman I, Yilmaz T, Şengul A, Salman S, Salman F, Uygur S, Baştar I, Tutuncu Y, Sargin M, Dinccag N, Karsidag K, Kalaca S, Ozcan C, King H, and the TURDEP Group (2002) Population-Based Study of Diabetes and Risk Characteristics in Turkey: Results of the Turkish Diabetes Epidemiology Study (TURDEP). Diabetes care. 25: 1551-1556.

[2] Satman I, Tutuncu Y, Gedik S, Dinccag N, Karsidag K, Yilmaz T, Omer B, Kalaca S, Telci A, Cakir B, Tuomilehto J (2011) Diabetes Epidemic in Turkey: Results of The

Second Population-Based Survey of Diabetes and Risk Characteristics in Turkey (TURDEP-II). 47th EASD Annual Meeting, 12-16 Sept. 2011, Lisbon. Diabetologia 54 (Suppl. 1): 324, PS 007.

[3] The Diabetes Control and Complications Trial Research Group (1993) The Effect of Intensive Treatment of Diabetes on the Development and Progression of Long-Term Complications in Insulin-Dependent Diabetes Mellitus. N. engl. j. med. 329: 977-986.

[4] UK Prospective Diabetes Study Group (1998) Tight Blood Pressure Control and Risk of Macrovascular and Microvascular Complications in Type 2 Diabetes: UKPDS 38. BMJ. 317: 703-713.

[5] Gaede P, Lund-Andersen H, Parving HH, Pedersen O (2008) Effect of a Multifactorial Intervention on Mortality in Type 2 Diabetes. N. engl. j. med. 358: 580-591.

[6] Dailey G (2011) Overall Mortality in Diabetes Mellitus: Where Do We Stand Today? Diabetes technol. ther. 13 (Suppl. 1): S65-74.

[7] Dailey G (2011) Early and Intensive Therapy for Management of Hyperglycemia and Cardiovascular Risk Factors in Patients with Type 2 Diabetes. Clin. ther. 33: 665-678.

[8] O'Connor PJ, Sperl-Hillen JM, Johnson PE, Rush WA, Blitz G (2007) Clinical Inertia and Outpatient Medical Errors. Advances in patient safety. 2: 293-308.

[9] Grol R, Buchan H (2006) Clinical Guidelines: What Can We Do to Increase their Use? Med. j. aust. 185: 301-302.

[10] Cabana MD, Rand CS, Powe NR, Wu AW, Wilson MH, Abboud PA (1999) Why Don't Physicians Follow Clinical Practice Guidelines? A Framework for Improvement. JAMA. 282: 1458-1465.

[11] Brown JB, Harris SB, Webster-Bogaert S, Wetmore S, Faulds C, Stewart M (2002) The Role of Patient, Physician and Systemic Factors in the Management of Type 2 Diabetes Mellitus. Fam. pract. 19: 344-349.

[12] Satman I, Imamoglu S, Yilmaz C, ve TEMD Diyabet Calisma Grubu (Editorler) (2008) Diabetes Mellitus ve Komplikasyonlarinin Tani, Tedavi ve Izlem Kilavuzu. 3. Baski, Muka Matbaasi, Istanbul.

[13] Satman I, Imamoglu S, Yilmaz C, and Diabetes Study Group of SEMT (2010) Clinical Practice Guidelines for Diagnosis, Treatment, and Follow-up of Diabetes Mellitus and its Complications. Updated 4th Edition. Turkish j. endocrinology and metabolism. (Turk Jem) 14 (Suppl. 1).

[14] Satman I, Imamoglu S, Yilmaz C, Akalin S ve TEMD Diabetes Mellitus Egitim ve Calisma Grubu (Editorler) (2011) Diabetes Mellitus ve Komplikasyonlarinin Tani, Tedavi ve Izlem Kilavuzu. 5. Baski, Bayt Matbaası, Ankara.

[15] ADA Clinical Practice Recommendations (2009). Diabetes Care 2009;32(Suppl.1):S13-61.

[16] Nathan DM, Buse JB, Davidson MB, et al. Medical management of hyperglycemia in type 2 diabetes -a consensus algorithm for the initiation and adjustment of therapy: a

consensus statement of the American Diabetes Association and the European Association for the Study of Diabetes. Diabetes Care 2009;32:1-11.

[17] Ratsep A, Oja I, Kalda R, Lember M (2007) Family Doctors' Assessment of Patient- and Health Care System-Related Factors Contributing to Non-Adherence to Diabetes Mellitus Guidelines. Prim. care. diabetes. 1: 93-97.

[18] Hetlevik I, Holmen J, Midthjell K (1997) Treatment of Diabetes Mellitus--Physicians' Adherence to Clinical Guidelines in Norway. Scand. j. prim. health care. 15: 193-197.

[19] Chan GC, Ghazali O, Khoo EM (2005) Management of Type 2 Diabetes Mellitus: Is It in Accordance with The Guidelines? Med. j. Malaysia. 60: 578-584.

[20] James PA, Cowan TM, Graham RP, Majeroni BA (1997) Family Physicians' Attitudes About and Use of Clinical Practice Guidelines. J. fam. pract. 45: 341-347.

[21] Larme AC, Pugh JA (1998) Attitudes of Primary Care Providers Toward Diabetes: Barriers to Guideline Implementation. Diabetes care. 21: 1391-1396.

[22] Zafar A, Davies M, Azhar A, Khunti K (2010) Clinical Inertia in Management of T2DM. Prim. care diabetes. 4: 203-207.

[23] Philips JC, Scheen AJ (2010) Clinical Inertia in the Management of Patients with Type 2 Diabetes: How to Solve it?. Rev. med. liege. 65: 318-325.

[24] Albisser AM, Inhaber F (2010) Automation of the Consensus Guidelines in Diabetes Care: Potential Impact on Clinical Inertia. Endocr. pract. 16: 992-1002.

[25] Borgermans L, Goderis G, Van Den Broeke C, Mathieu C, Aertgeerts B, Verbeke G, Carbonez A, Ivanova A, Grol R, Heyrman J (2008) A Cluster Randomized Trial to Improve Adherence to Evidence-based Guidelines on Diabetes and Reduce Clinical Inertia in Primary Care Physicians in Belgium: Study Protocol [NTR 1369]. Implement sci. 3: 42.

[26] Reach G (2008) Patient Non-adherence and Healthcare-provider Inertia are Clinical Myopia. Diabetes metab. 34(4 Pt 1): 382-385.

[27] Cook CB, Castro JC, Schmidt RE, Gauthier SM, Whitaker MD, Roust LR, Argueta R, Hull BP, Zimmerman RS (2007) Diabetes Care in Hospitalized Noncritically Ill Patients: More Evidence for Clinical Inertia and Negative Therapeutic Momentum. J. hosp. med. 2: 203-211.

[28] Ziemer DC, Doyle JP, Barnes CS, Branch WT Jr, Cook CB, El-Kebbi IM, Gallina DL, Kolm P, Rhee MK, Phillips LS (2006) An Intervention to Overcome Clinical Inertia and Improve Diabetes Mellitus Control in a Primary Care Setting: Improving Primary Care of African Americans with Diabetes (IPCAAD) 8. Arch. intern. med. 166: 507-513.

[29] Phillips LS, Branch WT, Cook CB, Doyle JP, El-Kebbi IM, Gallina DL, Miller CD, Ziemer DC, Barnes CS (2001) Clinical Inertia. Ann. intern. med. 135: 825-834.

[30] McKinlay JB, Link CL, Freund KM, Marceau LD, O'Donnell AB, Lutfey KL (2007) Sources of Variation in Physician Adherence with Clinical Guidelines: Results From a Factorial Experiment. J. gen. intern. med. 22: 289-296.

[31] Gerstein HC, Reddy SS, Dawson KG, Yale JF, Shannon S, Norman G (1999) A Controlled Evaluation of a National Continuing Medical Education Programme Designed to Improve Family Physicians' Implementation of Diabetes-Specific Clinical Practice Guidelines. Diabet med. 16: 964-969.

Chapter 8

Oestrogen Dependent Regulation of Gonadal Fate

Andrew John Pask

Additional information is available at the end of the chapter

http://dx.doi.org/10.5772/50701

1. Introduction

In mammals, the ovary has been historically viewed as the default gonadal state, such that in the absence of the Y-chromosome and the sex determining switch gene, *SRY*, an ovary would passively form (Wilhelm et al. 2007). This view was in stark contrast to our understanding of gonadal development in non-mammalian vertebrates, where the opposite appears to be true. Ovarian development is the active state, achieved in the presence of estrogen, while development of the testis appears to passively occur in the absence of estrogen signalling (Nagahama 2005) (Figure 1). Despite the different modes of achieving sex determination, recent research suggests that in fact, the role of estrogen may not be so different between non-mammalian and mammalian vertebrates.

Gonads are comprised of two primary cell types: the somatic cell lineages including the supporting cells and the germ cell lineage which gives rise to the haploid gametes. In testes, the supporting cells consist of the Sertoli cells, which support spermatogenesis, the Leydig cells, which produce testosterone, the peritubular myoid cells, which maintain the structure of the testis cord through the secretion of the basal lamina and the endothelial cells that form the vasculature. In the ovary, the supportings consist of the granulosa cells that support oogenesis, the theca cells that secrete hormones, and the stromal cells will form the connective tissue of the ovary. The germ cells will become the spermatozoa in the testes and oocytes in the ovary. The fate of the germ cells is dependent on the somatic cell environment, (ie, whether they are surrounded by Sertoli or granulosa cells) which, in turn, regulates the appropriate development of the gonad (Koubova et al. 2006; Bowles et al. 2006). Germ cells in the developing ovary will enter into meiotic arrest early in development, while testicular germ cells will arrest in mitosis. The regulation of germ cell entry into meiosis in the ovary is induced by retinoic acid (RA), which activates the expression of Stra8, a cytoplasmic protein required for pre-meiotic DNA replication

(Koubova et al. 2006). Early entry into meiosis in males is prevented by expression of *Cyp26b1* in the Sertoli cells, an enzyme in the cytochrome P450 family that degrades RA (Koubova et al. 2006; Bowles et al. 2006; Vernet et al. 2006). Thus, establishing somatic cell fate is key to regulating the overall development of the gonad.

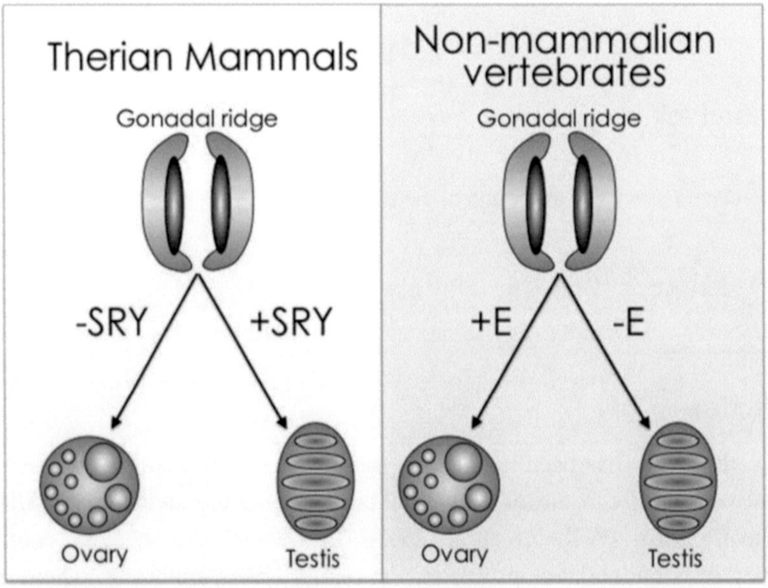

Figure 1. In most therian mammals (marsupials and eutherians; left panel), sex is determined by the presence or absence of the testis determining factor SRY, located on the Y-chromosome. When SRY is present, the gonad is activated to follow a testis pathway, while in its absence the ovary will develop. This is in contrast to most non-mammalian vertebrates (right panel) where sex appears to be determined by the presence or absence of oestrogen, which drives active ovarian development from the indifferent gonad when present. In the absence of oestrogen, the testis will form.

In the male gonad, it is the activation of *SOX9* (Sry-type HMG box number 9) in the somatic cells that directs Sertoli cell differentiation (Sinclair et al. 1990; Bishop et al. 2000). *SOX9* and its gonadal enhancer, TESCO (Testis-specific Enhancer of Sox9 Core element), are highly conserved in the tetrapods, suggesting they play a critical function in vertebrate testis development (Bagheri-Fam et al. 2010). SOX9 is initially present at low levels in the indifferent gonad and is localized to the cytoplasm of the somatic cell precursors. In developing testes, SOX9 translocates to the nucleus and is subsequently dramatically upregulated (de Santa Barbara et al. 2000; El Jamil et al. 2008; Morais da Silva et al. 1996). In mammals, it is the expression of the Y-linked sex-determining gene *SRY* (Sex-determining Region on the Y chromosome) that triggers *SOX9* upregulation in the male gonad (Sekido and Lovell-Badge 2008). SRY has been shown to bind directly to TESCO, leading to SOX9 activation. SOX9 then acts as a transcriptional activator of the testis differentiation pathway. The nuclear translocation of SOX9 is both necessary and sufficient for Sertoli cell development in mice (Qin et al. 2004; Bishop et al. 2000), and is the most critical step in the initiation of the testis pathway. However, even after testicular fate is established, the Sertoli cell phenotype remains plastic. In mice, expression of *Dmrt1* (Doublesex and mab-3 related transcription factor 1) is essential to maintain Sertoli cells (Matson et al. 2011). Loss of *Dmrt1* even in adult Sertoli cells, leads to upregulation of *FoxL2* (Forkhead box L2) and transdifferentiation in to a granulosa cell phenotype. Thus, development of the gonad requires a tightly regulated set of key factors to specify and then maintain gonadal cell identity.

2. Molecular control of ovarian differentiation

Since SRY is absent from the XX gonad, *SOX9* upregulation is not triggered, and SOX9 protein levels remain low and cytoplasmic in the somatic cells of the indifferent gonad. In the absence of nuclear SOX9, the testis differentiation pathway cannot be initiated and granulosa cell development is activated, leading ultimately to ovarian development. The precise mechanism preventing SOX9 from entering the nucleus and activating the Sertoli cell program in female gonads is unknown, but recent data suggest that oestrogen may play a key role in this process (Pask et al. 2010). The potential effect of estrogen on sex determination in mammals, including humans, is of great interest due to a recent increase in male reproductive abnormalities in humans and wildlife, resulting in lower sperm counts and quality and increased rates of hypospadias and testicular dysgenesis. The increase in these disorders is too rapid to be accounted for genetic factors, and instead has been attributed to an increased exposure to synthetic environmental endocrine disrupting compounds found in the environment (Giwercman et al. 1993; Carlsen et al. 1992). Defining how endogenous and exogenous estrogen affects gonadal development in mammals is essential for understanding the aetiology of such disorders.

The sex determining *SRY* gene was discovered in 1990 (Sinclair et al. 1990) and much of the subsequent research has focused on how it mediates testicular development. It is only in the past decade, that key ovary-promoting genes have been identified in mice and humans, which include the *WNT4* (Wingless-type MMTV Integration Site Family, Member 4), *RSPO1* (R-spondin-1) and *FOXL2* genes. Mutations in each of these genes is associated with a failure of normal ovarian formation in mice and humans (Chassot et al. 2008a; Chassot et al. 2008b; Heikkila et al. 2001; Uda et al. 2004; Vainio et al. 1999). In mice, Rspo1 activates the canonical beta-catenin signalling pathway required for female somatic cell differentiation (Chassot et al. 2008a; Chassot et al. 2008b). WNT4 suppresses the development of Leydig cells in the developing ovary and may act through follistatin (Fst) since mutations in both these gene result in a failure of the coelomic vessel to form (a key event in murine testis development) in XY mouse gonads and a loss of germ cells (Yao et al. 2004). The development of Leydig cells in *WNT4* mutant females results in masculinization and when the female germ cells are lost, seminiferous-like cords form (Heikkila et al. 2001; Vainio et al. 1999). Thus the germ cells play a central role in the development of a normal ovarian morphology (reviewed in (Whitworth 1998; Capel 2000; Brennan and Capel 2004)). While the loss of XX either mitotic or meiotic germ cells results in the formation of seminiferous-like cords in a developing ovary, loss of male germ cells has no effect on testicular formation

(Whitworth 1998; Burgoyne 1988; McLaren 1991; Whitworth et al. 1996). These findings suggest that XX germ cells actively participate in maintaining ovarian histology by inhibiting cord formation and highlight the importance of somatic cell-germ cell interactions in gonadal development.

FoxL2 is another gene that plays a central role in ovarian development by regulating female somatic cell fate. Ablation of FoxL2 in adult mouse ovaries leads to a loss of granulosa cell identity and instead the somatic cells develop a Sertoli cell phenotype and an show the upregulation of Sertoli cell markers such as *SOX9* (Uhlenhaut et al. 2009). FoxL2 appears to mediate somatic cell fate in the ovary by suppressing the male developmental program. It achieves this role through directly binding to the *SOX9* enhancer element, TESCO, suppressing *SOX9* transcription. Interestingly, FoxL2 achieves TESCO suppression in conjunction with activated oestrogen receptors (Uhlenhaut et al. 2009). The function of FOXL2 and activated oestrogen receptors in suppressing SOX9 appears to be highly conserved as the binding sites for both proteins are highly conserved in TESCO across mammals, including in the marsupials which last shared a common ancestor with the mouse over 160 million years ago (Luo et al. 2011) (Figure 2). Furthermore, FOXL2 has been shown to play a direct role in the upregulation of *CYP19* (Cytochrome P450 Aromatase; required for the synthesis of oestrogen from testosterone) in both the fish brain (Sridevi et al. 2011) and indifferent XX goat gonad, where it initiates the synthesis of oestrogen, promoting ovarian development (Pannetier et al. 2004).

3. Oestrogenic control of ovarian cell fate

Non-mammalian vertebrates trigger sex of the developing fetus in a variety of different ways. These can largely be grouped into either genetic sex determining mechanisms, where a sex specific gene triggers sex, or environmental sex determination, where extrinsic cues determine sex. Oestrogen is known to play an essential role in female sex determination in nonmammalian vertebrates regardless of the sex determining mechanism (Solari 1994; Nakamura 2010). The production of oestrogen in the indifferent gonad is controlled by the expression of *CYP19,* which encodes the aromatase enzyme and causes oestrogen production. In the presence of oestrogen, the indifferent gonad will follow an ovarian development pathway, while in its absence the gonad will become a testis (Solari 1994). As a result, exogenous oestrogen exposure to developing fish, reptile, amphibian and bird fetuses will trigger ovarian development, while exposure to oestrogen inhibitors causes testis development (Solari 1994; Ramsey and Crews 2009). This is in contrast to mammals where SRY triggers testis development and the ovary is the default state. However, in nonmammalian vertebrates, oestrogen appears to be the master regulator of ovarian development and in its absence the gonad will default to a testicular fate.

Despite the highly conserved role of oestrogen in nonmammalian vertebrates, its function in the development of the mammalian ovary remains less clear. Interestingly, expression of the oestrogen receptors, which mediate oestrogen actions within the cell, is maintained in the somatic cells of the indifferent gonads of mice, humans, goats, sheep and marsupials indicative of a highly conserved role for oestrogen in the early mammalian gonad (Calatayud et al. 2010). It was a surprising finding then, that oestrogen was not required for initial ovarian development in mice (Couse and Korach 1999). Mice deficient for both the alpha and beta oestrogen receptors or *CYP19*, have normal early ovarian differentiation (Britt and Findlay 2003; Britt et al. 2001). However, shortly after birth, germ cells are lost and the somatic cells take on a Sertoli cell phenotype (Fisher et al. 1998; Toda et al. 2001). These Sertoli-like cells express *SOX9* and show a characteristic Sertoli cell morphology, with tight junctions, and arrangement (Britt and Findlay 2003). Upon administration of oestrogen to aromatase deficient mice, ovarian histology is restored and *SOX9* levels are significantly decreased, along with several other testis markers, to normal female levels (Britt et al. 2004). Together these data show that the somatic cells of the ovary also retain a plasticity that, along with the genes regulating somatic cell differentiation, is directly responsive to oestrogen.

While mouse studies have been fundamental in developing a basic understanding of gonadal differentiation, there are differences in gene expression, responses to haploinsufficiency of critical genes and, most importantly, in the role of oestrogen in the fetal gonad between mice and other mammals (Wilhelm et al. 2007). Comparative analyses across multiple species can be particularly helpful in isolating critical regulatory networks required for developmental events from those that show species specific variations (Sanchez et al. 2011; Pounds et al. 2011; Crozat et al. 2010; Lu et al. 2009). Outside of the rodent lineage, upregulation of *CYP19* has been reported in the fetal ovary of many eutherian species including goats (Pannetier et al. 2004), sheep (Quirke et al. 2001) and cows (Garverick et al. 2010), suggesting oestrogen may play a central role in its early differentiation. Similarly, in humans, exposure of the developing fetus to potent synthetic oestrogenic compounds can dramatically affect male gonadal differentiation (Toppari 2008; Arai et al. 1983). Thus, it appears that gonadal development in rodents may be unusually resistant to a loss of oestrogen.

The ability for oestrogen to direct ovarian development in mammals has been demonstrated in marsupials (Pask et al. 2010; Coveney et al. 2001; Burns 1955). Marsupials have been evolving independently of humans and mice for around 160 million years (Figure 2) (Luo et al. 2011). Sexual differentiation occurs around the time of birth in marsupial, unlike in eutherian mammals where this process occurs *in utero*. Marsupials develop gonads that are identical in structure to human and mouse gonads and determine sex based on the presence/absence of the *SRY* bearing Y chromosome (Pask and Graves 2001). Development of the somatic cell lineages and germ cell entry into either meiotic or mitotic arrest is separated by several days in the tammar wallaby, similar to the developmental timing seen in human, goat, sheep and cow gonads, whereas in the mouse these events occur concurrently (Harry et al. 1995; Renfree et al. 1996). Thus in marsupials it is possible to examine the effects of exogenous oestrogen on the differentiation of the somatic cell lineages *ex utero*, uncomplicated by changes in germ cell development or the *in utero* environment.

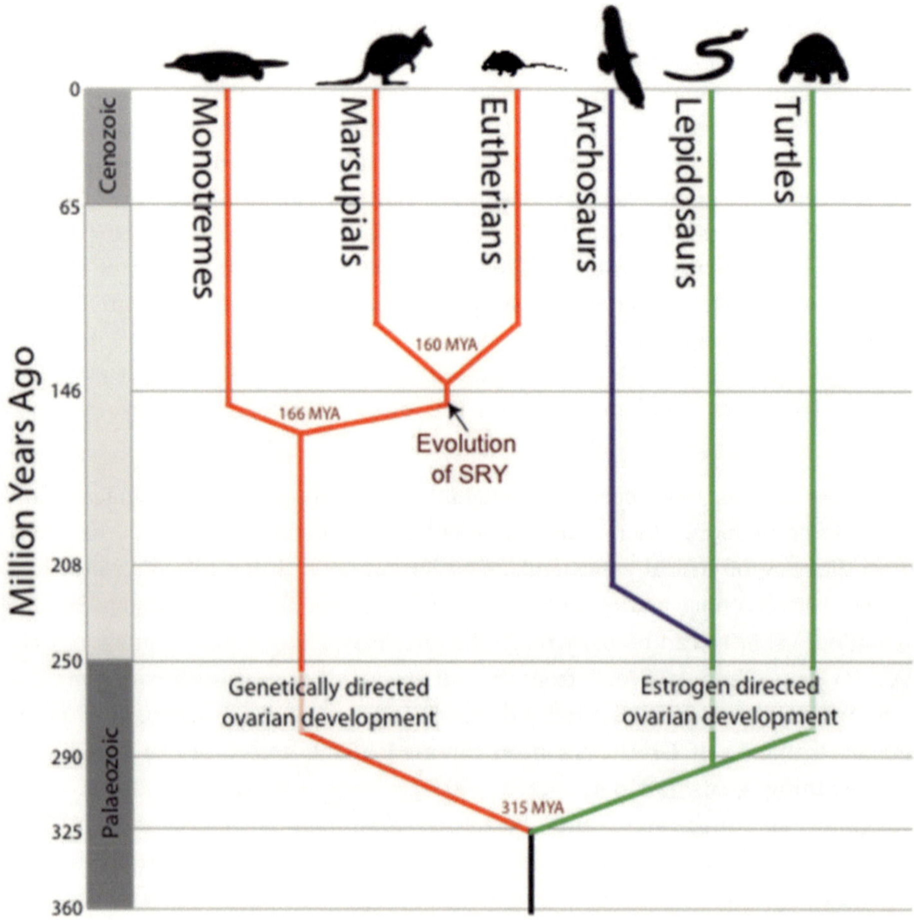

Figure 2. Alternative control of sex determination in amniotes. Amniotes split into the sauropsids (leading to birds and reptiles) and synapsids (leading to mammal-like reptiles). Both lineages have fundamentally different control of gonadal development. In the mammals (at least in marsupial and eutherian lineages) sex is controlled by the presence of the SRY gene on the Y. In non-mammalian amniotes, sex is primarily dependant on whether the gonad is exposed to estrogen or not in early development.

4. Oestrogen blocks male development by modulating SOX9

Administration of oestrogen to genetically male marsupial neonates causes ovarian development of the gonad (Pask et al. 2010; Coveney et al. 2001; Burns 1955). In the presence of oestrogen, key male differentiation genes fail to be up-regulated in the XY gonad and instead, key ovary-promoting genes are upregulated leading to ovarian development (Pask et al. 2010). Oestrogen appears to trigger sex reversal through the exclusion of SOX9 from entering the nucleus in the somatic cells of the developing gonad (Pask et al. 2010). In the absence of nuclear SOX9, Sertoli cell development cannot be initiated and the somatic cells follow a granulosa cell fate (Figure 3).

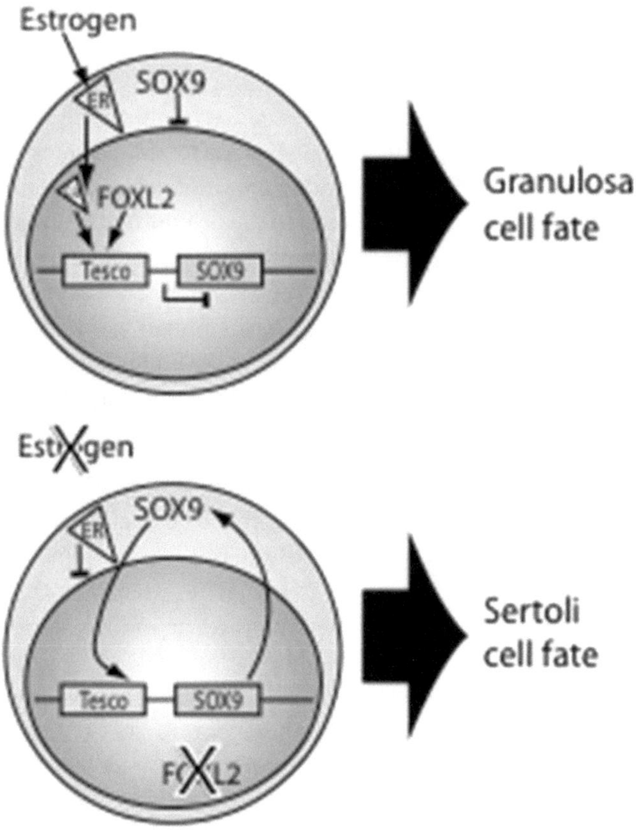

Figure 3. A potential model for the role of oestrogen in somatic cell determination and maintenance. In the presence of oestrogen (top panel), the activated oestrogen receptors direct gonadal somatic cells towards the granulosa cell pathway. Activated ERs (Oestrogen Receptors) work together with FOXL2 to suppress *TESCO* and *SOX9* transcription. Any SOX9 protein already produced within the cell fails to enter the nucleus. In the absence of nuclear SOX9, *AMH* fails to upregulate and ovarian genes are activated. Exogenous oestrogen retains the ability to direct XY bipotential somatic cells towards a granulosa cell fate. Oestrogen may act in a similar manner to maintain granulosa cell fate in mature eutherian ovaries, preventing basal levels of SOX9 protein from translocating to the nucleus and propagating its own upregulation. In normal XY gonads (bottom panel), the somatic cells upregulate *SRY*, which in turn upregulates *SOX9*. *SOX9* is translated and SOX9 protein can then translocate to the nucleus and activate the expression of *AMH* and direct Sertoli cell development.

A conserved role for oestrogen mediating SOX9 action is consistent with several observations in mammals. In mice, Sox9 is able to autoregulate by binding to its own promoter (Sekido and Lovell-Badge 2008). However, despite *Sox9* expression in the somatic cells of the adult mouse ovary, it does not become upregulated (Notarnicola et al. 2006). High levels of oestrogen could prevent the nuclear translocation of SOX9 in adult female gonads, preventing its own upregulation. Conversely, Sox9 is upregulated in the absence of oestrogen in aromatase-deficient mice ovaries, suggesting it can translocate to the nucleus to propagate its own transcription. However, when these mice are exposed to exogenous oestrogen the effect is reversible, and *Sox9* is repressed (Britt et al. 2002; de Santa Barbara et al. 2000). Data from marsupials would suggest this repression occurs by trapping SOX9 in the cytoplasm preventing its autoregulation. Furthermore, activated oestrogen receptors, in conjunction FoxL2, could directly suppress *SOX9* transcription through binding to TESCO (Uhlenhaut et al. 2009). Either way, in mammals oestrogen still remains a critical factor in maintaining ovarian somatic cell fate. This fundamental role of oestrogen is also consistent with observations in nonmammalian vertebrates. In the presence of oestrogen SOX9 remains cytoplasmic in the early developing gonads of many nonmammalian vertebrates permitting granulosa cell development (de Santa Barbara et al. 2000). However, in the absence of oestrogen, SOX9 becomes nuclear and Sertoli cell development is initiated (Sim et al. 2008). Therefore, the ability of oestrogen to mediate the subcellular localization of SOX9 and directly mediate its transcription, could explain the primary mechanism by which oestrogen establishes sex in nonmammalian vertebrates.

Further investigations are needed to determine how oestrogen mediates the subcellular localization of SOX9 within the somatic cells. SOX9 contains two defined nuclear localization signals (NLS) found in the C- and N-termini that are 100% conserved between mouse, human and the wallaby (Pask et al. 2002). Active transport through nucleopore complex is facilitated in part by importin-β, binding directly to the C-terminal NLS (Sim et al. 2008). This binding is enhanced by phosphorylation of SOX9 by phosphokinase A, facilitating increased nuclear import (Malki et al. 2005). The N-terminal NLS binds calmodulin, another factor that facilitates nuclear transport of SOX9 (Argentaro et al. 2003). SOX9 is also subject to SUMOylation and ubiquitination (Sim et al. 2008). SUMOylation has been shown to regulate nucleocytoplasmic trafficking of several proteins while ubiquitination marks proteins for degradation. SUMOylation of SOX9 in COS7 cells has been shown to alter its subnuclear localisation and transcriptional activity (Hattori et al. 2006). Oestrogen may affect one or many of these different pathways to regulate the subcellular localization and activity of SOX9.

5. Conclusions

5.1. A conserved model for determining vertebrate somatic cell fate

While the switch mechanisms that trigger the development of the ovary or testis pathways vary widely among vertebrates, the fundamental control mechanisms regulating somatic cell fate share many commonalities. This suggests a highly conserved and antagonistic relationship between SOX9 and oestrogen driving Sertoli cell and granulosa cell differentiation respectively. In mammals, the somatic cell decision is initially determined by the presence or absence of SRY. When SRY is present, *SOX9* is upregulated and can translocate to the nucleus to activate Sertoli cell differentiation. In females, in the absence of *SRY*, *SOX9* is not upregulated and the granulosa cell program is initiated. While it is yet to be shown if oestrogen plays a critical role in early mammalian ovary formation outside of the rodent lineage, oestrogen is essential for maintaining granulosa cell fate in the mature gonads, possibly by ensuring that any SOX9 protein produced remains trapped in the cytoplasm. In nonmammalian vertebrates, the primary sex determining mechanism, be it genetic sex determination or environmental sex determination, leads to either the presence or absence of *CYP19* expression. In the presence of aromatase and oestrogen, basal SOX9 cannot enter the nucleus and the Sertoli cell program is blocked. In the absence of aromatase and oestrogen, SOX9 can translocate to the nucleus, trigger its own upregulation and initiate Sertoli cell development. More work is needed to confirm this model and determine the precise mechanism by which activated oestrogen receptors mediate the subcellular localization of SOX9. However, these findings provide a simple explanation for the dramatic switch in vertebrate sex determination mechanisms from primarily hormonal control to primarily genetic control, converging through the modulation of SOX9.

Author details

Andrew John Pask
Department of Molecular and Cell Biology, The University of Connecticut, Storrs, USA

6. References

Arai Y, Mori T, Suzuki Y, Bern HA (1983) Long-term effects of perinatal exposure to sex steroids and diethylstilbestrol on the reproductive system of male mammals. Int Rev Cytol 84:235-268

Argentaro A, Sim H, Kelly S, Preiss S, Clayton A, Jans DA, Harley VR (2003) A SOX9 defect of calmodulin-dependent nuclear import in campomelic dysplasia/autosomal sex reversal. J Biol Chem 278 (36):33839-33847. doi:10.1074/jbc.M302078200 M302078200 [pii]

Bagheri-Fam S, Sinclair AH, Koopman P, Harley VR (2010) Conserved regulatory modules in the Sox9 testis-specific enhancer predict roles for SOX, TCF/LEF, Forkhead, DMRT, and GATA proteins in vertebrate sex determination. Int J Biochem Cell Biol 42 (3):472-477. doi:S1357-2725(09)00193-9 [pii] 10.1016/j.biocel.2009.07.001

Bishop CE, Whitworth DJ, Qin Y, Agoulnik AI, Agoulnik IU, Harrison WR, Behringer RR, Overbeek PA (2000) A transgenic insertion upstream of sox9 is associated with dominant XX sex reversal in the mouse. Nat Genet 26 (4):490-494. doi:10.1038/82652

Bowles J, Knight D, Smith C, Wilhelm D, Richman J, Mamiya S, Yashiro K, Chawengsaksophak K, Wilson MJ, Rossant J, Hamada H, Koopman P (2006) Retinoid signaling determines germ cell fate in mice. Science 312 (5773):596-600. doi:1125691 [pii] 10.1126/science.1125691

Brennan J, Capel B (2004) One tissue, two fates: molecular genetic events that underlie testis versus ovary development. Nat Rev Genet 5 (7):509-521. doi:10.1038/nrg1381 nrg1381 [pii]

Britt KL, Drummond AE, Dyson M, Wreford NG, Jones ME, Simpson ER, Findlay JK (2001) The ovarian phenotype of the aromatase knockout (ArKO) mouse. J Steroid Biochem Mol Biol 79 (1-5):181-185. doi:S0960076001001583 [pii]

Britt KL, Findlay JK (2003) Regulation of the phenotype of ovarian somatic cells by estrogen. Mol Cell Endocrinol 202 (1-2):11-17. doi:S0303720703000558 [pii]

Britt KL, Kerr J, O'Donnell L, Jones ME, Drummond AE, Davis SR, Simpson ER, Findlay JK (2002) Estrogen regulates development of the somatic cell phenotype in the eutherian ovary. FASEB J 16 (11):1389-1397. doi:10.1096/fj.01-0992com 16/11/1389 [pii]

Britt KL, Stanton PG, Misso M, Simpson ER, Findlay JK (2004) The effects of estrogen on the expression of genes underlying the differentiation of somatic cells in the murine gonad. Endocrinology 145 (8):3950-3960. doi:10.1210/en.2003-1628 en.2003-1628 [pii]

Burgoyne PS (1988) Role of mammalian Y chromosome in sex determination. Philos Trans R Soc Lond B Biol Sci 322 (1208):63-72

Burns RK (1955) Experimental Reversal of Sex in the Gon Ads of the Opossum Didelphis Virginiana. Proc Natl Acad Sci U S A 41 (9):669-676

Calatayud NE, Pask AJ, Shaw G, Richings NM, Osborn S, Renfree MB (2010) Ontogeny of the oestrogen receptors ESR1 and ESR2 during gonadal development in the tammar wallaby, Macropus eugenii. Reproduction 139 (3):599-611. doi:REP-09-0305 [pii] 10.1530/REP-09-0305

Capel B (2000) The battle of the sexes. Mech Dev 92 (1):89-103. doi:S0925477399003275 [pii]

Carlsen E, Giwercman A, Keiding N, Skakkebaek NE (1992) Evidence for decreasing quality of semen during past 50 years. BMJ 305 (6854):609-613

Chassot AA, Gregoire EP, Magliano M, Lavery R, Chaboissier MC (2008a) Genetics of ovarian differentiation: Rspo1, a major player. Sex Dev 2 (4-5):219-227. doi:000152038 [pii] 10.1159/000152038

Chassot AA, Ranc F, Gregoire EP, Roepers-Gajadien HL, Taketo MM, Camerino G, de Rooij DG, Schedl A, Chaboissier MC (2008b) Activation of beta-catenin signaling by Rspo1 controls differentiation of the mammalian ovary. Hum Mol Genet 17 (9):1264-1277. doi:ddn016 [pii] 10.1093/hmg/ddn016

Couse JF, Korach KS (1999) Estrogen receptor null mice: what have we learned and where will they lead us? Endocr Rev 20 (3):358-417

Coveney D, Shaw G, Renfree MB (2001) Estrogen-induced gonadal sex reversal in the tammar wallaby. Biol Reprod 65 (2):613-621

Crozat K, Guiton R, Guilliams M, Henri S, Baranek T, Schwartz-Cornil I, Malissen B, Dalod M (2010) Comparative genomics as a tool to reveal functional equivalences between human and mouse dendritic cell subsets. Immunol Rev 234 (1):177-198. doi:IMR868 [pii] 10.1111/j.0105-2896.2009.00868.x

de Santa Barbara P, Moniot B, Poulat F, Berta P (2000) Expression and subcellular localization of SF-1, SOX9, WT1, and AMH proteins during early human testicular development. Dev Dyn 217 (3):293-298.

El Jamil A, Kanhoush R, Magre S, Boizet-Bonhoure B, Penrad-Mobayed M (2008) Sex-specific expression of SOX9 during gonadogenesis in the amphibian Xenopus tropicalis. Dev Dyn 237 (10):2996-3005. doi:10.1002/dvdy.21692

Fisher CR, Graves KH, Parlow AF, Simpson ER (1998) Characterization of mice deficient in aromatase (ArKO) because of targeted disruption of the cyp19 gene. Proc Natl Acad Sci U S A 95 (12):6965-6970

Garverick HA, Juengel JL, Smith P, Heath DA, Burkhart MN, Perry GA, Smith MF, McNatty KP (2010) Development of the ovary and ontongeny of mRNA and protein for P450 aromatase (arom) and estrogen receptors (ER) alpha and beta during early fetal life in cattle. Anim Reprod Sci 117 (1-2):24-33. doi:S0378-4320(09)00120-1 [pii] 10.1016/j.anireprosci.2009.05.004

Giwercman A, Carlsen E, Keiding N, Skakkebaek NE (1993) Evidence for increasing incidence of abnormalities of the human testis: a review. Environ Health Perspect 101 Suppl 2:65-71

Harry JL, Koopman P, Brennan FE, Graves JA, Renfree MB (1995) Widespread expression of the testis-determining gene SRY in a marsupial. Nat Genet 11 (3):347-349. doi:10.1038/ng1195-347

Hattori T, Eberspaecher H, Lu J, Zhang R, Nishida T, Kahyo T, Yasuda H, de Crombrugghe B (2006) Interactions between PIAS proteins and SOX9 result in an increase in the cellular concentrations of SOX9. J Biol Chem 281 (20):14417-14428. doi:M511330200 [pii] 10.1074/jbc.M511330200

Heikkila M, Peltoketo H, Vainio S (2001) Wnts and the female reproductive system. J Exp Zool 290 (6):616-623. doi:10.1002/jez.1112 [pii]

Koubova J, Menke DB, Zhou Q, Capel B, Griswold MD, Page DC (2006) Retinoic acid regulates sex-specific timing of meiotic initiation in mice. Proc Natl Acad Sci U S A 103 (8):2474-2479. doi:0510813103 [pii] 10.1073/pnas.0510813103

Lu Y, Huggins P, Bar-Joseph Z (2009) Cross species analysis of microarray expression data. Bioinformatics 25 (12):1476-1483. doi:btp247 [pii] 10.1093/bioinformatics/btp247

Luo ZX, Yuan CX, Meng QJ, Ji Q (2011) A Jurassic eutherian mammal and divergence of marsupials and placentals. Nature 476 (7361):442-445. doi:nature10291 [pii] 10.1038/nature10291

Malki S, Nef S, Notarnicola C, Thevenet L, Gasca S, Mejean C, Berta P, Poulat F, Boizet-Bonhoure B (2005) Prostaglandin D2 induces nuclear import of the sex-determining factor SOX9 via its cAMP-PKA phosphorylation. EMBO J 24 (10):1798-1809. doi:7600660 [pii] 10.1038/sj.emboj.7600660

Matson CK, Murphy MW, Sarver AL, Griswold MD, Bardwell VJ, Zarkower D (2011) DMRT1 prevents female reprogramming in the postnatal mammalian testis. Nature 476 (7358):101-104. doi:nature10239 [pii] 10.1038/nature10239

McLaren A (1991) Development of the mammalian gonad: the fate of the supporting cell lineage. Bioessays 13 (4):151-156. doi:10.1002/bies.950130402

Morais da Silva S, Hacker A, Harley V, Goodfellow P, Swain A, Lovell-Badge R (1996) Sox9 expression during gonadal development implies a conserved role for the gene in testis differentiation in mammals and birds. Nat Genet 14 (1):62-68. doi:10.1038/ng0996-62

Nagahama Y (2005) Molecular mechanisms of sex determination and gonadal sex differentiation in fish. Fish Physiol Biochem 31 (2-3):105-109. doi:10.1007/s10695-006-7590-2

Nakamura M (2010) The mechanism of sex determination in vertebrates-are sex steroids the key-factor? J Exp Zool A Ecol Genet Physiol 313 (7):381-398. doi:10.1002/jez.616

Notarnicola C, Malki S, Berta P, Poulat F, Boizet-Bonhoure B (2006) Transient expression of SOX9 protein during follicular development in the adult mouse ovary. Gene Expr Patterns 6 (7):695-702. doi:S1567-133X(06)00005-6 [pii] 10.1016/j.modgep.2006.01.001

Pannetier M, Mandon-Pepin B, Copelli S, Fellous M (2004) Molecular aspects of female and male gonadal development in mammals. Pediatr Endocrinol Rev 1 (3):274-287

Pask A, Graves JA (2001) Sex chromosomes and sex-determining genes: insights from marsupials and monotremes. EXS (91):71-95

Pask AJ, Calatayud NE, Shaw G, Wood WM, Renfree MB (2010) Oestrogen blocks the nuclear entry of SOX9 in the developing gonad of a marsupial mammal. BMC Biol 8 (1):113. doi:1741-7007-8-113 [pii] 10.1186/1741-7007-8-113

Pask AJ, Harry JL, Graves JA, O'Neill RJ, Layfield SL, Shaw G, Renfree MB (2002) SOX9 has both conserved and novel roles in marsupial sexual differentiation. Genesis 33 (3):131-139. doi:10.1002/gene.10096

Pounds S, Gao CL, Johnson RA, Wright KD, Poppleton H, Finkelstein D, Leary SE, Gilbertson RJ (2011) A Procedure to Statistically Evaluate Agreement of Differential Expression for Cross-Species Genomics. Bioinformatics. doi:btr362 [pii] 10.1093/bioinformatics/btr362

Qin Y, Kong LK, Poirier C, Truong C, Overbeek PA, Bishop CE (2004) Long-range activation of Sox9 in Odd Sex (Ods) mice. Hum Mol Genet 13 (12):1213-1218. doi:10.1093/hmg/ddh141 ddh141 [pii]

Quirke LD, Juengel JL, Tisdall DJ, Lun S, Heath DA, McNatty KP (2001) Ontogeny of steroidogenesis in the fetal sheep gonad. Biol Reprod 65 (1):216-228

Ramsey M, Crews D (2009) Steroid signaling and temperature-dependent sex determination-Reviewing the evidence for early action of estrogen during ovarian determination in turtles. Semin Cell Dev Biol 20 (3):283-292. doi:S1084-9521(08)00117-1 [pii] 10.1016/j.semcdb.2008.10.004

Renfree MB, O WS, Short RV, Shaw G (1996) Sexual differentiation of the urogenital system of the fetal and neonatal tammar wallaby, Macropus eugenii. Anat Embryol (Berl) 194 (2):111-134

Sanchez DH, Pieckenstain FL, Szymanski J, Erban A, Bromke M, Hannah MA, Kraemer U, Kopka J, Udvardi MK (2011) Comparative functional genomics of salt stress in related model and cultivated plants identifies and overcomes limitations to translational genomics. PLoS One 6 (2):e17094. doi:10.1371/journal.pone.0017094

Sekido R, Lovell-Badge R (2008) Sex determination involves synergistic action of SRY and SF1 on a specific Sox9 enhancer. Nature 453 (7197):930-934. doi:nature06944 [pii] 10.1038/nature06944

Sim H, Argentaro A, Harley VR (2008) Boys, girls and shuttling of SRY and SOX9. Trends Endocrinol Metab 19 (6):213-222. doi:S1043-2760(08)00089-1 [pii] 10.1016/j.tem.2008.04.002

Sinclair AH, Berta P, Palmer MS, Hawkins JR, Griffiths BL, Smith MJ, Foster JW, Frischauf AM, Lovell-Badge R, Goodfellow PN (1990) A gene from the human sex-determining region encodes a protein with homology to a conserved DNA-binding motif. Nature 346 (6281):240-244. doi:10.1038/346240a0

Solari AJ (1994) Sex chromosomes and sex determination in vertebrates. CRC Press, Boca Raton

Sridevi P, Chaitanya RK, Dutta-Gupta A, Senthilkumaran B (2011) FTZ-F1 and FOXL2 up-regulate catfish brain aromatase gene transcription by specific binding to the promoter motifs. Biochim Biophys Acta. doi:S1874-9399(11)00179-9 [pii] 10.1016/j.bbagrm.2011.10.003

Toda K, Takeda K, Okada T, Akira S, Saibara T, Kaname T, Yamamura K, Onishi S, Shizuta Y (2001) Targeted disruption of the aromatase P450 gene (Cyp19) in mice and their ovarian and uterine responses to 17beta-oestradiol. J Endocrinol 170 (1):99-111. doi:JOE04026 [pii]

Toppari J (2008) Environmental endocrine disrupters. Sex Dev 2 (4-5):260-267. doi:000152042 [pii] 10.1159/000152042

Uda M, Ottolenghi C, Crisponi L, Garcia JE, Deiana M, Kimber W, Forabosco A, Cao A, Schlessinger D, Pilia G (2004) Foxl2 disruption causes mouse ovarian failure by pervasive blockage of follicle development. Hum Mol Genet 13 (11):1171-1181. doi:10.1093/hmg/ddh124 ddh124 [pii]

Uhlenhaut NH, Jakob S, Anlag K, Eisenberger T, Sekido R, Kress J, Treier AC, Klugmann C, Klasen C, Holter NI, Riethmacher D, Schutz G, Cooney AJ, Lovell-Badge R, Treier M (2009) Somatic sex reprogramming of adult ovaries to testes by FOXL2 ablation. Cell 139 (6):1130-1142. doi:S0092-8674(09)01433-0 [pii] 10.1016/j.cell.2009.11.021

Vainio S, Heikkila M, Kispert A, Chin N, McMahon AP (1999) Female development in mammals is regulated by Wnt-4 signalling. Nature 397 (6718):405-409. doi:10.1038/17068

Vernet N, Dennefeld C, Rochette-Egly C, Oulad-Abdelghani M, Chambon P, Ghyselinck NB, Mark M (2006) Retinoic acid metabolism and signaling pathways in the adult and developing mouse testis. Endocrinology 147 (1):96-110. doi:en.2005-0953 [pii] 10.1210/en.2005-0953

Whitworth DJ (1998) XX Germ Cells: The Difference Between an Ovary and a Testis. Trends Endocrinol Metab 9 (1):2-6. doi:S1043-2760(98)00002-2 [pii]

Whitworth DJ, Shaw G, Renfree MB (1996) Gonadal sex reversal of the developing marsupial ovary in vivo and in vitro. Development 122 (12):4057-4063

Wilhelm D, Palmer S, Koopman P (2007) Sex determination and gonadal development in mammals. Physiol Rev 87 (1):1-28. doi:87/1/1 [pii] 10.1152/physrev.00009.2006

Yao HH, Matzuk MM, Jorgez CJ, Menke DB, Page DC, Swain A, Capel B (2004) Follistatin operates downstream of Wnt4 in mammalian ovary organogenesis. Dev Dyn 230 (2):210-215. doi:10.1002/dvdy.20042

Chapter 9

Role of Corticosteroids in Treatment of Vitiligo

Nooshin Bagherani

Additional information is available at the end of the chapter

http://dx.doi.org/10.5772/48384

1. Introduction

Vitiligo is the most frequent pigmentary disorder (Bagherani et al., 2011; Nazer et al., 2011;Yaghoobi et al., 2011a; as cited in Wolff et al., 2007). It is an acquired, idiopathic and progressive skin disease (Bagherani et al., 2011; Shameer et al., 2005; Yaghoobi et al., 2011a), characterized by sharply demarcated depigmented lesions on any part of the body (Van Geel et al., 2004). This disease can also affect hair and mucosal areas such as mouth and genitalia (Gawkrodger et al., 2010).

Vitiligo usually begins after birth (Gawkrodger et al., 2010). Regarding the studies retrieved from PubMed since 1995, it has been shown that approximately 50% of the vitiligo cases have its onset before the age of 20 years and 25% before the age of 14 years (Kakourou, 2009).

The incidence rate of vitiligo is between 0.1-2% of the world population (Bagherani et al., 20011; Yaghoobi et al., 2011a,b; as cited in Alkhateeb et al., 2003). Its incidence in those with racially pigmented skin is higher, although reliable figures are not available (Burns et al., 2004; Howitz et al., 1977) . The prevalence has been reported as high as 4% in some South Asian, Mexican and American populations (Parsad et al., 2003; Sehgal & Srivastava, 2007; Szczurko & Boon, 2008).

Both sexes are equally afflicted by vitiligo (Krϋger et al., 2011; Njoo & Westerhof, 2001; Wolf et al.,2007) . In some studies, a female preponderance has been reported (Burns at al., 2004; Howitz et al. 1977; Wolf et al., 2007), but the discrepancy can be attributed to a presumed increase in reporting of cosmetic concerns by female patients (Wolf et al.,2007).

This disorder afflicts all races and has a long history (Koranue& Sachdeva, 1988). Vitiligo was first described more than 3,000 years ago in pre-Hindu Vedic and ancient Egyptian texts (Mahmoud et al., 2008; as cited in Millington& Level, 2007). It has been introduced based on its visual phenotype (Yaghoobi et al., 2011a,b; as cited in Birlea et al., 2008; Howitz et al., 1977).

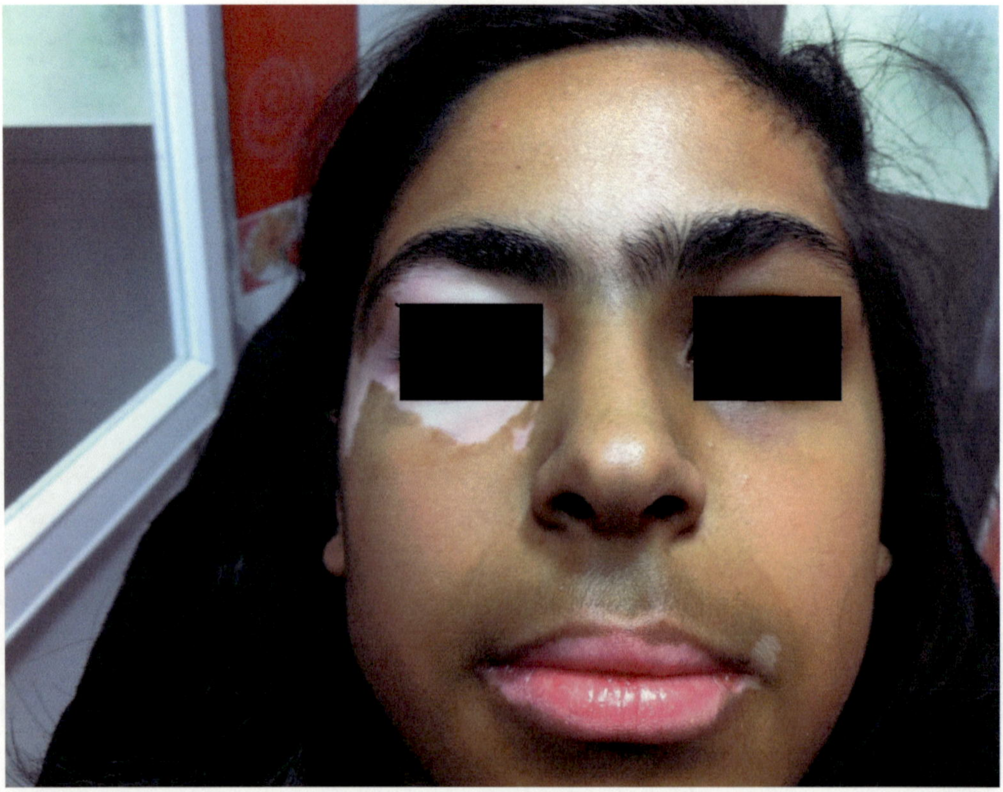

Figure 1. Vitiligo can affect skin, hair and mucous membranes

Studies have shown that approximately 20% of vitiligo patients have at least one first-degree relative with this disorder; so, it seems that the relative risk for first-degree relatives of vitiligo patients is increased by 7- to 10- fold (Wolff et al., 2007; Yaghoobi et al., 2011b). Only a few vitiligo susceptibility genes have been introduced with certainty. Currently, there is strong support for HLA, PTPN22, NALP1 and perhaps CTLA4. All of these genes are associated with autoimmune susceptibility (Spritz, 2008; Boisy & Spritz, 2009).

Although vitiligo is not painful or life-threatening, its disfiguring manifestation has a devastating effect on patient's psychosocial wellbeing. Patients often complain from stigmatization such as curiosity by other people, rejection and discrimination at work, low self-esteem, embarrassment, impaired quality of life, and higher prevalence of sexual difficulties, especially in women (Krϋger et al., 2011).Hence, treatment of vitiligo seems important.

2. Clinical manifestation of vitiligo

Vitiligo is categorized as a depigmentation disorder, where the loss of active melanocytes causes the appearance of white patches on the skin (Whitton et al.,2008 ; Yaghoobi et al., 2011b). These patches are of various sizes and shapes. Involvement often is symmetrical (Yaghoobi et al., 2011b).

Vitiligo lesions present as one or more amelanotic macules or patches that appear chalk- or milk-white in color, surrounded by normal or hyperpigmented border. Sometimes, the lesions have a red inflammatory border (Yaghoobi et al., 2011b).

Vitiligo lesions enlarge centrifugally with an unpredictable rate and can involve any body site (Wolff et al., 2007). Initial lesions appear most frequently on the hands, forearms, feet and face (Tonsi, 2004; Wolff et al., 2007). The most affected sites are face, upper chest, dorsal part of hands, axillae and groin. It has a tendency to involve the skin around orifices. Lesions also appear at trauma sites (James et al., 2006; Yaghoobi et al., 2011b).Vitiligo lesions are sensitive to ultraviolet light and burn readily (Lotti et al., 2008b).

Vitiligo is currently classified in to two subtypes: a) segmental (type B), and b) non-segmental (type A) (Le Poole et al., 1993a; Yaghoobi et al., 2011b). Type B is more rare and characterized by focal lesions restricted to a segment. This type has a rapid onset and a stable course (Lotti et al., 2008b; Yaghoobi et al., 2011b).Type A is more common and has a potential lifelong evolution. Köbner phenomenon and autoimmune diseases are more associated with this subtype of vitiligo (Lotti et al., 2008b; Yaghoobi et al., 2011b).

In another view, vitiligo is classified based on distribution and extension of lesions (Nodlund classification) (Table-1) (Nordlund & Lerner, 1982; Lotti et al., 2008b; Yaghoobi et al., 2011b). In this classification, generalized vitiligo is the most common type of vitiligo in both adults and children (Kakourou, 2009).

Localized	
Focal	One or more macules with casual distribution
Unilateral	One or more macules are localized in a unilateral body region, with a dermatometric distribution
Mocosal	Unique involvement of mucous membranes
Generalized	
Vulgaris	Presence of scattered stains extensively disseminated
Acrofacialis	Patches are localized on distal extremities and face
Mixed	Coexistence of acrofacialis and vulgaris forms
Universalis	Depigmented lesions completely or almost completely (≥80% of body surface) cover the skin surface

Table 1. Nordlund clinical classification of vitiligo (Kakourou, 2009; Nordlund & Lerner, 1982; Lotti et al., 2008b; Yaghoobi et al., 2011b).

3. Diagnosis and differential diagnosis of vitiligo

Diagnosis of vitiligo is based on its clinical manifestation (Lotti et al., 2008b; Yaghoobi et al., 2011b). Wood's light is 365 nm, used commonly for diagnosing and confirming diagnosis of some dermatologic diseases (James et al., 2006). Vitiligo diagnosis can be confirmed with Wood's lamp examination. Its lesions are enhanced with this examination (Wolf et al., 2007).

The differential diagnoses of vitiligo have been listed in Table-2.

Aquired disoreders
Post inflammatory hypopigmentation
Chemical leukoderma
Tinea versicolor
Pityriasis alba
Lichen sclerosus et atrophicus
Morphea
Sarcoidosis
Leprosy
Tertiary stage of pinta
Congenital disorders and syndromes
Nevus depigmentosus
Hypomelanotic macules of tuberus sclerosis
Piebaldism
Albinism
Vogt-Kianagi syndrome
Waardenburg's syndrome
Ziprkowski-Margolis syndrome

Table 2. List of differential diagnoses of vitiligo(Burns et al., 2004; James et al., 2006; Kakourou, 2009; Wolff et al., 2007; Yaghoobi et al.,2011b)

4. Etiology and pathogenesis of vitiligo

Vitiligo is a multifactorial disorder. It is related to both genetic and nongenetic factors (Bagherani et al., 2011; Bolognia, et al., 2008). Regarding the observed variation in its clinical manifestation, it seems likely that its pathogenesis may differ among patients (Bagherani et al., 2011; as cited in Boisy & Spritz, 2009).

Genes certainly play important role in vitiligo pathogenesis (Bagherani et al., 2011; spritz, 2008). It seems that this disorder is part of a broader, genetically determined, autoimmune, and autoinflammatory diathesis (Bagherani et al., 20011; Lebwohl et al., 2006; spritz, 2008). HLA types associated with vitiligo include in A2, DR4, DR7, and Cw6 (Bagherani et al., 2011; James et al., 2006). There are linkage signals on chromosome 1, 7, and 17 in Caucasian families with generalized vitiligo and autoimmune diseases (Bagherani et al., 2011; Jin et al., 2010). Studies have shown that HLA, PTPN22, NALP1 and CTLA4 are associated with autoimmune susceptibility in vitiligo patients (Spritz, 2008; Boisy & Spritz, 2009). Mutation is another pathogenesis suggested for vitiligo (Le Poole et al., 1993a).

Autoimmunity is the most popular hypothesis for vitiligo pathogenesis (Daneshpazhooh et al., 2006; Yaghoobi et al., 2011b). Regarding the autoimmune hypothesis, antibodies develop against melanocyte surface antigens (Mahmoud et al., 2008). Many patients with generalized vitiligo have serum autoantibodies and circulating autoreactive T cells against melanocytes and their components (Yaghoobi et al., 2011b). In a study, an elevated ratio of $CD4^+/CD8^+$ T cells was seen, which was a sign of imbalanced lymphocyte immune response (Pichler et al., 2009). In another study, small amount of IgG and C3 deposits in the basement-membrane zone and keratinocytes were seen in vitiligo lesions (Uda et al., 1984).

The melanocytes of vitiligo patients are susceptible to environmental triggers or other stressors. These events can possibly result in melanocyte death by necrosis, apoptosis or pyroptosis, consequent presentation of tolerogens and loss of immune tolerance, and ultimately autoimmunity directed against melanocytes (Boisy & Spritz, 2009; Mahoney & Rosen, 2005).

Increased level of soluble IL-2 receptor, IL-6 and IL-8 in vitiligo patients suggests that T cell activation may be a component in vitiligo pathogenesis (Mandelcorn-Monson et al 2003; Namazi, 2005). The detection of significantly higher expression of IL-6 and TNF-α in vitiligo skin, compared with healthy skin indicates an imbalance of epidermal cytokines at sites of lesions (Moretti et al., 2002).

Oxidant stress may also play an important pathogenic role in vitiligo (Wolff et al., 2007). It is suggested that the imbalance in the oxidant-antioxidant system rather than oxidative stress might play such role in this disease (Helmy et al., 2004).

As another probable pathogenesis, it is suggested that carious factors including localized trauma, stress and autoimmune predisposition can act synergistically to disappear melanocytes from the epidermis (Gauthier et al., 2003; Yaghoobi et al., 2011b)

Melanocyte growth factor deficiency is another hypothesis about vitiligo pathogenesis (Hossani-Madani & Halder, 2010; Njoo & Westerhof, 2001).

In human melanocytes, there is expression of 1,25-dihydroxy-vitamine D3 receptor. Defect in calcium uptake has been seen in keratinocytes and melanocytes of vitiligo lesions. This defect can inhibit melanogenesis via downregulation of tyrosinase activity (Lotti et al., 2008b).

The melanocytorrhagy is a hypothesis which was described by Gauthier and colleagues for the first time. According to this hypothesis, melanocyte detachment from the basal layer and transepidermal migration can trigger melanocyte death in vitiligo (Gauthier et al., 2003).

Zinc α-2-glycoprotein is a plasma glycoprotein which regulates melanin production by normal and malignant melanocytes (Bagherani et al., 2011; Hale, 2002). For the first time, as a hypothesis, Bagherani and colleagues suggested that there might be association between this glycoprotein and vitiligo, which should be confirmed (Bagherani, 2011, 2012a, b; Bagherani et al., 2011; Yaghoobi et al., 2011a).

Other etiopathogeneses which have been suggested for vitiligo are summarized in: accumulation of toxic compounds, impaired melanocyte migration and/ or proliferation, altered cellular environment, infection, neural and autocytotoxic factors (Yaghoobi et al., 2011b).

Whatever its etiology or pathogeneseis, it seems that stress or certain life events such as loss of close relations, bereavement, moving home, giving birth or losing a job can trigger the onset or progression of vitiligo. On the other hand, in one study, Krüger and colleagues showed that there is no difference in levels of cortisol and β-endorphin between patients and controls, indicating that stress per se is not a significant contributor in vitiligo (Krüger et al. 2011).Hence, the role of stress in onset and progression of vitiligo should be assessed.

The probable pathogeneses of vitiligo have been summarized in Scheme 1.

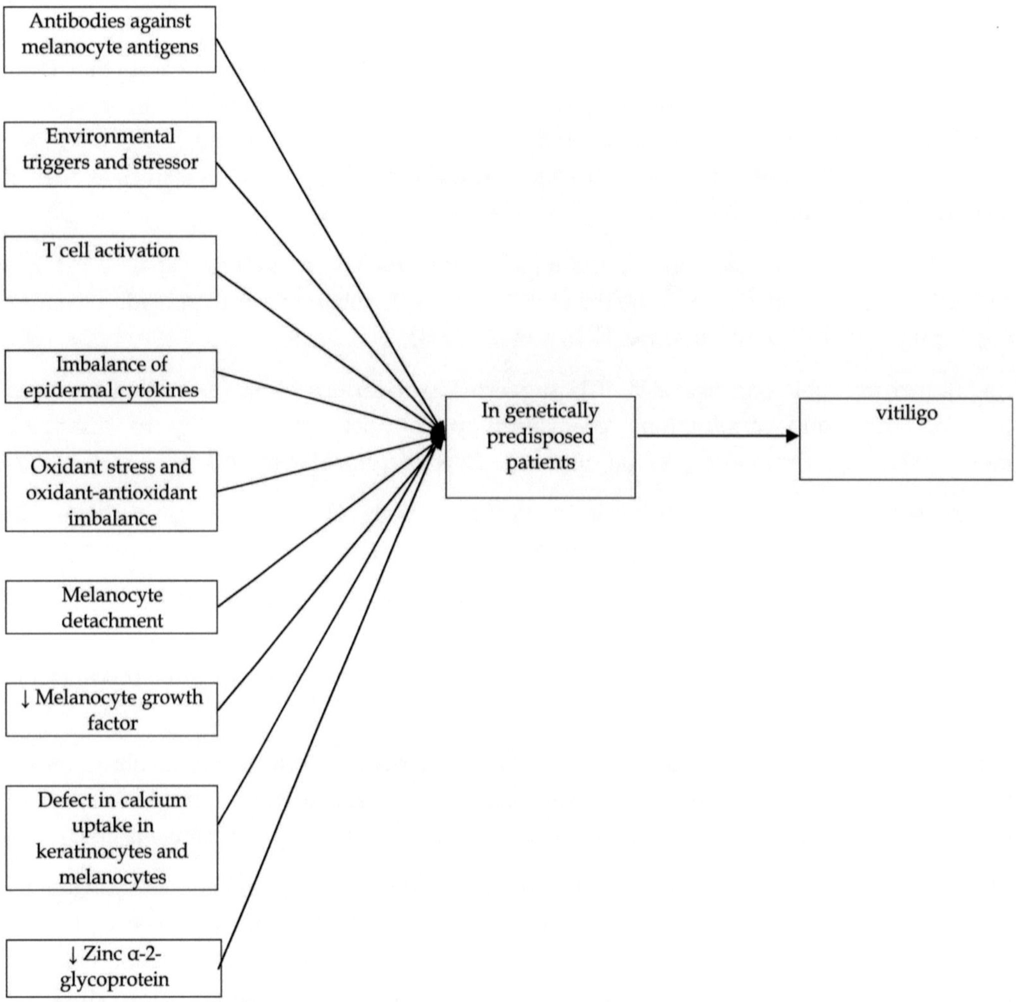

Scheme 1. The probable pathogeneses of vitiligo

5. Pathology of vitiligo

Histopathologically, the most prominent feature of vitiligo is the alteration of melanocytes in the dero-epidermal junction (Elder et al., 2009; Yaghoobi et al., 2011b). Most of the studies confirm the complete absence of melanocytes in the fully depigmented skin in vitiligo; thus, it seems that only hair follicles can act as a reservoir (Dogra & Bhusahan, 2005; Le Poole et al., 1993).

There is inconstant lymphonuclear infiltrate in the advancing margins of lesions (Ogg et al., 1998; Lotti et al., 2008b). In the outer border of lesions, melanocytes are often prominent which show long dendritic processes filled with granules of melanin (Moellman et al., 1982).

In this disorder, melanocytes are degenerated and seem to be replaced by Langerhans cells Lotti et al., 2008b). In addition, the epidermis of regions around the margins of vitiligo has abnormality of keratinocytes (Burn et al., 2004). In long-lasting lesions, there are degenerative changes in nerves and adnexal structures of the skin (Elder et al., 2009).

6. Association between vitiligo and other disorders

Disorders associated with vitiligo have been listed in Table-4. Hashimoto's thyroiditis is the most common associated disorder in children vitiligo; so, thyroid function test should be screened annually in all children with vitiligo (Kakourou, 2009).

Autoimmune disorders
Autoimmune thyroid disease (particularly Hashimoto thyroiditis and Graves disease)
Pernicious anemia
Systemic lupus erythematosus
Lichen sclerosis
Morphea
Scleroderma
Diabetes mellitus
Adrenal insufficiency (Addison's disease)
Alopecia areata
Hypoparathyroidism
Myasthenia gravis
Gonadal failure
Inflammatory bowel disease
Rheumatoid arthritis
Psoriasis
Chronic urticaria
Autoimmune polyglandular syndrome
Sutton or halo nevus
Others
Malignant melanoma
Asthma

Table 3. Disorders associated with vitiligo (Alkhateeb et al., 2003; Birlea et al., 2008; Bolognia et al, 2008; Burn's et al., 2004; Daneshpazhooh et al., 2006; James et al., 2006; Lebwohl et al., 2006; Pichler et al., 2009; Yaghoobi et al., 2011b; Zhang et al., 2009)

7. Treatment of vitiligo

The disfigurement related to vitiligo causes emotional stress for the patient and his or her family, which necessitates treatment (Lebwol et al., 2006; Yaghoobi et al., 2011b). Although vitiligo is generally resistant to most of treatments, spontaneous repigmentation can occur in more than 10-20% of patients (Lotti et al., 2008b; Yaghoobi et al., 2011b).

Emotional stress can induce and exacerbate vitiligo and vice versa (Kakourou, 2009). On the other hand, it seems that poor patient satisfaction can cause poor adherence to treatment with consequently poor response. Studies have shown that the likelihood of dermatological patient satisfaction is increased by the physician's ability to exhibit empathy (Boehncke et al., 2002); thus, at the beginning of treatment, psychological interventions are important and suggested as a way of improving quality of life (Gawkrodger et al., 2010).

The aim of vitiligo treatment is stopping the disease progress and restoring the loss of melanocytes in the lesions (Gawkrodger et al., 2010; Njoo et al., 1999).Some treatments can achieve both aims (Gawkrodger et al., 2010).

Although a variety of therapeutic modalities have been introduced for treatment of vitiligo, there is still no universally effective and safe therapy (Njoo et al., 1999). However, sunscreens and camouflage products should be offered to all patients (Gawkrodger et al., 2010).

Almost all therapy modalities for vitiligo have borrowed from therapies whose prime target has been another disease (Gawkrodger et al., 2010). Till 2010, 68 treatments for vitiligo had been evaluated in clinical trials during 43 years (Eleftheriadou et al., 2011; as cited in Whitton et al., 2010).

7.1. Topical corticosteroids

In many instances, the first line therapy for vitiligo is topical medicaments. Regarding topical therapy that might be effective in treatment of vitiligo, topical corticosteroids are the usual first line treatment (Gawkrodger et al., 2010). The ease of application, high rate of compliance, and low cost are the advantages of topical corticosteroid therapy for vitiligo (Coskun et al., 2005; Kostovic et al., 1999).

According to the high incidence of corticosteroid side effects in children, recommended treatments for children with vitiligo differ slightly from those for adults (Gawkrodger et al., 2010). In generalized vitiligo, the use of topical steroids is impractical because of associated side effects (Mahmoud et al., 2008).

Topical corticosteroids are available in a variety of potencies and preparations (Ference & Last, 2009). Studies have shown that use of highly potent or potent topical corticosteroids can repigment vitiligo, but only in a small proportion of cases (Clayton, 1977; Gawkrodger et al., 2010; Kandil, 1974). In another study, the responses to corticosteroid therapy in vitiligo patients range between 20% and 90% improvement, usually not be a complete cure (Clayton, 1977; Kandil, 1974; Lepe et al., 2003; Njoo et al., 1998).

Studies have shown that clobetasol is the most effective topical corticosteroid for treatment of vitiligo because it can very often produce pigmentation (Lepe et al., 2003).

7.2. Topical calcineurin inhibitors

Regarding the autoimmune hypothesis of vitiligo pathogenesis due to humoral and cellular dysfunction, the topical use of immunomodulating calcineurin inhibitors such as tacrolimus and pimecrolimus, in addition to corticosteroids which are also immunosuppressive, appears reasonable for treatment of this disease (Coskun et al., 2005). They act at the level of gene expression and suppress proinflammatory cytokines such as interleukins TNF-α and INF (Berti et al., 2009 ; Mahmoud et al., 2008).

The efficacy of topical calcineurin inhibitors in treatment of vitiligo is comparable with topical corticosteroids (Mahmoud et al., 2008). They can be used as a treatment of choice for the vitiligo lesions on the head and neck, especially when the disease is long lasting (Berti et al., 2009). The treatment response of segmental vitiligo is appropriate to calcineurin inhibitors (Kakouro, 2009; Silverberg et al., 2004).

These agents have no side effects seen in long-term use of corticosteroids (Lebwohl et al., 2003; Mahmoud et al., 2008). Pruritus, burning sensation, and erythema are the adverse reactions of topical cacineurin inhibitors (Lepe, et al, 2003). Although topical application of these agents is not related to immunosupression, the long-time risk from their application to the skin is still unknown (Berti et al., 2009)

7.3. Phototherapy

Phototherapy has been mainstay treatment for vitiligo for several years (Gawkrodger et al., 2010). It is appropriate for extensive vitiligo, especially active one (Gawkrodger et al., 2010). Ultraviolet (UV)-based therapy includes photo therapy [ultraviolet B (UVB)], photochemotherapy [psoralen plus ultraviolet A (UVA) or PUVA], and targeted phototherapy (excimer laser and excimer lamp) (Hamzavi et al., 2012).

The efficacy of phototherapy is related to lesional location. While face and neck lesions show good responses to phototherapy, acral lesions are resistant (Lee et al., 2010).

Photosensitizers used in photochemotherapy either increase the sensitivity of the skin (psoralen) or increase the sensitivity of melanocytes (khellin) via activating melanocytes and melanosomes and inducing IL-1 synthesis (Mahmoud et al. 2008).

The risk of skin cancer in PUVA- treated vitiligo patients is not clear (Gawkrodger et al., 2010). In a cohort study, Nijsten and Stern showed that exposure to PUVA increased the risk of nonmelanoma skin cancer dramatically (Nijsten & Stern, 2003).

In a retrospective study on 97 patients during 10 years, Kwok and colleagues concluded that response to PUVA is often followed by relapse. They emphasized that careful patient counseling before PUVA therapy is necessary, because this treatment seldom causes extensive repigmentation which is cosmetically acceptable (Kwok et al., 2002).

UVB, in the form of narrow band (NB-UVB) (311nm-313nm) or broad band (BB-UVB) (290nm-320nm), can inhibit cytokines induction and secretion , and stimulate inactive melanocytes of the outer root sheath of hair follicles for migrating to vitiligo lesions (Mahmoud et al. 2008).

NB-UVB uses the effective part of ultraviolet B and excludes erythema-inducing ray; so it has a definite edge over BB-UVB. The Excimer light is a NB-UVB source for treating localized areas (Gawkrodger et al., 2010).

The advantages of NB-UVB are shorter sessions of phototherapy and suitability in pregnancy and children. In addition, it causes no phototoxicity, xerosis, or hyperkeratosis as seen with PUVA (Rath et al., 2008). Treatment with NB-UVB can produce approximately 42.9% repigmentation in vitiligo patients after 6 months of therapy (Hamzavi et al., 2004). One clinical trial showed that segmental vitiligo was resistant to NB-UVB. In this study, Anbar and colleagues showed that response to UVB was better in earlier lesions especially lesions on the face, trunk and limb (Anbar et al., 2006).

Studies have revealed that NB-UVB is superior to PUVA when comparing the rate of pigmentation. In addition, these studies showed that UVB results in improved color-matched repigmentation and has lower incidence of side effects, comparing to PUVA (Parasad et al., 2006; Yones et al., 2007). In a meta-analysis of studies on generalized vitiligo, the highest mean success rates were achieved orderly with NB-UVB (63%; 95% CI, 50-76%), BB-UVB (57%; 95% CI, 29-82%), and PUVA phototherapy (51%; 95% CI, 46%-56%). This analysis also revealed that PUVA is associated with the highest rates of side effects. On the other hand, El Mofty and colleagues showed that NB-UVB photo therapy had a similar repigmentary effect as PUVA (El Mofty et al., 2006). By comparing these findings, NB-UVB is choice treatment for extensive vitiligo.

Combination of NB-UVB and calcipotriol has no increase in efficacy comparing to NB-UVB alone, because calcipotriol is rapidly degraded (>90%) by UV (Mahmoud et al, 2008; Sitek et al., 2007). Findings have shown that combination of PUVA and calcipotriol is more effective than PUVA alone (Mahmoud et al., 2008).

Some studies have shown a synergistic activity in combination therapy with topical tacrolimus and UVB phototherapy. In addition, Tacrolimus can prevent UVB-induced erythema by suppressing early-phase events of the inflammatory process. But this combination may increase the risk of skin cancer because findings in animals have shown that topical calcineurin inhibitors have no effect on the clearance of DNA photoproducts (Mahmoud et al., 2008).

Excimer laser is another treatment option for vitiligo, which has a wavelength of 308 nm. Its efficacy in treatment of vitiligo lesions on face, neck and genitalia is good (>70% repigmentation) (Mahmoud et al., 2008).

Low- energy helium-neon laser (632.8 nm) is effective in treatment of vitiligo. This kind of laser has a biostimulation effect rather than thermal effect. In vitro study on cultured keratinocytes and melanocytes conducted by Yu and colleagues showed that helium-neon laser could stimulate proliferation and migration of melanocytes. Their study on the efficacy of this kind of laser on patients with segmental vitiligo revealed positive responses (> 50% repigmentation in 60% of patients with segmental vitiligo) (Yu et al., 2003).

7.4. Vitamin D derivatives

Calcipotriol is a vitamine D3 analogue that inhibits T-cell activation. It also stimulates growth and differentiation of keratinocytes and melanocytes, induces melanogenesis by reducing the disturbed calcium influx into melanocytes, and restores calcium homeostasis (Lebwohl et al., 2003; Mahmoud et al., 2008).

Several studies have shown that calcipotriol, as a monotherapy has little or no treatment response in vitiligo patients (Mahmoud et al., 2008). Some another studies have shown that calcipotriol is 77% effective in treating adults with vitiligo (Ermis et al., 2001; Lepe et al., 2003).

Katayama and colleagues showed that clinical response to tacalcitol [1α24(OH)2D3] was unfavoprable in treatment of vitiligo, but it in combination with solar irradiation had favorable responses (Katayama et al., 2003).

7.5. Systemic immunosuppressive agents

Systemic immunosuppressive is another option for treatment of vitiligo (Dogra& Bhusahan, 2005; Gawkrodger et al., 2010; Kovacs& Missouri, 1998). Systemic corticosteroids and azathioprine are immunosuppressives with well-known efficacy in treatment of this disorder (Gawkrodger et al., 2010).

The efficacy of intralesional and oral corticosteroids have been assessed in limited trials with unknown significance (Whitton et al., 2008; Yaghoobi et al., 2011b). Dogra and Bhushan reported a patient with vitiligo universalis concurrent with pemphigus vulgaris, treated with dexamethasone-cyclophosphamide pulse therapy. Their patient showed repigmentation on the face after 37 years (Dogra& Bhusahan, 2005).

Azathioprine in combination with PUVA can produce earlier and greater repigmentation in adults with symmetrical vitiligo lesions (Radmanesh & Saedi, 2006).

The efficacy of methotrexate in treatment of vitiligo was assessed for the first time by Nazer and colleagues. They revealed that its efficacy was comparable with NB-UVB and systemic corticosteroids (Nazer et al., 2011).

7.6. Surgical modalities

Surgical modalities are only appropriate for stable vitiligo (Njoo et al., 1999; as cited in Falabella et al., 1995; Hatchome et al., 1990). They are appropriate for cosmetically sensitive sites such as face and back of hands. These modalities are not recommended in children (Gawkrodger et al., 2010).

Surgical treatments have the advantage of rapid and desirable amounts of repigmentation. Patients with positive history of Köbner phenomenon, postinflammatory hyperpigmentation, keloids, or hypertrophic scars are not suitable candidate for surgical interventions (Mahmoud et al., 2008).

The different procedures of surgical modalities include in tattooing, organ-cultured fetal skin allografting, epidermal culture grafting, melanocyte culture grafting, autologous noncultured melanocyte-keratinocyte cell transplantation, epidermal blister grafting, thin Thiersch split skin grafting and miniature punch grafting (Mahmoud et al., 2008).

Among the several surgical modalities for treatment of vitiligo, the highest mean success rates are achieved with split skin grafting and epidermal blister grafting (Njoo et al., 1998). Sometimes multiple modalities are needed for getting to desirable responses (Mahmoud et al., 2008).

Dermabrasion is another treatment option for vitiligo (Hossani-Madani& Halder, 2010; Mahmoud et al., 2008).

7.7. Other complementary modalities

For the first time, Bagherani and colleagues revealed that oral zinc can be effective in treatment of vitiligo (Bagherani et al.,2011; Yaghoobi et al., 2011a).

Oral supplementation with antioxidant pools containing α-lipoic acid before and during NB-UVB significantly improves the clinical effectiveness of phototherapy and reduces vitiligo-associated oxidative stress (Dell'Anna et al., 2007).

Oral sex steroid-thyroid hormone is also effective in treatment of generalized vitiligo. This efficacy is related to the stimulatory effect of melanocyte proliferation and melanin production via alpha-MSH (Ichimiya, 1999; Muto et al., 1995; Nagai et al, 2000).

Levamisole is another option for treatment of vitiligo. It is safe and effective in controlling the activity of the disease process in limited slow-spreading vitiligo. Combination of levamisole with topical corticosteroids can produce faster rate of repigmentation (Pasricha & Khera, 1994).

A rather uncommon, but effective, treatment modality is the combination of pseudocatalase and balneo/climatotherapy at the Dead sea (Krüger et al., 2011; as cited in Schallreuter et al., 2002). Krüger and colleagues showed in their study that group therapy had a strong and long- lasting positive effects in quality of life in vitiligo patients (Krüger et al., 2011).

Ginkgo biloba (Szczurko et al., 2011) , oral L-phenylalanine (Whitton et al., 2008), topical fluorouracil(Tsuji & Hamada, 1983), topical prostaglandin E (PGE2), topical melagenina I and II, minoxidil, homeopathy,placental extract in combination with light exposure (Majid, 2010), ayurvedic medicine, climtologic, and balneologic therapies (Lotti et al., 2008b). are as alternative therapies for vitiligo. As a hypothesis, phenytoin can be effective in treatment of vitiligo (Namazi, 2005).

7.8. Depigmenting agents

Depigmentation can be recommended to adults severely affected by vitiligo (Gawkrodger et al., 2010). It can be achieved with monobenzyl ether of hydroquinone and monomethyl ether of hydroquinone at 20% concentration, either alone or in combination with Q-switched ruby laser (Mahmoud et al., 2008).

8. History of vitiligo treatment with corticosteroids

In human body, inflammatory immune reactions are regulated by endogenous glucocorticoids such as cortisol (Wolverton, 2007). For more than 50 years, steroids have been introduced to be involved in various physiological responses (Falkenstein et al.,2000 ; as cited in Beato et al., 1996; Beato and Klug, 2000).

For the first time, Kendall described compound E (cortisone) in 1935. In 1948, a Mayo Clinic group described primarily the use of cortisone and adrenocorticotropic hormone (ACTH) in patients with rheumatoid arthritis (Wolverton, 2007; as cited in Lester, 1989).

Several stronger corticosteroids are now available since their first introduction. They are used as monotherapy or in combination with other agents for increasing efficacy (Tadicherla et al., 2009).

Corticosteroids with a keton group at the C11 position such as cortisone must be reduced to their 11-hydroxyl analogs (hydrocortisone) to be active. This process cannot occur effectively in the skin (Wolverton, 2007). Thus, early attempts to use cortisone failed until 1951, when Sulzberger and colleagues described the use of cortisone and ACTH in a variety of inflammatory dermatoses for the first time (Wolverton, 2007; as cited in Sulzberger et al., 1951).Their success was a cornerstone in dermatology (Wolverton, 2007). Now days, topical corticosteroids are the most commonly prescribed agents in treatment of dermatologic conditions (Tadicherla et al., 2009).

Almost all treatments of vitiligo have borrowed from therapies whose prime targets have been another diseases (Gawkrodger et al., 2010). Topical corticosteroids have been indicated and used during the last three decades for treatment of limited area of vitiligo (Coskun et al., 2005; Hartmann et al., 2004). For two decades, monotherapy with topical corticosteroids has been the most common treatment for vitiligo in children (Lepe et al., 2003; Njoo et al., 1998).

The search for substances, such as calcipotriol and tacrolomus, with the benefits of topical steroids without serious side effects has made big advances in treatment of vitiligo (Lepe et al., 2003; as cited in Assmann et al., 2000).

9. Place of corticosteroids in treatment of vitiligo

Many skin disorders are treated with topical corticosteroids, but evidence of effectiveness has been published only for a small number of disorders (Ference & Last, 2009). For concerning specific indications for topical corticosteroids, skin diseases should be clarified in which: a) topical corticosteroids are first choice treatment; b) topical corticosteroids are efficacious as alternative or adjuvant treatment; c) the proposed use of topical corticosteroids to be confirmed as effective; and d) topical corticosteroids can be prescribed for symptomatic relief (Giannotti& Pimpinelli, 1992).

In addition to vitiligo, topical corticosteroids are effective for treatment of psoriasis (Ference & Last, 2009), atopic dermatitis, aczema, infantile seborrhoeic eczema, pompholyx, contact dermatitis (Harper, 1988), lichen sclerosus, bullous pemphiguid, pemphigus foliaceus, alopecia areata, phimosis, and radiation dermatitis. Topical corticosteroids may also be effective in other conditions, but data supporting their use in these conditions are from low-level studies. Melasma, chronic idiopathic urticaria, infantile acropustulosis and prepubertal labial adhesions are included in the latter category (Ference & Last, 2009).

Systemic corticosteroid is useful in treatment of skin diseases. In addition to vitiligo, it is also effective in treatment of acute hypersensitivity diseases, connective tissue diseases, and immunological blistering diseases (Barnetson & White, 1992).

Assessment of different vitiligo treatment options is difficult because there is no standardized scoring system for vitiligo (Mahmoud et al. 2008). Some studies concluded that topical corticosteroids and narrowband UVB monotherapy were the most effective and safest forms of treatment for localized and generalized vitiligo, respectively (Whiton et al., 2008).

The ease of application, high rate of compliance, and low cost are the advantages of topical corticosteroid therapy (Coskun et al., 2005; Kostovic et al., 1999) which take it as a first choice in treatment of localized forms of vitiligo (Coskun et al., 2005). A study conducted by AlGhamdi showed that the most two common treatment modalities for vitiligo were topical corticosteroids and NB-UVB in Saudi Arabia (AlGhamdi, 2009).

Clobetasol is the most effective topical corticosteroid for treatment of vitiligo because it can often produce pigmentation where other topical steroids have failed (Lepe et al., 2003).

Fluticasone propionate is the first carbothioate corticosteroids, classified as a potent, characterized by high lipophilicity, high glucocorticoid receptor binding and activation, and a rapid metabolic turnover in skin; thus, it has low cutaneous and systemic side effects, even in sensitive areas such as face, the eyelids and intertriginous regions (Kumaran, 2006). It seems that it can be a good treatment option for vitiligo.

Mometasone furoate is a non fluorinated topical corticosteroid. It has high potency and safety profile. Masuria and colleagues have shown that this corticosteroid was a suitable option for treatment of vitiligo in children. In their study, 90-100% repigmentation was echieved in more than 80% of cases with lesions on the face, and more than 60% of patients with vitiligo on the other parts of the body (Masuria et al., 1999).

Several studies have reported use of topical corticosteroids with varying degrees of efficacy in treatment of vitiligo (Coskun et al., 2011; Ongenae et al., 2004). Some of them have shown that the responses to corticosteroid therapy in vitiligo patients range between 20% and 90% improvement, usually not be a complete cure (Lepe et al., 2003; Njoo et al., 1998).A study assessing intermittent topical clobetasol propionate, conducted by Kumari and colleagues showed 90-100% repigmentation in more than 80% of patients with vitiligo of the face and more than 40% of patients with vitiligo on other parts of the body (Kumari, 1984). Moderate- to high-potency topical corticosteroids are also effective for children vitiligo, but may be associated with systemic absorption (Kwinter et al., 2007).

Repigmentation in vitiligo can be labeled as marginal, perifollicular, diffuse, and combined. Parsad and colleagues, during a study on repigmentation patterns in 352 vitiliginous patches, showed that Perifollicular repigmentation was the most prevalent type of repigmentation. In their study, marginal pattern was the most stable one (93.3%), followed by perifollicular (91.7%) and combined type (84.4%). Diffuse pattern of repigmentation was the least stable (78.5%). They revealed that PUVA predominantly exhibited a perifollicular pattern and topical or systemic corticosteroids produced diffuse one. The majority (80%) of marginal pattern was seen in systemic PUVA and calcipotriol. They also showed that the repigmentation speed was much faster when the initial pigmentation was of diffuse pattern. Hence, corticosteroid in comparison with PUVA and calcipotriol induce faster, but less stable repigmentation (Parsad et al., 2004). In addition, it seems that combination therapies with producing a variety of repigmentation patterns can be remarkably more effective than monotherapy.

Combination of topical and systemic corticosteroids is effective in treatment of vitiligo. During a clinical trial, Majid and colleagues showed that more than 90% of children with rapidly progressive vitiligo went to complete remission after the start of the therapy with combination of methylprednisolone oral minipulse therapy (0.8 mg/kg body weight on two consecutive days every week) and topical fluticasone. In addition, 65% of these children achieved good to excellent repigmentation at the end of six months of therapy (majid et al, 2009).

Westerhof and colleagues, in probably the best controlled study to date of topical medications in vitiligo treatment, assessed the efficacy of topical fluticasone propionate alone or in combination with UVA in 135 adults during 9 months. They revealed that fluticasone alone induced mean repigmentation of only 9% (compared to UVA alone of 8%), whereas fluticasone-UVA combination resulted in mean repigmentation of 31%. They found no corticosteroid atrophy in users (Westerhof et al., 1999).

In a study, Lotti and colleagues showed that monotherapy with NB-UVB and topical betamethasone dipropionate were more effective than topical immunomodulators, calcipotriol and topical phenylalanine. They also revealed that combination of betamethasone dipropionate and NB-UVB resulted in the highest repigmentation rate (Lotti et al, 2008). In other study, Sassi and colleagues also showed that combination of excimer laser and topical hydrocortisone was effective in treatment of recalcitrant vitiligo of the face and neck (Sassi, 2008).

Kumaran, in one sudy revealed that combination therapy with topical corticosteroids and calcipotriol produced a significantly faster onset of repigmentation along with better stability of repigmentation (Kumaran, 2006).

In one clinical trial, Yaghoobi and colleagues showed that topical corticosteroids plus oral zinc was more effective than topical corticosteroid alone in treatment of vitiligo, but this difference was not statistically significant. It seems that more robust long-term randomized controlled trials with more patients, maybe with higher doses of oral zinc are necessary to confirm the efficacy of oral zinc in treatment of vitiligo (Yaghoobi et al., 2011a).

In a study by Lee and colleagues, it was shown that combination treatment of high-dose methylprednisolone therapy and PUVA may represent a highly effective therapeutic option for generalized vitiligo. In this study, they administered intravenous methylprednisolone for 3 day followed by PUVA twice weekly. This manner of corticosteroid administration can minimize the side effects of corticosteroids (Lee et al., 2007).

Lepe and colleagues have shown that there was no significant difference between the efficacy of clobetasol and tacrolimus used topically for treatment of vitiligo. Their study showed that with clobetasol, perifollicular islands of pigment were observed after 3 weeks of treatment. Because tacrolimus does not produce atrophy or other adverse effects, it may be very useful for younger patients and sensitive areas of the skin such as eyelids. It also can be considered as a replacement therapy for long-term corticosteroid therapy (Lepe et al., 2003).

During a prospective study on 10 patients, Coskun and colleague also showed that topical pimecrolimus was as effective as topical clobetasol to restore skin discoloring in vitiligo (Coskun et al., 2005). On the other side, during a review comparing topical corticosteroids and immunomodulators in treatment of vitiligo, Choi and colleagues showed that the duration from the start of treatment to onset of repigmentation was significantly shorter in the topical immunomodulator. They also concluded that topical immunomodulators can be considered as an alternative to topical corticosteroids in vitiligo treatment (Choi et al., 2008).

In a double-blind randomized trial comparing the efficacy of topical betamethasone and catalase/dismutase superoxide in treatment of vitiligo, Sanclemente and colleagues showed that there was no statistically significant difference on the rate of repigmentation between two agents (Sanclemente et al., 2008).

Camacho and Mazuecos in one study assessed the efficacy of oral and topical L-phenylalanine in combination with sunlight in days and topical clobetasol at nights. They showed that this combination was effective in treatment of vitiligo, with no side effect. Hence, this combination can be recommended to the patients with vitiligo on face and children (Camacho & Mazuecos, 2002).

Systemic corticosteroids can arrest the progression of vitiligo and lead to repigmentation (Mahmoud et al., 2008), but they may produce unacceptable side effects (Lee et al., 2007). There have been few reports on the efficacy of systemic corticosteroids in treatment of vitiligo (Mahmoud et al., 2008).

With using oral corticosteroids, repigmentation can become evident within 4 weeks in most cases (Imamura & Tagami, 1976). In a study on 81patients with actively spreading vitiligo , it has been shown that low daily dose of oral prednisolone (0.3 mg/kg) arrested disease progression in 87.7% and repigmentation in 70.4% of cases. Results of other study also confirmed this rate of efficacy (Mahmoud et al., 2008).Seiter and colleagues in two separated studies concluded that high-dose methylprednisolone pulse therapy was effective in treatment of patients with generalized rapid progressive vitiligo (Seiter et al., 1999,2000).Kim and colleagues also revealed that low-dose daily oral prednisolone (0.3 mg/kg) was effective in preventing the progression and inducing repigmentation of actively spreading vitiligo, which was resistant to topical corticosteroids or photochemotherapy. They also showed that this dose of prednisolone had no side effect (Kim et al., 1999). In other study, Pasricha and Khaitan showed that oral mini pulse treatment with betamethasone (5 mg as a single oral dose on 2 consecutive days per week) was effective to arrest the vitiligo progression and induce repigmentation (Pasricha & Khaitan, 1993).On the other hand, Rath and colleagues in one study showed that oral minipulse betamethasone (0.1 mg/kg body weigh twice weekly on two consecutive days) had only adjunct value and had no efficacy by itself (Rath, 2008).

In one study, Vasistha and Singh showed that there was no significant difference in efficacy of intralesional corticosteroid versus placebo in treatment of vitiligo . In addition, atrophy, telangiectasia, infection and intradermal hemorrhage were some of the side effects of this treatment (Vasistha &Singh, 1979).

The possibility of Köbner phenomenon always exists with any surgical procedure in vitiligo patients. When combined with systemic corticosteroids, this possibility will decrease. In a study, the efficacy of combination of low-dose oral betamethasone and melanocyte – keratinocyte transplantation was assessed in treatment of vitiligo. Mulekar in this study showed that this combination was able to induce complete repigmentation in patients with large vitiliginous areas (Mulekar, 2006). Another study by Barman and colleague also showed that the efficacy of punch grafting in combination with topical corticosteroids was comparable with its combination with PUVA (Barman et al., 2004).

It should be noticed that brand-name corticosteroids may be more expensive, which may reduce patient's compliance. On the other hand, some generic formulation may be less or more potent than their brand-name equivalent (Ference & Last, 2009; as cited in Oslen, 1991).

10. Suggested guideline for treatment of vitiligo

To choose the best therapy for vitiligo with the highest probability of success for an individual patient, identifying the disease characteristics which help predict the therapy outcome is important (Njoo et al., 1999).Thus, beside age, duration of disease, disease localization, extent of depigmentation, and current disease activity should also be considered for clinical decision making (Giannotti & Pimpinelli, 1992; Njoo, et al., 1999; as cited in Antoniou & Katsambas, 1992; Drake et al., 1996). As a rule, it should be noticed that targeted combination therapies in vitiligo are remarkedly more effective than single treatments (Lotti et al., 2008a).

In adults and children with skin type I and II, in the consultation, it is better to consider no active treatment. The use of sunscreens and camouflages products are all the things which they need (Gawkrodger et al., 2010).

In adults and children with recent onset of vitiligo and limited involvement, treatment with topical modalities should be considered (Gawkrodger et al., 2010). In vitiligo involvement less than 20% skin surface area, a potent or highly potent topical corticosteroid or topical cacineurin inhibitors are the first choice for a trial period of no more than 2 months. In these situations, combination of topical corticosteroids with excimer laser or UVA is more effective than corticosteroids alone (Hossani-Madani& Halder, 2010).

Treatment with corticosteroids for more than 2 months should be monitored closely for well-known side effects (Gawkrodger et al., 2010).Treatment with corticosteroids should be discontinued if there is no clinical improvement after 2 months of therapy (Mahmoud et al., 2008).

Once- or twice-daily application is recommended for most corticosteroid preparations (Drake et al., 1996; Ference & Last, 2009). More frequent administration does not produce better results (Ference & Last, 2009; as cited in du Vivier, 1976).

When prescribing topical corticosteroids, in addition to its potency, it is important to notice delivery vehicle, frequency of administration, duration of treatment, and side effects. It also is important to that hydration can promote corticosteroid penetration, so applying it after a shower or bath improves effectiveness (Ference & Last, 2009). Topical corticosteroids may differ in potency as well as side effects based on the vehicle in which they are formulated (Ference & Last, 2009; as cited in Pariser, 1991).

Calcineurin Inhibitors such as tacrolimus and pimecrolimus can be considered as an alternative to a topical steroid especially in children because of better safety profile (Gawkrodger et al., 2010).

One study showed that combination therapy with topical corticosteroids and calcipotriol produced a significantly faster onset of repigmentation along with better stability of repigmentation. They also showed that this combination is able to minimize corticosteroid side effects (Kumaran et al, 2006). In other study, Travis and Siverberg revealed that calcipotriene in combination with corticosteroids could repigment vitiligenous lesions, even in those with previous treatment failure with corticosteroids (Travis & Siverberg, 2004).

Extensive vitiligo (involvement more than 50%) in dark-skinned patients, especially with involvement of cosmetically sensitive areas such as hands and face can produce a severe social disability. In this instance, complete depigmentation of the affected areas might be beneficial. This procedure should be undertaken only by a specialist dermatology unit (Gawkrodger et al., 2010). Because of the psychological and cultural problems following the depigmentation and because of the increased risk of skin cancer in this condition, this procedure is better to be suggested to patients more than 50 years of age.

Surgical treatments are offered to patients with stable vitiligo, who are refractory to medical therapy (Mahmoud et al., 2008); so, these procedures should be suggested only if the disease has been inactive for 6-12 months (Gawkrodger et al., 2010). Segmental vitiligo, characterized by rapid progression followed by stabilization, is the best candidate for surgical interventions (Mahmoud et al., 2008).

According to the above-mentioned statements about vitiligo and the efficacy of the whole options for treatment of this disorder, the author suggests a vitiligo treatment guideline which has been summarized in the Schemes of 2 to 5.

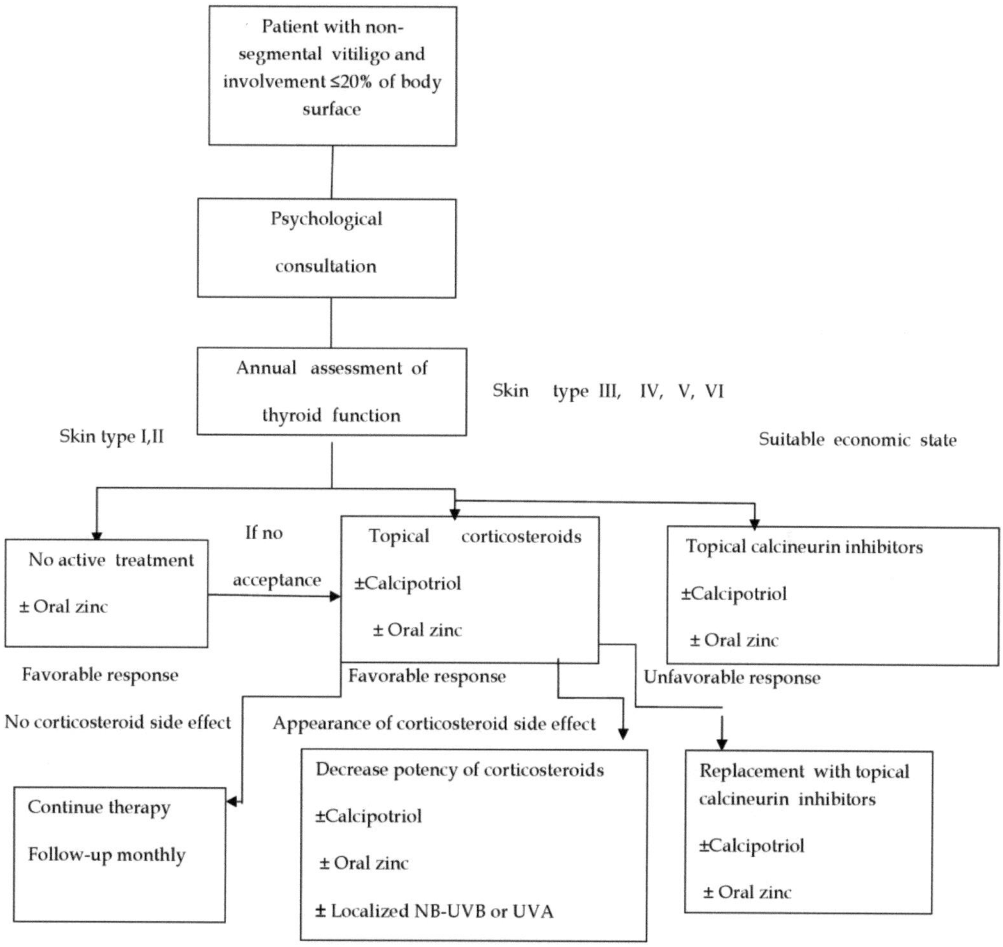

Notice to the following notes:
- In patients under treatment with oral zinc, serum zinc level must be checked every 1-2 months.
- The first visit after beginning treatment is done after 2 months, and next visits are done every month.

Scheme 2. Suggested treatment guideline for patients with non-segmental vitilgo and involvement ≤20% of body surface

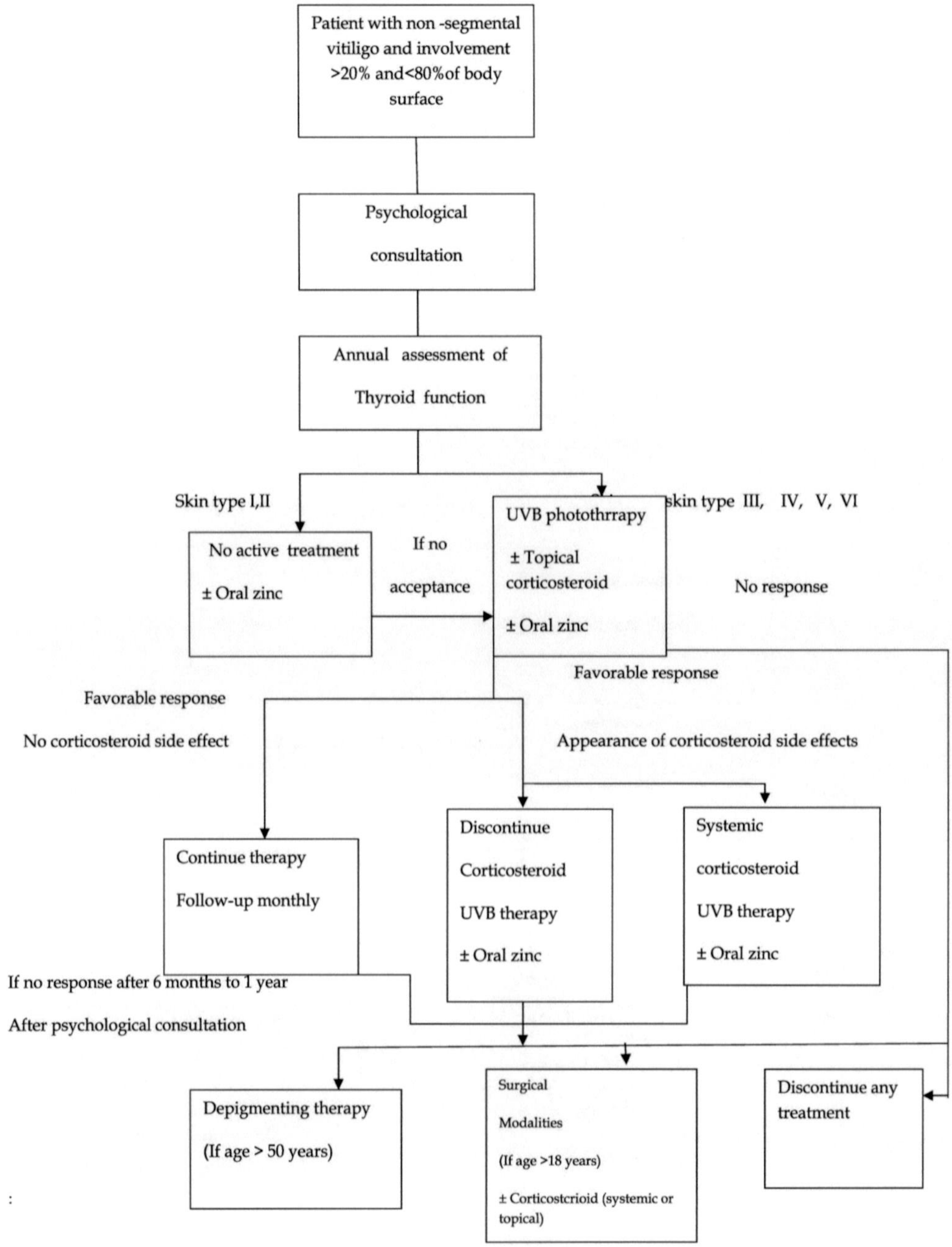

Notice to the following notes:
-In patients under treatment with oral zinc, serum zinc must be checked every 1-2 months.
-The first visit after beginning treatment is done after 2 months, and next visits are done every month.
-Topical corticosteroids should be administered for the limited parts especially for exposed areas, for getting better response , while presenting less systemic side effects.

Scheme 3. Suggested treatment guideline for patients with non-segmental vitilgo and involvement >20% and <80% of body surface

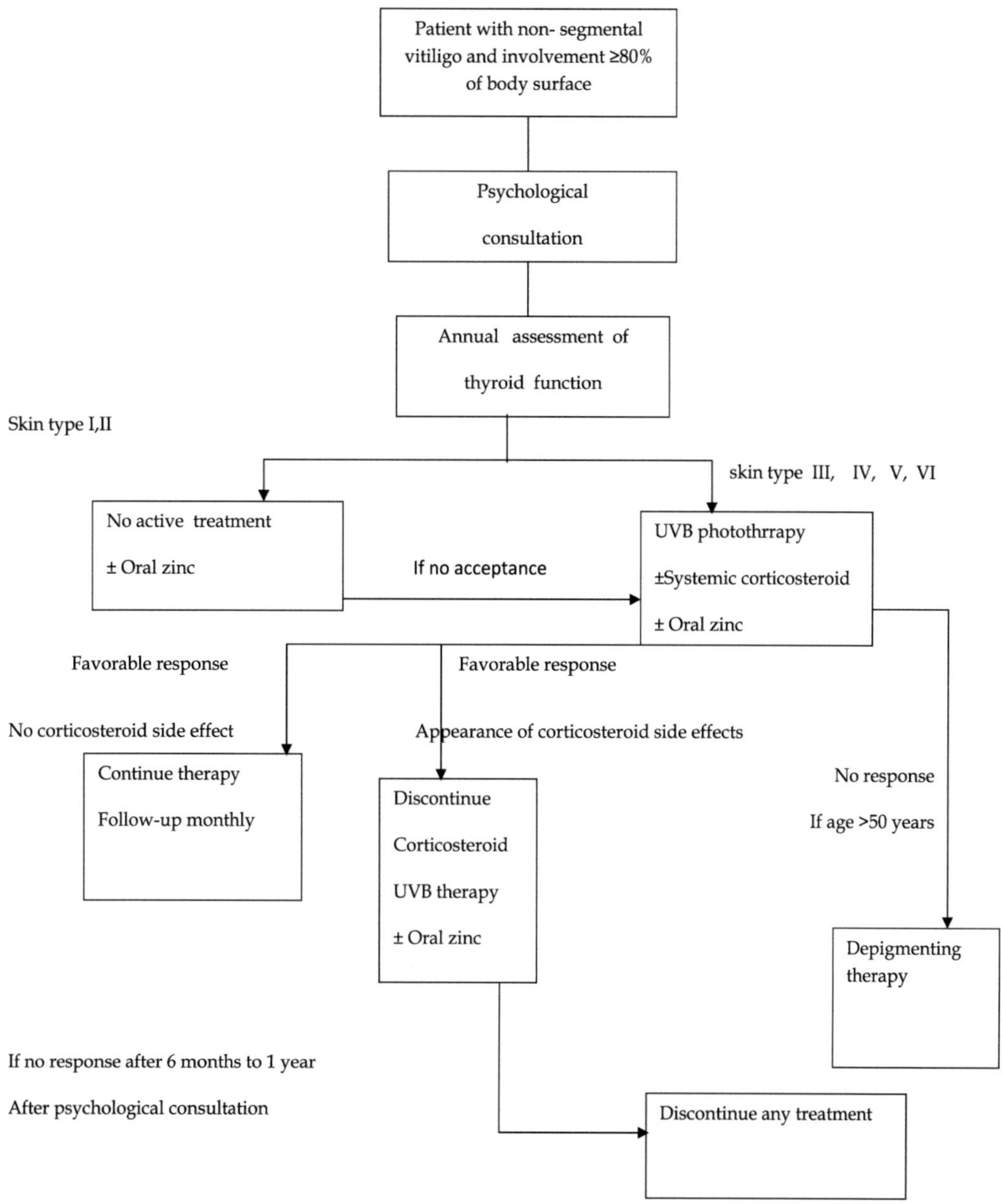

Notice to the following notes:
-In patients under treatment with oral zinc, serum zinc must be checked every 1-2 months.
-The first visit after beginning treatment is done after 2 months, and next visits are done every month.

Scheme 4. Suggested treatment guideline for patients with non-segmental vitilgo and involvement ≥80% of body surface

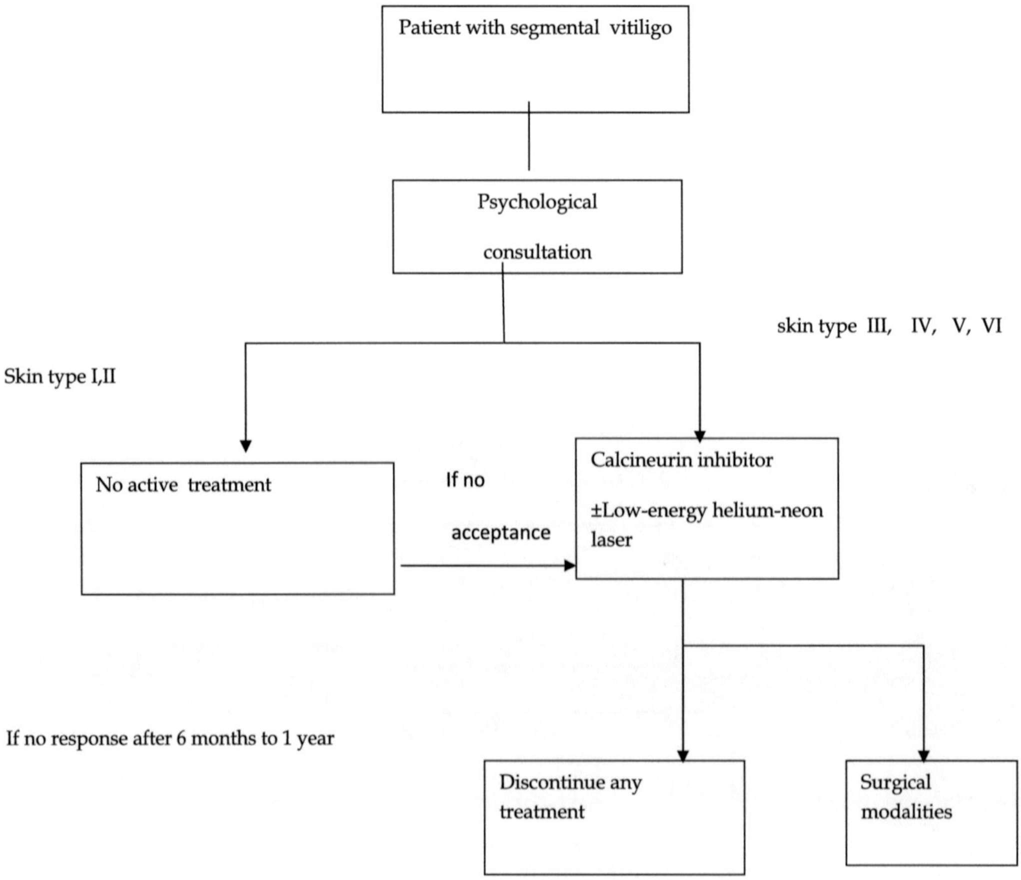

Scheme 5. Suggested treatment guideline for patients with segmental vitiligo

11. Assessment of vitiligo

In the first step, the diagnosis of vitiligo should be confirmed. Often its diagnosis is straightforward, although it is not always so. In vitiligo, the skin texture is usually normal. In the next step, the effect of vitiligo on the patients must be assessed; so the examination should include record of the disease distribution, extent and involvement of mucous membrane (Gawkrodger et al., 2010).

The definition of active or stable vitiligo is not the same in different clinicians' viewpoints. To date, disease activity is mainly assessed based on medical history and physical examination. Thus, the size of lesions along with their number and the grade of repigmentation are recorded using photographic tools in any follow-up visit (Njoo et al., 1999).

One of the vitiligo-associated skin manifestations is Köbner phenomenon, defined as " the development of vitiligo lesions at sites of specifically traumatized skin". Some epidemiological studies have shown that this phenomenon occurs in most patients with vitiligo (Njoo et al., 1999). Its clinical relevance is not established; however it seems that Köbner may indicate disease activity (Table-2)(Njoo et al., 1999; as cited in Hatchome et al., 1990). Njoo and colleagues have concluded that experimental Köbner phenomenon can function as a valuable clinical factor to assess disease activity (Njoo et al., 1999).

Disease activity	VIDA Score
Active, in the past 6 weeks	+4
Active, in the past 3 months	+3
Active, in the past 6 months	+2
Active, in the past 1 year	+1
Stable, for at least 1 year	0
Stable, for at least 1 year and spontaneous repigmenting	-1

*Active refers to expansion of existing lesions or appearance of new lesions; stable refers to condition when these symptoms are not present.

Table 4. Vitiligo disease activity (VIDA) score based on the patient's own opinion (Njoo et al., 1999).

Assessment of different vitiligo treatment options is difficult because there is no standardized scoring system for vitiligo (Mahmoud et al. 2008). The percentage of depigmentation in association with total body surface can be estimated by using the hand-palm rule,i.e., a lesion in the size of the patient's palm is equal to 1% of the total body surface (Kakourou, 2009) . Vitiligo Area Scoring Index or VASI can be achieved by this rule. For each body region, the VASI is determined by the hand unite rule. The total body VASI is calculated by the following formula by considering the contribution of all body regions (possible rang: 0-100) (Hamzavi et al., 2004):

$$VASI= \sum [\text{Hand Unites}] \times [\text{Residual Depigmentation}]$$

Because VASI is not accurate, Van Geel and colleagues have introduced a more accurate manner so-called a digital image analysis system for assessing vitiligo lesion surfaces both before and after different therapeutic modalities (Van Geel et al., 2004).

Patients with vitiligo have a high prevalence of autoimmune thyroid disease or other autoimmune diseases; so, thyroid function should be checked in these patients (Gawkrodger et al., 2010).

12. Probable mechanisms of corticosteroid function in treatment of vitiligo

Regarding the classic genomic theory of action, in human body, steroids such as glucocorticoids bind to specific receptors, which are intracellular transcription factors, and exert positive or negative effects on the expression of target genes (Falkenstein et al.,2000 ; as cited in Beato et al., 1996; Beato and Klug, 2000). These effects are mediated by a specific delay and sensitivity toward inhibitors of transcription and translations (Falkenstein et al.,2000 ; as cited in Beato, 1989; Evans, 1988; Fuller, 1991).

In addition to the delayed genomic actions, steroids also have rapid nongenomic effects (Falkenstein et al.,2000).These nongenomic effects on cellular function involve conventional second messenger cascades, include in phospholipase C (PLC) (Falkenstein et al.,2000; as cited in Civitelli et al., 1990), phosphoinositide turnover (Falkenstein et al.,2000; as cited in Morelli et al., 1993; Morley et al., 1992), intracellular pH (Falkenstein et al.,2000; as cited in Jenis et al., 1993), free intracellular calcium (Ca^{2+}) (Falkenstein et al.,2000; as cited in de Boland& Norman, 1990), and protein kinase C (PKC) (Falkenstein et al.,2000).

Topical corticosteroids like human steroid hormones exert their effects through both direct and indirect mechanisms, which are mediated via the glucocorticosteroid receptors. These drugs affect every aspect of cutaneous inflammatory cells and immunologic mediators. They can reduce the number of lymphocytes and epidermal antigen- presenting cells. These drugs also can reduce the synthesis and secretion of IL-1, IL-2 , IFN-γ and TNF (Wolverton, 2007).

Topical corticosteroids are effective for disorders characterized by hyperproliferation, inflammation, and immunologic involvement (Ference & Last, 2009).

Corticosteroids can effective in treatment of vitiligo via the following mechanisms:

1. Corticosteroids can reduce the number of epidermal antigen- presenting cells so-called Langerhans' cells. They also decrease the cellular receptors of Langerhans' cells, indicating decreased antigen –presenting function (Wolverton, 2007). On the other hand, melanocytes in vitiligo lesions are replaced by Langerhan's cells (Lotti et al., 2008b). It seems that this increasing in the number of Langerhans' cells in vitiligo may be responsible for introducing unknown antigens to immune system in this disorder; thus, it appears that corticosteroid with decreasing these antigen –presenting cells in vitiligo lesions can suppress the process of its appearance.
2. Corticosteroids are able to reduce the number of lymphocytes and its antibody-dependent cellular toxicity (Wolverton, 2007). In vitiligo, the number of lymphocytes are increased in the progressing border of vitiligo lesions (Ogg et al., 1998; Lotti et al., 2008b). On the other hand, increased level of soluble IL-2 receptor, IL-6 and IL-8 in vitiligo patients suggests that T cell activation may be responsible in vitiligo pathogenesis (Mandelcorn-Monson et al 2003; Namazi, 2005). It is concluded that corticosteroids can treat vitiligo by decreasing the number of lymphocytes and their actions.
3. Topical corticosteroid can reduce the synthesis and secretion of IL-1, IL-2 , IFN-γ and TNF (Wolverton, 2007). The detection of significantly higher expression of IL-2, IL-6 and TNF-α in vitiligo indicates an imbalance of epidermal cytokines at sites of lesions (Mandelcorn-Monson et al 2003; Moretti et al., 2002; Nazer et al., 2011).Thus, it seems that corticosteroids via decreasing these cytokines are able to suppress the vitiligo activity.
4. Studies have shown that patients with a positive Köbner phenomenon respond significantly better to topical corticosteroids (Njoo et al., 1999). Because the positive Köbner phenomenon is indicator of active vitiligo (Njoo et al., 1999; as cited in Xunquan

et al., 1990), it reveals that corticosteroids may act by suppressing abnormal immune responses present in actively spreading lesions of this disorder.

5. Systemic corticosteroids can reduce complement-mediated cytotoxicity by autoantibodies to melanocytes and antibody titer to surface antigens of melanocytes in serum of users (Han et al., 1993; Mahmoud et al., 2008). On the other hand, there is positive correlation between the presence of autoantibodies and the efficacy of topical corticosteroids (Takei et al., 1984). Thus, these findings suggest that corticosteroid can be effective in treatment of vitiligo via decreasing the rate of autoantibodies-associated melanocyte cytotoxicity.
6. In a study, Bleehen showed that the melanocytes in the steroid-treated repigmented areas were more dentritic and dopa-positive. They also contained more melanosome of normal size, shape and melanization, when comparing to pigmented margins of untreated lesions (Bleehen, 1976).
7. As a hypothesis, Bagherani suggested that the level of zinc α-2 glycoprotein in vitiligo lesions decreases (Bagherani, 2011, 2012a,b). On the other hand, studies have shown that corticosteroids are able to increase ZAG expression. Regarding these findings, it seems that corticosteroids are effective in treating vitiligo via enhancing ZAG (Bagherani, 2011, 2012a,b; Russell & Tisdale, 2005).

   The mechanisms of corticosteroids in treatment of vitiligo has been summarized in Scheme 6.

13. Prognostic factors effective in treatment of vitiligo

The course of vitiligo is unpredictable, but progressive. In some patients, vitiligo can be stable for many years; while in others lesions can increase in size and number. Segmental vitiligo has a stable course and resistant to treatment (Yaghoobi et al., 2011b).

Spontaneous repigmentation can appear in more than 10-20% of patients with vitilgo . This repigmentation is partial, and occurs mainly in children and in sun-exposed areas (Yaghoobi et al., 2011b).

Beside patient's age, duration, localization, extent and current activity of the disease are important for predicting the outcome of therapy in vitiligo (Njoo, et al., 1999; as cited in Antoniou & Katsambas, 1992; Drake et al., 1996). Studies have shown that younger or darker skinned patients and also those with vitiligo of the face and neck seem to respond better to therapy (Wolverton, 2007; as cited in Cockayne et al., 2002). The treatment result in Asian patients is better (Kumari, 1984). Lesions in the exposed areas response better to treatment (Imamura & Tagami, 1976). Lesions on the thorax also responded better than those on the abdomen, legs and hands (Gawkrodger et al., 2010).

It has been revealed that long lasting disease is relatively resistant to local corticosteroid, probably because of the depletion of melanocytic reserves in the hair follicles (Njoo et al., 1999; as cited in Geraldez& Gutierrez, 1987).

Takei and colleagues have shown that there is positive correlation between the antibodies and positive microsome test, thyroid test, DNA test and the efficacy of topical corticosteroids (Takei et al., 1984).

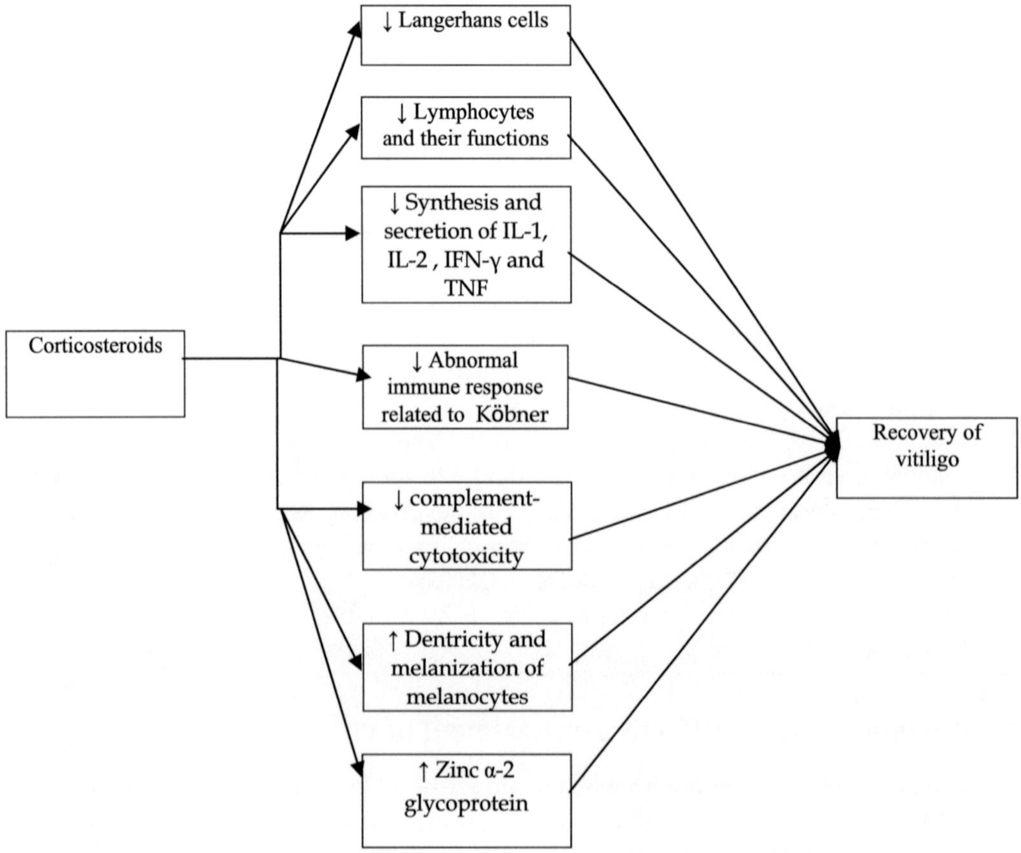

Scheme 6. The mechanisms of corticosteroids in treatment of vitiligo

In a study comparing the efficacy of clobetasol and tacrolimus in treatment of vitiligo, Lepe and colleagues have revealed that with both treatments, new pigments were conserved and the best effects of repigmentation were observed in the face and areas with greater density of hair follicules. During this 2-month study, no pigment on the dorsum of hands or areas devoid of hair follicules was seen (Lepe et al., 2003).

Kim and colleagues in one study on the efficacy of low-dose oral corticosteroid in treatment of vitiligo, showed that the response rate was statistically significant in male sex, patient age of 15 years or under, and a disease duration of 2 years or less (Kim et al., 1999).

Although it has been frequently reported that the Köbner phenomenon may be indicative of vitiligo activity, it is not clear whether patients with a positive Köbner have a different prognosis than patients with the negative one. In one study, Njoo and colleagues showed that experimental Köbner phenomenon might predict responsiveness to local corticosteroid therapy but not to UVB therapy. They revealed that patients with a positive experimental Köbner responded significantly better to topical corticosteroid combined with UVA therapy than do those with a negative one, suggesting this therapy is most effective when administered during the active stage of vitiligo (Njoo et al., 1999).

Studies have shown that patients with a good response to corticosteroid-UVA combination therapy have significantly shorter disease duration than do those with a poor response to this combination therapy (Njoo et al., 1999; as cited in Geraldez & Gutierrez, 1987).

Medical therapies are equally effective in active and stable vitiligo, while surgical procedures are only appropriate for stable one (Njoo et al., 1999; as cited in Falabella et al., 1995; Hatchome et al., 1990).

14. Side effects of corticosteroids in vitiligo patients

For the first time, Hench and colleagues presented a report concerning the side effects and toxicity of corticosteroids (Wolverton, 2007; as cited in Hench et al., 1950).It is difficult to quantify the incidence rate of side effects caused by topical corticosteroids (Ference & Last, 2009; Henge et al., 2006).

The usefulness and side effects of topical corticosteroids are a direct result of their anti-inflamatory properties. They are also dependent on the frequency of administration, duration of treatment, and where on the body the drug is used (Ference & Last, 2009). Prolonged use of topical corticosteroids may cause side effects (Ference & Last, 2009; Hengge et al. 2006). When low- to high-potency corticosteroids are used for less than three months, side effects are rare with the exception of intertriginous areas, face and neck or when occlusion is used (Drake et al., 1996; Ference & Last, 2009).

Young age (infancy/children), liver disease, renal disease, hypothyroidism, obesity, lack of physician supervision, amount and potency of topical corticosteroids are risk factors which increase the chance of systemic side effects of topical corticosteroids. Young age, potency of corticosteroids and site (face, neck, axillae, groin and upper inner thighs) can enhance local side effects of topical corticosteroids (Wolverton, 2007).

Recurrence after cessation of corticosteroid therapy and their side effects including skin atrophy, telangiectasia, striae, (Coskun et al., 2005; Kostovic et al., 1999), hypopigmentation, and hypertrichosis (Ference & Last, 2009; Henge et al., 2006) are the most limiting factors in treatment of vitiligo with corticosteroids. These potential side effects must be monitored closely especially in children.

Skin atrophy is a common complication of topical corticosteroids after only 2 months treatment (Gawkrodger et al., 2010; as cited in Whitton et al., 2010). In one study conducted by Clayton on 23 vitiligo patients, skin atrophy was seen in all users of clobetasol propionate (used for 8 weeks) (Clayton, 1977). In other study on 23 vitiligo patients with betamethasone valerate, Kandil noted hypertrichosis in 2, and acne in 4 subjects (Kandil, 1974). Hypopigmentation is more apparent in darker skin. Repigmentation often occurs after corticosteroids discontinuing (Ference & Last, 2009; Henge et al., 2006).

Chronic application of topical corticosteroids can result in tolerance and tachyphylaxis (Drake et al., 1996; Ference & Last, 2009; Wolverton, 2007). Other less common, but important, side effects of topical corticosteroid include in: purpura, psedoscars, ulceration, delayed wound healing, aggravation of cutaneous infection, hyperpigmentation, , perioral dermatitis, contact dermatitis (allergic or irritant), photosensitization, rebound flare, stroid-induced acne, steroid-induced rosacea, folliculitis, miliaria, granuloma gluteal infantum, reactivation of Kaposi's sarcoma and ocular effects (cataracts and glaucoma) (Ference & Last, 2009; Henge et al., 2006; Wolverton, 2007).

Topical high- and ultra-high- potency corticosteroids can be absorbed enough to cause systemic manifestations such as Cushing syndrome, Hypothalamic-pituitary-adrenal suppression, aseptic necrosis of the femoral head, decreased growth rate, hypertension, hyperglycemia, and peripheral edema (Ference & Last, 2009; Henge et al., 2006; Wolverton, 2007).

Birth defects have been reported in animals, when used large amounts of topical corticosteroids; but this effect has not yet been reported in humans (Drake, 1996; Ference & Last, 2009). Topical corticosteroids are classified by the U.S. Food and Drug Administration as pregnancy category C (Ference & Last, 2009).

It is not reported whether topical corticosteroids can be excreted in breast milk; thus it is better to use topical corticosteroids to the breast immediately following nursing (Ference & Last, 2009).

Topical corticosteroids may differ in potency as well as side effects based on the vehicle in which they are formulated. Topical corticosteroids in ointment vehicle can cause maceration and folliculitis in intertriginous areas (e.g., groin, gluteal cleft, axilla). In addition, their greasy nature may result in poor patient's satisfaction and compliance (Ference & Last, 2009).

Corticosteroids in cream base are able to vanish into skin, make them cosmetically appealing. Although creams are generally less potent than ointments of the same medication and so have less side effects, skin irritation, stinging, and allergic reactions are more with creams because they often contain preservatives. Contact dermatitis also is seen more with non-fluorinated steroids (e.g., hydrocortisone and budesonide) (Ference & Last, 2009; Henge et al., 2006).

Occlusion increases penetration of topical corticosteroids; so it can increase their side effects. Irritation, folliculitis, and infection can develop rapidly from occlusive dressings (Drake et al., 1996; Ference & Last, 2009).

Side effects are common with systemic corticosteroids in vitiligo patients, include weight gain, acne, menstrual irregularity and hypertrichosis (Radakovic et al., 2001).

15. Prevention and treatment of corticosteroid side effects in vitiligo patients

Multiple daily applications of corticosteroids do not lead to better and faster response. It only increase incidence rate of side effects. Intermittent therapy with steroid-free intervals can be as effective as continuous treatment (Giannotti, 1988). For the first time, Reichling and Kligman suggested alternate-day corticosteroid use in 1961 (Wolverton, 2007; as cited in Reichling & Kligman, 1961). This is an important way for decreasing side effects of corticosteroids. In addition, this alternate-day use can maintain significant anti-inflammatory effect over the 48- hour period between doses (Wolverton, 2007).

Topical corticosteroid therapy requires physician's close supervision to optimize benefits and minimize adverse effects. The follow-up visit is the most effective form of supervision (Wolverton, 2007).

For decreasing the side effects, choosing the least potent topical corticosteroids necessary to achieve an appropriate response and then tapering the potency as quickly as possible is a key point (Wolverton, 2007).

If longer duration is needed, corticosteroid should be gradually tapered to avoid rebound symptoms, and treatment should be resumed after a steroid-free period of at least one week. This schedule can be repeated chronically, until the condition resolves (Drake et al., 1996; Ference & Last, 2009).

For preventing tolerance and tachyphylaxis to topical corticosteroids, ultra-high-potency corticosteroids should not used for more than 3 weeks continuously (Drake et al, 1996; Ference & Last, 2009).

Occlusion can increase corticosteroid penetration. A simple plastic dressing is able to increase corticosteroid penetration several folds. Thus occlusion should not be applied to the face or intertriginous areas (Drake et al., 1996; Ference & Last, 2009).

Adjunctive therapy with other immunosuppressive drugs and pulse therapy are another ways for decreasing the side effects of corticosteroids. These advances in corticosteroid therapy occurred during the 1970s and 1980s (Wolverton, 2007). Topical immunomodulator calcineurin inhibitors such as tacrolimus and pimecrolimus don't produce atrophy or other side effects of corticosteroids (Coskun et al., 2005; Gawkrodger et al., 2010) , so they can be very useful for patients with vitiligo involvement in sensitive areas of the skin such as eyelids, and also they should be considered in other skin disorder currently treated with topical corticosteroids for prolonged periods (Coskun et al., 2005).

Combination therapy with corticosteroid and calcipotriol, not only produces faster onset of repigmetion in vitiligo patients, but also decreases the incidence rate of side effects (Kumaran, 2006).

Treatment with combination of corticosteroids and retinoids can prevent corticosteroid-induced atrophy (Lepe, 2003).

As a hypothesis, phenitoin by stimulating collagen production and inhibiting its breakdown can prevent corticosteroid-induced skin atrophy (Namazi, 2005).

16. Conclusion

The exact etiology and pathogenesis of vitiligo are unclear; thus, discovery of biological pathways of vitiligo pathogenesis will result in novel therapeutic and prophylactic targets in treatment of this disease (Bagherani et al., 2011).

Several factors have effects on the choice of treatment for vitiligo. The best treatment chosen should be individualized for each patient based on the extent, distribution and the rate of progression of the lesions (Mahmoud et al., 2008). Topical corticosteroids and narrowband

UVB monotherapy were the most effective and safest forms of treatment for localized and generalized vitiligo, respectively (Whiton et al., 2008).

Author details

Nooshin Bagherani
Dr. Nooshin Bagherani's Office, Khoramshahr, Khuzestan province, Iran

17. References

AlGhamdi, KM. (2009). A survey of vitiligo management among dermatologists in Saudi Arabia. *J Eur Acad Dermatol Venereol*, Vol. 23, N. 11, pp. 1282-1288.

Alkhateeb, A., Fain, PR., Thody, A., Bennett, DC.,& Spritz, RA. (2003). Epidemiology of vitiligo and associated autoimmune diseases in Caucasian probands and their families. *Pigment Cell Res*, Vol. 16, pp. 208-214.

Anbar, TS., Westerhof, W., Abdel-Rahman, AT.,& El-Khayyat, MA. (2006). Evaluation of the effects of NB-UVB in both segmental and non-segmental vitiligo affecting different body sites. *Photodermatol, Photoimmunol & Photo med*, Vol. 22, N. 3, pp. 157-163.

Antoniou, C.,& Katsambas, A. (1992). Guildelines for the treatment of vitiligo. *Drug*, Vol. 43, pp. 490-498.

Assmann, T., Homey, B.,& Ruzicka, T. (2000). Applications of tacrolimus for treatment of skin disorders. *Immunopharmacol*, Vol. 47, pp. 203-213.

(Bagherani, N.(2012a) The newest Hypothesis about vitiligo.Most of the suggested pathogeneses of vitiligo can be attributed to lack of one factor: Zinc- α2-glycoprotein. *Current Medicinal Chemistry, 4th international conference on drug discovery & therapy*, Dubi, Feb, 2012

Bagherani, N.(2012b) The newest hypothesis about vitiligo. Most of the suggested pathogeneses about vitiligo can be attributed to lack of one factor: Zinc-α2-glycoprotein. ISRN J. www.isrn.com/journals/dermatology/aip/405268

Bagherani, N. (2011). Two Important Discoveries. *International drug discovery science and technology*, china, Nov, 2011

Bagherani, N., Yaghoobi, R.,& Omidian, M. (2011). Hypothesis: Zinc can be effective in treatment of vitiligo. *Indian J Dermatol*, Vol. 56, N.5, pp. 480-484.

Barman, KD., Khaitan, BK.,& Verma, KK. (2004). A comparative study of punch grafting followed by topical corticosteroid versus punch grafting followed by PUVA therapy in stable vitiligo. *Dermatol Surg*, Vol. 30, N. 1, pp. 49-53.

Barnetson, RS.,& White, AD. (1992). The use of corticosteroids in dermatological practice. *Med J Aust*, Vol. 156, N. 6, pp. 428-431.

Beato, M. (1989). Gene regulation by steroid hormones. *Cell*, Vol. 56, pp. 335-344.

Beato, M., Chavez, S.,& Truss, M. (1996). Transcriptional regulation by steroid hormones. *Steroids*, Vol. 61, pp. 240-251.

Beato, M.,& Klug, J. (2000). Steroid hormone receptors: An update. *Hum Reprod Update*, Vol. 6, pp. 225-236.

Berti, S., Buggiani, G.,& Lotti, T.(2009). Use of tacrolimus ointment in vitiligo alone or in combination therapy. *Skin Therapy Lett,* Vol. 14, N. 4, pp.5-7.

Birlea, SA., Fain, PR.,& Spritz RA (2008). A Romanian population isolate with high frequency of vitiligo and associated autoimmune disease. *Arch Dermatol,* Vol. 144, pp.310-316.

Bleehen, SS. (1976). The treatment of vitiligo with topical corticosteroids. Light and electronmicroscopic studies. *Br J Dermatol,* Vol. 94, N. 12 (Suppl), pp. 43-50.

Boehncke, WH., Ochsendorf, F., Paeslack, I., Kaufmann, R.,& Zollner, TM. (2002). Decorative cosmetics improve the quality of life in patients with disfiguring skin diseases. *Eur J Dermatol,* Vol. 12, N.6, pp. 577-580.

Boisy, RE. Spritz, RA. (2009). Frontiers and controversies in the pathobiology of vitiligo: separating the wheat from chaff. *Exp Dermatol,* Vol. 18, pp. 583-585.

Bolognia, JL., Jorizzo, JL., & Rapini, R. (2008). (Ed.2). (2008). *Dermatology.* Philadelphia, Mosby Elsevier. USA.

Burns, T., Breathnach, S., Cox, N.,& Griffiths C. (Ed. 7). (2004). *Rook's Textbook of Dermatology.* Oxford Blackwell Science. UK.

Camacho, F., & Mazuecos, J. (2002). Oral and topical L-phenylalanine, clobetasol propionate, and UVA/sunlight- a new study for the treatment of vitiligo. *J Drugs Dermatol,* Vol. 1, N. 2, pp. 127-131.

Choi, CW., Chang, SE., Bak, H., Choi, JH., Park, HS., Huh, CH., Kim, CW., Kim, SE., Mun, SK., Kim, BJ.,& Kim, MN. (2008). Topical immunomodulators are effective for treatment of vitiligo. *J Dermatol,* Vol.35, N. 8, pp. 503-507.

Civitelli, R., Kim, YS., Gunsten, SL., Fujimori, A., Huskey, M., Avioli, LV.,& Hruska, KA. (1990). Nongenomic activation of the calcium message system vitamin D metabolites in osteoblast-like cells. *Endocrinology,* Vol. 127, N., pp. 2253-2262.

Clayton, R. (1977). A double-blind trial of 0.05% clobetasol propionate in treatment of vitiligo. *Br J Dermatol,* Vol.96, pp.71-73.

Cockayne, SE., Messenger, AG.,& Gawkrodger DJ. (2002). Vitiligo treated with topical corticosteroid: Children with head and neck involvement respond well. *J Am Acad Dermatol,* Vol. 46, N.6, pp. 964-965.

Coskun, B., Saral, Y.,& Turgut, D. (2005). Topical 0.05% clobetasol propionate versus 1% pimecrolimus ointment in vitiligo. *Eur J Dermatol,* Vol. 15, N. 2, pp-88-91.

Daneshpazhooh, M., Mostofizadeh, GM., Behjati, J., Akhyani, M.,& Mahmoud Robati R. (2006). Anti-thyroid peroxidase antibody and vitiligo: a controlled study. *BMC Dermatol,* Vol6, N. 3.

de Boland, AR., & Norman, AW. (1990). Influx of extracellular calcium mediates 1,25-dihydroxyvitamin D_3-dependent transcaltachia (the rapid stimulation of duodenal Ca2+ transport). *Endocrinol,* Vol. 127, pp. 2475-2480.

Dell'Anna, ML., Mastrofrancesco, A.,Sala, R., Venturini, M., Ottaviani, M., Vidolin, AP., Leone, G., Calzavara, PG., Westerhof,W.,& Picardo, M. (2007). Antioxidants and narrow band-UVB in the treatment of vitiligo: a double-blind placebo controlled trial. *Clin Exp Dermatol,* Vol.32, N.6, pp.631-636.

Dogra, S.,& Bhushan, K. (2005). Repigmentation in vitiligo universalis: role of melanocyte density, disease duration, and melanocyte reservoir. *Dermatology Online Journal,* Vol. 11, N.3, pp.30.

Drake, LA., Dinehart, SM., Farmer, ER., Goltz, RW., Graham, GF., Hordinsky, MK., Lewis, CW., Pariser, DM., Skouge, JW., Turner, ML., Webster, SB., Whitaker, DC., Lowery, BJ.,

Nordlund, JJ., Grimes, PE., Halder, RM.,& Minus HR. (1996). Guidelines of care for vitiligo. *J Am Acad Dermatol*, Vol. 35, N., pp. 620-626.

Du Vivier, A. Tachyphylaxis to topically applied steroids. *Arch Dermatol*, Vol.112, N. 9, pp.1245-1248.

Elder, DE., Elenitsas, R., Johnson, BL JR., Murphy, GF.,& Xu, X.(2009).(Ed. 10) *Lever's Histopathology of the skin*, Lippincott Williams& Wilkins, New York.

Eleftheriadou, V., Whitton, ME., Gawkrodger, DJ., Batchelor, J., Corne, J., Lamb, B,. Ersser, S., Ravenscroft, J.,& Thomas, KS. (2011). Future research into treatment of vitiligo: where should our priorities lie? Results of the vitiligo priority setting partnership. *British Journal of Dermatology*, Vol. 164, pp. 530-536.

El Mofty, M., Mostafa, W., Esmat, S., Youssef, R., Azzam, O., Hunter, N., El Hanafi, G.,& Fawzi, M. (2006). Narrow band ultraviolet B 311 nm in the treatment of vitiligo: two right-left comparison studies. *Photodermatol Photoimmunol & Photomed*. Vol. 22, N. 1, pp.6-11

Ermis, O., Alpsoy, E., Cetin, L.,& Yilmaz, E. (2001). Is the efficacy of psoralens plus ultraviolet A therapy for vitiligo enhanced by concurrent topical calcipotriol? A placebo-controlled double-blind study. *Br J Dermatol*, Vol.145, pp. 472-475.

Evans RM. (1988). The steroid and thyroid hormone receptor superfamily. *Science*, Vol. 240, pp. 889-895.

Falabella, R., Arrunategui, A., Barona, MI.,& Alzate, A. (1995). The minigrafting test for vitiligo: detection of stable lesions for melanocyte transplantation. *J Am Acad Dermatol*, Vol. 32, pp.228-232.

Falkenstein, E., Tillmann, HC., Feuring, M.,& Wehling, M.(2000) Multiple actions of steroid hormones- A focus on rapid, nongenomic effects. *Pharmacol* Rev, Vol. 52, N.4, pp.513-556.

Ference, JD., & Last, AR. (2009). Choosing topical corticosteroids. *American Family Physician*, Vol. 79, N. 2, pp. 135-140.

Gauthier, Y., Cario, AM.,& Taieb, A. (2003). A critical appraisal of vitiligo etiologic theories. Is melanocyte loss a melanocytorrhagy? *Pigment Cell Res*, Vol. 16, N. 4,pp. 322-332.

Gawkrodger, DJ., Ormerod, AD., Shaw, L,. Mauri-Sole, I., Whitton, ME., Watts, MJ., Anstey, AV,. Ingham, J., & Young, K. (2010). Vitiligo: concise evidence based guidelines on diagnosis and management. *Postgrad Med J*, Vol.86, N. 1018, pp. 466-471.

Geraldez, CB.,& Gutierrez, GT. (1987). A clinical trial of clobetasol propionate in Filipino vitiligo patients. *Clin Ther*, Vol. 9, pp. 474-482.

Giannotti B. (1988). Current treatment guildlines for topical corticosteroids. *Drugs*, Vol. 36, N. 5 (Suppl), pp. 9-14.

Giannotti, B.,& Pimpinelli, N. (1992). Topical corticosteroids. Which drug and when? *Drugs*, Vol. 44, N. 1, pp. 65-71.

Hamzavi, IH., Jain, H., McLean, D., Shpiro, J., Zeng, H., & Lui, H. (2004). Parametric modeling of narrowband UV-B phototherapy for vitiligo using a novel quantitative tool. *Arch Dermatol*, vol. 140, pp.677-683.

Hamzavi, IH., Lim, HW., & Syed, ZU. (2012). Ultraviolet-based therapy for vitiligo: What's new? *Indian J Dermatol Venereol Leprol*, Vol. 78, N. 1, pp. 42-48.

Hann, SK., Kim, HI., Im, S., Park, YK., Cui, J., & Bystryn, JC. (1993). The change of melanocyte cytotoxicity after systemic steroid treatment in vitiligo patients. *J Dermatol Sci*, Vol. 6, N. 3, pp. 201-205.

Harper, J. (1988). Topical corticosteroids for skin disorders in infants and children. *Drugs*, Vol. 36, N. 5 (suppl), pp. 34-37.

Hartmann, A., Brocker, EB.,& Becker, JC. (2004). Hypopigmentary skin disorders: current treatment options and future directions. *Drug*, Vol. 64, pp. 89-107.

Hatchome, N., Kato, T., & Tagamit, H. (1990). Therapeutic success of epidermal grafting in generalized vitiligo is limited by the Koebner phenomenon. *J Am Acad Dermatol*, Vol. 22, pp.87-91.

Helmy, M I., Gayyar, EIMA., Hawas, S.,& Eissa, EA.(2004). Role of oxidative stress in the pathogenesis of vitiligo. *J Pan-Arab League Dermatologist*, Vol: 15, pp. 97-105.

Hench, PS., Kendall, ES., Slocumb, CH.,& Polley, HF. (1950). Effects of cortisone acetate and pituitary ACTH on rheumatoid arthritis, rheumatic fever, and certain other conditions; study in clinical physiology. *Arch Intern Med*, Vol.85, N.4, pp. 545-556.

Hengge, UR., Ruzicka, T., Schwartz, RA., & Cork, MJ. (2006). Adverse effects of topical glucocorticosteroids. *J Am Acad Dermatol*, Vol.51, N.1, pp.1-15.

Hossani-Madani, AR.,& Halder, RM. (2010). Topical treatment and combination approaches for vitiligo: a new insights, new developments. *G Ital Dermatol Venereol*, Vol. 145, N.1, pp. 57-78.

Howitz, J., Brodthagen, H., Schwartz, M., & Thomsen, K. (1977).Prevalence of vitiligo. *Arch Dermatol*, Vol. 113, pp. 47-52.

Howitz, J., Brodthagen, H., Schwartz, M.,& Thomsen, K. (1977). Prevalence of vitiligo. *Archives Dermatology?*, Vol. 113, pp. 47-52.

Ichimiya, M. (1999). Immunohistochemical study of ACTH and alpha-MSH in vitiligo patients successfully trated with a sex steroid-thyroid hormone mixture. *J Dermatol*, Vol. 26, N. 8, pp. 502-506.

Imamura, S., & Tagami, H. (1976). Treatment of vitiligo with oral corticosteroids. *Dermatologica*, Vol. 153, N. 3, pp. 179-185.

James, WD., Berger, TG., & Elston DM. (Ed 10). (2006). *Andrews disease of the skin. Clinical Dermatology*. Philadelphia: Saunders Elsevier, USA.

Jenis, LG., Lian, JB., Stein, GS., Baran, DT. (1993). 1α, 25-dihydroxy vitamin D_3-induced changes in intracellular pH in osteoblast-like cells modulate gene expression. *J Cell Biochem*, Vol. 53, pp. 234-239.

Jin, Y., Riccardi, SL., Gowan, K., Fain, PR., & Spritz, RA. (2010). Fine-mapping of vitiligo succeptibility loci on chromosomes 7 and 9 and interactions with NLPR1 (NALP1). *J Invest Dermatol*, Vol. 130, pp.774-783.

Kakourou, T. (2009). Vitiligo in children. *World J Pediatr*, Vol. 5, N. 4, pp. 265-268.

Kandil, E. (1974). Treatment of vitiligo with 0.1 per cent betamethasone 17-valerate in isopropyl alcohol- a double-blind trial. *Br J Dermatol*, Vol. 91, pp. 257-460.

Katayama, I., Ashida, M., Maeda, A., Eishi, K., Murota, H., & Bae, SJ. (2003). Open trial of topical tacalcitol [$1\alpha24(OH)2D3$] and solar irradiation for vitiligo vulgaris: upregulation of c-Kit mRNA by cultured melanocytes. *Eur J Dermatol*, Vol. 13, N. 4, pp. 372-376.

Kim, SM., Lee, HS., & Hann, SK. (1999). The efficacy of low-dose oral corticosteroids in the treatment of vitigo patients. *Int J Dermatol*, Vol. 38, N. 7, pp. 546-550.

Koranue, RV. , &Sachdeva, KG. (1988). Vitiligo. *International Journal of Dermatology*, Vol. 27, pp. 676-681.

Kostovic, K., Nola, I., Bucan, Z., & Situm, M. (2003). Treatment of vitiligo: current methods and new approaches. *Acta Dermatovenerol Croat*, Vol. 11, pp. 163-17.

Kovacs, SO., & Missouri, SF. (1998). Vitiligo. J *Am Acad Dermatol*, Vol. 38, pp. 647-666.

Krüger, Ch., Smythe, JW., Spencer, JD., Hasse, S., Panske, A., Chiuchiarelli, G. ,& Schallreuter, KU. (2011). Significant immediate and long- term improvement in quality of life and disease coping in patients with vitiligo after group climatotherapy at Dead sea. *Acta Derm Venereol*, Vol.91, pp. 152-159.

Kumaran, MS., Kaur, I., & Kumar, B. (2006). Effect of topical calcipotriol, betamethasone dipropionate and their combination in the treatment of localized vitiligo. *J Eur Acad Dermatol Venereol*, Vol. 20, N. 3, pp. 269-273.

Kumari, J. (1984). Vitiligo treated with topical clobetasol propionate. *Arch Dermatol*, Vol. 120, pp.631-635.

Kwinter, J., Pelletier, J., Khambalia, A., & Pope, E. (2007). High-potency steroid use in children with vitiligo: a retrospective study. *J Am Acad Dermatol*, Vol. 56, N. 2, pp. 236-241.

Kwok, YKC., Anstey, AV., & Hawk, JLM. (2002). Psoralen photochemotherapy (PUVA) is only moderately effective in widespread vitiligo: a 10-year retrospective study. *Clin Exp Dermatol*, Vol.27, N. 2, pp.104-110.

Lebwohl, MG. ,Heymann, WR. ,Berth-Jones, J., & Coulson, I. (Ed. 2). (2006). *Treatment of skin disease. Comprehensive therapeutic strategies*. Philadelphia Mosby Elsevier, USA.

Lebwohl, M. Quijije, J. Gilliard, J. Rollin, T., & Watts, O. (2003). Topical calcitriol is degraded by ultraviolet light. *J Invest Dermatol*, Vol. 121, N. 3, pp.594-595.

Lee, DY., Kim, CR., & Lee, JH. (2010). Recent onset vitiligo on acral areas treated with phototherapy: need of early treatment. *Photodermatol Photoimmunol Photomed*, Vol. 26, N. 5, pp. 266-268.

Lee, Y., Seo, YJ., Lee, JH.,& Park, JK. (2007). High-dose prednisolone and psoralen ultraviolet A combination therapy in 36 patients with vitiligo. *Clin Exp Dermato*l, Vol. 32, N. 5, pp. 499-501.

Lepe, V., Moncada, B., Castanedo-Cazares, JP. ,Torres-Alvarez, MB., Ortiz, CA.,& Torres-Rubalcava, AB. (2003). A double-blind randomized trial of 0.1% tacrolimus vs 0.05% clobetasol for the treatment of childhood vitiligo. *Arch Dermatol*, Vol. 139, No.5, pp. 581-585.

Le Poole, IC., Das, PK., Van den Wijngaard, RM., Bos, JD.,& Westerhof, W. (1993a). Review of the etiopathomechanism of vitiligo: a convergence theory. *Exp Dermatol*, Vol. 2, pp.145-153.

Le Poole, IC.ﻭVan den Wijngaard, RM., Westerhof, W., Dutrieux, RP., & Das, PK. (1993b). Presence or absence of melanocytes in vitiligo : an immunohistochemical investigation. *J Invest Dermatol*, Vol.100, pp.816-822.

Lester, RS. Corticosteroids. (1989). *Clin Dermatol*, vol. 7, N. 3, pp. 80-97.

Long, CC., & Finaly, AY. (1991). The finger-tip unit- a new practical measure. *Clin Exp Dermatol*, Vol. 16, N. 6, pp. 444-447.

Lotti, T., Buggiani, G., Troiano, M., Assad, GB., Delescluse, J., De Giorgi, V.,& Hercogova, J. (2008a). Targeted and combination treatments for vitiligo. Comparative evaluation of different current modalities in 458 subjects. *Dermatol Ther*, Vol.21, N. 1(Suppl), pp. s20-26.

Lotti, T., Gori, A., Zanieri, F., Colucci, R., Moretti, S. Vitiligo: new and emerging treatment. Dermatol Ther, vol.21, pp.110-117.

Mahmoud, BH., Hexsel, CL. , & Hamzavi, IH. (2008). An update on new and emerging options for the treatment of vitiligo. *Skin Therapy Lett*, Vol. 13, N.2, pp. 1-6.

Majid, I., Masood, Q., Hassan, I., Khan, D.,& Chisti, M. (2009). Childhood vitiligo: Reponse to methylprednisolone oral minipulse therapy and topical fluticasone combination. *Indian J Dermatol*, Vol. 54, N. 2, pp. 124-127.

Majid, I. (2010). Topcal placental extract: Does it increase the efficacy of narrowband UVB therapy in vitiligo? *Indian J Dermatol Venereol Leprol*, Vol. 76, N. 3, pp. 254-258.

Mandelcorn-Monson, RL., Shear, NH., Yau, E. Sambhara, S., Barber, BH., Spaner, D., & DeBenedette, MA(2003). Cytotoxic T lymphocyte reactivity to gp100, melan A/MART I, and tyrosinase, in HLA-A2-positive vitiligo patients. *J Invest Dermatol*, Vol. 121,pp. 550-556.

Masuria, BL., Batra, A., Kothiwala, RK., & Khuller, R. (1999). Topical mometasone furoate for the treatment of childhood vitiligo. *Indian J Dermatol Venereol Leprol*, Vol.65, N.5, pp.219-221.

Millington, GW., & Levell, NJ. (2007).Vitiligo. The historical curse of depigmentation. *Int J Dermatol*, Vol. 46, N.9, pp. 990-995.

Moellmann, G., Klein-Angerer, S., & Scollay, DA. (1982). Extracellular granular material and degeneration of keratinocytes in the normally pigmented epidermis of patients with vitiligo. *J Invest Dermatol*, Vol. 79, pp. 321-330.

Morelli, S., de Boland, AR. & Boland, RL. (1993). Generation of inositol phosphates, diacylglycerol and calcium fluxes in myoblasts treated with 1, 25-dihydroxyvitamine D_3. *Biochem J*, Vol. 289, pp. 675-679.

Moretti, S., Spallanzani, A., Amato, L. ,Hautmann, G., Gallerani, I., Fabianini, M., & Fabbri , P. (2002). New insights into the pathogenesis of vitiligo: imbalance of epidermal cytokines at sites of lesions. *Pigment Cell Res*, Vol.15, pp. 87-92.

Morley, P., Whitfield, JF., Vanderhyden, BC., Tsang, BK., & Schwartz, JL. (1992). A new, nongenomic estrogen action: The rapid release of intracellular Ca^{2+}. *Endocrinol*, Vol. 131, pp. 1305-1312.

Mulekar, SV. (2006). Stable vitiligo treated by a combination of low-dose oral pulse betamethasone and autologous, noncultured melanocyte-keratinocyte cell transplantation. *Dermatol Surg*, Vol. 32, N. 4, pp. 536-541.

Muto, M., Furumoto, H., Ohmura, A., & Asagami, C. (1995). Successful treatment pf vitilgo with a sex steroid-thyroid hormone mixture. *J dermatol*, Vol. 22, N. 10, pp. 770-772.

Nagai, K., Ichimiya, M., Yokoyama, K,. Hamamoto, Y., & Muto, M. (2000). Successful treatment of non-segmental vitiligo: systemic therapy with sex hormone-thyroid powder mixture. *Horm Res*, Vol. 54, N. 5-6, pp. 316-317.

Namazi, MR. (2005). Phenytoin as a novel anti-vitiligo weapon. *J Autimmune Dis*, Vol.2, N.11.

Nazer, HEI., Emam, H., Abdel Hamid, MF., Aly, D., Shehata, H., Hussein, M., Raafat, M., Salama, I., Abdel Ghaffar, N., Fathy, A., Kotb, A., & Sadek, M. (2011). The effectiveness of narrow-band phototherapy, corticosteroid, and methotrexate on clinical picture and serum level of soluble interleukin-2 receptors among vitiligo patients. *Medical Research Journal*, Vol.10, N.1, pp.18-22.

Nijsten, TEC., & Stern, RS. (2003). The increased risk of skin cancer is persistent after discontinuation of psoralen+ultraviolet A: a cohort study. *J Invest Dermatol*, Vol. 121, pp. 252-258.

Njoo, MD., Das, PK., Bos, JD., & Weserhof, W. (1999). Association of the Köbner phenomenon with disease activity and therapeutic responsiveness in vitiligo vulgaris. *Arch Dermatol*, Vol. 135, pp. 407-413.

Njoo, MD., Spuls, PI., Bos, JD., Westerhof, W., & Bossuyt, PM. (1998). Nonsurgical repigmentation therapies in vitiligo. *Arch Dermatol*, Vol. 134, pp. 1532-1540.

Njoo, MD., Weserhof, W., Bos, JD.,& Bossuyt, PM. (1998). A systemic review of autolougous transplantation methods in vitiligo. *Arch Dermatol*. Vol. 134, pp. 1543-1549.

Njoo, MD., & Westerhof, W. (2001). Vitiligo. Pathogenesis and treatment. *Am J Clin Dermatol*. Pathogenesis and treatment, Vol. 2, N. 3, pp. 167-181.

Nordlund, JJ. Lerner, AB. (1982). Vitiligo. It is important. *Arch Dermatol*, Vol.118, pp.5-8.

Ogg, GS., Dunbat, PR., Romero, P., Chen, JL., & Cerundulo, V. (1998). High frequency of skin homing melanocyte-specific cytotoxic T lymphocytes in autoimmune vitiligo.*J Exp Med*, Vol. 188, pp. 1203-1208.

Ongenae, K., Van Geel, N., De Schepper, S., Vander Haeghen, Y., & Naeyaert, JM. (2004). Management of vitiligo patients and attitude of dermatologists toward vitiligo. *Eur J Dermatol*, Vol. 14, N. 3, pp. 177-181.

Oslen, EA. (1991). A double-blind controlled comparison of generic and trade-name topical steroids using the vasoconstriction assay. *Arch Dermatol*, Vol. 127, N.2, pp.197-201.

Pariser, DM. (1991). Topical steroids: a guide for use in the elderly patient. *Geriatrics*, Vol. 46, N. 10, pp. 51-54, 57-60, 63.

Parsad, D., Kanwar, AJ., & Kumar, B. (2006). Psoralen-ultaviolet A vs. narrow-band ultraviolet B phototherapy for the treatment of vitiligo. *J Eur Acad Dermatol Venereol*, Vol. 20, N. 2, pp. 175-177.

Parsad, D., Pandhi, R., Dogra, S., & Kumar, B. (2004). Clinical study of repigmentation patterns with different treatment modalities and their correlation with speed and stability of repigmentation in 352 vitiliginnous patches. *J Am Acad Dermatol*, Vol. 50, N. 1, pp. 63-67.

Parsad, D., Pandhi, R., & juneja, A. (2003).Effective of oral Ginkgo biloba in treating limited, slowly spreading vitiligo. *Clinic Exp Dermatol*, Vol. 28, pp.285-287.

Pasricha, JS. Khaitan, BK. (1993). Oral mini pulse therapy with betamethasone in vitiligo patients having extensive or fast-spreading disease. *Int J Dermatol*, Vol. 32, N. 10, pp. 753-757.

Pasricha, JS., & Khera, V. (1994). Effect of prolonged treatment with levamisole on vitiligo with limited and slow-spreading disease. *Int J Dermatol*, Vol. 33, N. 8, pp. 584-587.

Pichler, R., Sfetsos, K., Badics, B., Gutenbrunner, S., Berg, J., & Auböck, J. (2009). Lymphocyte imbalance in vitiligo patients indicated by elevated CD4+/CD8+ T-cell ratio. *Wien Med Wochenschr*, Vol. 159, pp. 337-341.

Radakovic, FS., Furnsinn, FA., Honigsmann, H., & Tanew, A. (2001). Oral dexamethasone pulse treatment for vitiligo. *J Am Acad Dermatol*, Vol. 44, N. 5, pp. 814-817.

Radmanesh, M., & Saedi, K. (2006). The efficacy of combined PUVA and low-dose azathioprine for early and enhanced repigmentation in vitiligo patients. *J Dermatol Treat*, Vol. 17, pp. 151-153.

Rath, N., Kar, HK., & Sabhnani, S. (2008). An open labeled, comparative clinical study on efficacy and tolerability of oral minipulse of steroid (OMP) alone, OMP with PUVA and broad/narrow band UVB phototherapy in progressive vitiligo. *Indian J Dermatol Venereol*, Vol. 74, N.4, pp.357-360.

Roeder, A., Schaller, M., Schäfer-Korting, M., & Korting, HS. (2005). Safty and efficacy of fluticasone propionate in the topical treatment of skin diseases. *Skin Pharmacol Physiol*, Vol. 18, N. 1, pp.3-11.

Sanclemente, G., Garcia, JJ., Zuleta, JJ., Diehl, C., Correa, C. , & Falabella, R. (2008). A double-blind, randomized trial of 0.05% betamethasone vs. topical catalase/dismutase superoxide in vitiligo. *J Eur Acad Dermatol Venereol*, Vol.22, N. 11, pp. 1359-1364.

Sassi, F., Cazzaniga, S., Tessari, G., Chatenoud, L., Reseghetti, A., Marchesi, L., Girolomoni, G., & Naldi, L. (2008). Randomized controlled trial comparing the effectiveness of 308-nm excimer laser alone or in combination with topical hydrocortisone 17-butyrate cream in treatment of vitiligo of the face and neck. *Br J Dermatol*, Vol. 159, N. 5, pp. 1186-1191.

Schallreuter, KU., Moore, J., Behrens-Williams, S., Panske, A., & Harari, M. (2002). Rapid initiation of repigmentation in vitiligo with Dead Sea climatotherapy in combination with pseudocatalase (PC-KUS). *Int J Dermatol*, Vol. 41, pp. 482-487.

Sehgal, VN., & Srivastava G. (2007). Vitiligo: compendium of clinico-epidemiological features. *Indian J Dermatol Venereol Leprol*, Vol. 73, pp.149-156.

Seiter, S., Ugurel, S., Pföhler, C., Tilgen, W., & Reinhold, U. (1999). Successful treatment of progressive vitiligo with high-dose intravenous methylprednisolone 'pulse' therapy. *Dermatol*, Vol. 199, N. 3, pp. 261-262.

Seiter, S., Ugurel, S., Tilgen, W., & Reinhold, U. (2000). Use of high-dose methylprednisolone pulse therapy in patients with progressive and stable vitiligo. *Int J Dermatol*, Vol. 39, N. 8, pp. 624-627.

Shameer, P. Prasad, PVS. Kaviarasan, PK.(2005). Serum zinc level in vitiligo: a case control study. *Indian Journal of Dermatology, venereology and leprology*, Vol. 71, pp.206-207.

Silverberg, N., Lin, P., Travis, L., Farley-Li, J, Mancini, AJ., Wagner, AM., Chamlin, SL., & Paller, AS (2004). Tacrolimus ointment promotes repigmentation of vitiligo in children: a review of 57 cases. *J Am Acad Dermatol*, Vol.51, N. 5, pp.760-766.

Sitek, JC., Loeb, M., & Ronnevig, JR. (2007). Narrowband UVB therapy for vitiligo: does the repigmentation last?*J Euir Acad Dermatol Venereol*, Vol.21, N. 7, pp.891-896.

Spritz, RA. (2008). The genetics of generalized vitiligo. *Curr Dir Autoimmune*, Vol. 10, pp. 244-257.

Sulzberger, MB., Witten, VH., & Yaffe, SN. (1951). Cortisone acetate administered orally in dermatologic therapy. *Arch Dermatol Syphilol*, Vol. 64, pp.573-578.

Szczurko, O. Boon, HS. (2008). A systematic review of natural heath product treatment for vitiligo. *BMC Dermatol*, Vol.8, N.2.

Szczurko, O.Shear, N. Taddio, A. Boon, H. (2011). Ginkgo biloba for the treatment of vitiligo vulgaris: an open label pilot clinical trial. *BMC Complementary Alternative Medicine*, Vol. 11, N. 21.

Tadicherla, S., Ross, K., Shenefelt, PD., & Fenske, NA. (2009). Topical corticosteroids in dermatology. *J Drugs Dermatol*, Vol.8, N. 12, pp.1093-1105.

Takei, M., Mishima, Y., & Uda H. (1984). Immunopathology of vitiligo vulgaris, Sutton's leukoderma and melanoma-associated vitiligo in relation to steroid effects. I. Curculating antibodies for cultured melanoma cells. *J Cut Pathol*, Vol. 11, N. 2, pp. 107-113.

Russell, ST.,& Tisdale MJ. (2005). The role of glucocorticoids in the induction of zinc- α2-glycoprotein expression I adipose tssue in cancer cachexia. *British J Cancer,* Vol.92, pp.876-881.

Tonsi, A. (2004). Vitiligo and its management update: a review. *Pak J Med Sci,* Vol. 20, pp. 242-247.

Travis, LB., & Silverberg, NB. (2004). Calcipotriene and corticosteroid combination therapy for vitiligo. *Peddiatr Dermatol,* Vol. 21, N. 4, pp. 495-498.

Tsuji, T., & Hamada, T.(1983). Topically administered fluorouracil in vitiligo. *Arch Dermatol,* Vol. 119, pp. 722-727.

Uda, H., Takei, M., & Mishima, Y. (1984). Immunopathology of vitiligo vulgaris, Sutton's leukoderma and melanoma-associated vitiligo in relation to steroid effects. II. The IgG and C3 deposits in the skin. *J Cutan Pathol,* Vol. 11, N. 2, pp. 114-124.

Van Geel, N., Vander Haeghen, Y.,Ongenae, K., & Naeyaert, JM. (2004). A new digital image analysis system useful for surface assessment of vitiligo lesions in transplantation studies. *European Journal of Dermatology*? Vol. 14, N. 3, pp. 150-155.

Vasistha, LK.,& Singh, G. (1979). Vitiligo and intralesional steroids. *Indian J Med Res,* Vol. 69, pp. 308-311.

Westerhof, W., Nieuweboer-Krobotova, L. Mulder, PGH.,& Glazenburg EJ. (1999). Left-right comparison study of the combination of fluticasone propionate and UV-A vs either fluticasone propionate or UV-A alone for the long-term treatment of vitiligo. *Arch Dermatol,* Vol. 135, pp. 1061-1066.

Whitton, ME., Ashcrft, DM., & González, U. (2008). Therapeutic intervention for vitiligo. J *Am Acad Dermatol,* Vol. 59, pp. 713-717.

Whitton, M. Pinart, M. Batchelor, J....(2010). Interventions for vitiligo. *Cochrane Database Sys Rev,* 1, CD003263

Wolff, K., Goldsmith, LA., Katz, SI., Gilchrest, BA., Paller, AS.,& Leffell, DJ. (Ed. 7). (2007). *Fitzpatrick's Dermatology in General Medicine,* Mac Graw Hill, ISBN. 978-0-07-146690-5.USA.

Wolverton, SE. (Ed. 2). (2007). *Comprehensive Dermatologic Drug Therapy,* Saunders Elsevier, ISBN-10:978-1-4160-2471-2.USA.

Xunquan, L., Changgeng, S., Peiying, J., Huaiqu, W., Gan-yun, Y., & Yawalkar, S. (1990). Treatment of localized vitiligo with ulobetasol cream. *Int J Dermatol,* Vol. 29, pp. 295-297.

Yaghoobi, R., Omidian, M.,& Bagherani, N. (2011a). Comparison of therapeutic efficacy of topical corticosteroid and oral zinc sulfate-topical corticosteroid combination in the treatment of vitiligo patients: a clinical trial. *BMC Dermatology,* Vol. 11, N. 7.

Yaghoobi, R., Omidian, M., & Bagherani, N. (2011b). Vitiligo: A review of the published work. *The Journal of Dermatology,* Vol.38, No. 5, pp. 419-431.

Yones, SS., Palmer, RA., Garibaldinos, TM., Et al. (2007). Randomized double-blind trial of treatment of vitiligo: efficacy of psoralen- UVA therapy vs. narrowband- UVB therapy. *Arch Dermatol,* Vol. 143, N. 5, pp. 578-584.

Yu, HS., Wu, ChSh., Yu,ChL., Kao, YH., & Chiou, MH. (2003). Helium-neon laser irradiation stimulates migration and proliferation in melanocytes and induces repigmentation in segmental-type vitiligo. *J Invest Dermatol,* Vol. 120, pp.56-64.

Zhang, Z., Xu, SX., Zhang, FY., Yin, XY., Yang, S., Xiao, FL., Du, WH., Wang, JF., Lv, YM., Tang, HY., & Zhang XJ.(2009). The analysis of genetics and associated autoimmune disease in Chinese vitiligo population. *Arch Dermatol Res,* Vol. 301, pp. 167-173.